EFFECTS OF DRUGS
ON CELLULAR CONTROL MECHANISMS

BIOLOGICAL COUNCIL

The Co-ordinating Committee for Symposia
on Drug Action

A Symposium on

EFFECTS OF DRUGS
ON CELLULAR CONTROL MECHANISMS

Edited by

B. R. RABIN

*Department of Biochemistry,
University College,
London*

and

R. B. FREEDMAN

*Biology Laboratory,
University of Kent
at Canterbury*

UNIVERSITY PARK PRESS
BALTIMORE • LONDON • TOKYO

First published 1972

THE MACMILLAN PRESS LTD
*London and Basingstoke
Associated companies in New York Melbourne
Toronto Dublin Johannesburg and Madras*

Published in North America by
UNIVERSITY PARK PRESS
Chamber of Commerce Building
Baltimore, Maryland 21202

Library of Congress Cataloging in Publication Data
Main entry under title:

A Symposium on effects of drugs on cellular control
mechanisms.

At head of title: Biological Council: the Co-
ordinating Committee for Symposia on Drug Action.

Held Mar. 29-30, 1971, at Middlesex Hospital Medical School, London.

Includes bibliographies.

1. Drug metabolism—Congresses. 2. Cytochemistry
—Congresses. I. Rabin, Brian Robert, 1927-   ed. II.
Freedman, R. B., ed. III. London. University. Middlesex
Hospital Medical School. IV. Biological Council.
Coordinating Committee for Symposia on Drug Action.
V. Title: Effects of drugs on cellular control mechanisms.
QP901.S94   615'.7   71-171248
ISBN 0-8391-0646-7

PRINTED IN GREAT BRITAIN

PREFACE

The Biological Council sponsors annually a Symposium on drug action and this book records the proceedings of the 1971 Symposium, the organisation of which was made possible by generous help from the Wellcome Trust and CIBA Foundation.

The first day of the Symposium was devoted to a discussion of the Role of Steroid Hormones in Control Processes under the chairmanships of J. R. Tata and T. F. Slater. The coverage is very wide and ranges from physicochemical studies of the interaction of steroid hormones with macromolecules and membranes to the role of steroid hormones in development and gene expression. The second day of the Symposium was devoted to Cyclic AMP. The morning session, chaired by B. R. Rabin, covered some basic biochemical aspects and the afternoon session, chaired by H. O. Schild, covered material of more direct pharmacological interest. Many of the papers on both days provoked lively discussion, much of which is recorded in this book. The meeting was truly interdisciplinary and this book shows very clearly how thoroughly inter-related pharmacology and biochemistry have become. It is our hope that this book will encourage others to cross the constraining boundaries of their individual specialisms.

B.R.R.
R.B.F.

SYMPOSIUM ORGANISATION

BIOLOGICAL COUNCIL

Co-ordinating Committee for Symposia on Drug Action

EFFECTS OF DRUGS ON CELLULAR CONTROL MECHANISMS

Report of a Symposium held on 29 and 30 MARCH 1971

in

London

at The Middlesex Hospital Medical School

Sponsored by
British Pharmacological Society
and
Biochemical Society
British Society for Cell Biology
British Society for Immunology
Nutrition Society
Pharmaceutical Society of Great Britain
Physiological Society
Royal Society of Medicine
Society for Drug Research
Society for Endocrinology
Society for Experimental Biology

Organised by a Symposium Committee consisting of:
B. R. Rabin (*Chairman and Hon. Secretary*)
D. H. Jenkinson   J. L. Mongar
A. Korner   T. F. Slater

CONTENTS

Contents

LIST OF CONTRIBUTORS

Dr A. C. Allison, Clinical Research Centre, Watford Road, Harrow, Middx.

Dr E. S. K. Assem, Department of Pharmacology, University College London, WC1E 6BT

Mr T. Atkins, Department of Biological Sciences, University of Aston in Birmingham, Birmingham

Dr A. W. Bennett, Department of Surgery, King's College Hospital Medical School, London S.E.5

Dr Carol A. Blyth, Department of Biochemistry, University College London, Gower Street, London WC1E 6BT

Professor G. V. R. Born, Department of Pharmacology, Royal College of Surgeons, Lincoln's Inn Fields, London W.C.2

Dr R. W. Butcher, University of Massachusetts Medical School, Department of Biochemistry, 419 Belmont Street, Worcester 01604, Mass., U.S.A.

Dr M. J. Clemens, National Institute of Medical Research, The Ridgeway, Mill Hill, London NW7 1AA

Dr N. R. Cohen, The Open University, Walton Hall, Milton Keynes, Bletchley, Bucks.

Dr B. M. Cox, Department of Pharmacology, Chelsea College of Science and Technology, Manresa Road, London S.W.3

Dr P. Davies, Clinical Research Centre, Watford Road, Harrow, Middx.

Dr M. Delma Doherty, Biochemistry Department, University of Queensland, St Lucia, Brisbane 4067, Queensland, Australia

Dr I. R. Falconer, Department of Applied Biochemistry and Nutrition, University of Nottingham

Dr I. A. Forsyth, National Institute for Research in Dairying, Shinfield, Reading, Berks.

Dr R. B. Freedman, Biology Laboratory, University of Kent at Canterbury, Canterbury, Kent

Dr J. D. P. Graham, Department of Pharmacology, Welsh National School of Medicine, Heath Park, Cardiff CF4 4XW

Dr D. G. Grahame-Smith, Medical Unit, St Mary's Hospital Medical School, London W.2

Professor J. K. Grant, Department of Steroid Biochemistry, University of Glasgow, Glasgow Royal Infirmary, Glasgow C.4

Dr R. J. Haslam, I.C.I. Ltd (Pharmaceuticals Division), Alderley Park, Macclesfield, Cheshire

Professor P. J. Heald, Department of Biochemistry, University of Strathclyde, Glasgow C.2

Dr K. J. Hittelman, Department of Biochemistry, School of Medicine, University of Massachusetts, Worcester, Mass., U.S.A.

B. Hughes, Beecham Research Laboratory, The Pinnacles, Harlow, Essex

Dr K. D. Jaitly, Royal Netherlands Fermentation Industries Ltd., Delft, Holland

Dr J. S. Jenkins, St George's Hospital, London S.W.1

Dr Brian Ketterer, Courtauld Institute of Biochemistry, Middlesex Hospital Medical School, London W.1

Dr R. J. B. King, Department of Hormone Biochemistry, Imperial Cancer Research Fund, Lincoln's Inn Fields, London WC2A 3PX

Professor H. W. Kosterlitz, Department of Pharmacology, University Medical Buildings, Foresterhill, Aberdeen AB9 22D

Dr Ilse Lasnitzki, Strangeways Laboratory, Cambridge

Professor G. Litwack, Department of Biochemistry, Fels Research Institute, Temple University, Health Sciences Center, School of Medicine, Philadelphia, Penn. 19140, U.S.A.

Professor H. McIlwain, Department of Biochemistry, Institute of Psychiatry, De Crespigny Park, London S.E.5

Dr W. J. Marshall, King's College Hospital Medical School, Department of Chemical Pathology, London S.E.5

Dr J. Matthews, Chemical Sciences Research Department, Boots Pure Drug Co., Pennyfoot Street, Nottingham

Dr R. H. Mitchell, Department of Biochemistry, University of Birmingham, Birmingham

Dr D. Monard, Friedrich Miescher Institute, P.O. Box 273, CH-4002 Basel, Switzerland

Dr K. S. Morey, California State Polytechnic College, San Luis Obispo, California, U.S.A.

Dr R. Neher, Friedrich Miescher Institute, P.O. Box 273, CH-4002 Basel, Switzerland

Dr T. Oka, Department of Health, Education and Welfare, Public Health Service, National Institute of Health, Bethesda, Maryland 20014, U.S.A.

Professor J. A. Olson, Department of Biology, Middlesex Hospital Medical School, Cleveland Street, London W.1

Professor D. V. Parke, Biochemistry Department, University of Surrey, Guildford, Surrey

Professor V. R. Pickles, Physiology Department, University College, Cardiff

Dr G. Powis, Department of Pharmacology, Glasgow University, Glasgow W.2

Professor B. R. Rabin, Department of Biochemistry, University College London, Gower Street, London WC1E 6BT

Dr I. Rabinowitz, Alza Corporation, 950 Page Hill Road, Palo Alto, California 94304, U.S.A.

Dr P. Ramwell, Alza Corporation, 950 Page Hill Road, Palo Alto, California 94304, U.S.A.

Dr R. Rodnight, Department of Biochemistry, Institute of Psychiatry, De Crespigny Park, London S.E.5

Dr Anne Roobol, Tropical Metabolism Research Unit, University of the West Indies, Mona, Kingston 7, Jamaica

Professor H. O. Schild, F.R.S., Department of Pharmacology, University College London, Gower Street, London WC1E 6BT

Dr D. Schlessinger, Washington University School of Medicine, Department of Microbiology, 4550 Scott Avenue, St Louis, Missouri 63110, U.S.A.

Dr J. G. Schofield, Biochemistry Department, Medical School, University Walk, Bristol

Professor T. F. Slater, Department of Biology, Brunel University, Kempton Lane, Hillingdon, Uxbridge, Middx.

Mr H. Smith, Beecham Research Labs, Brockham Park, Betchworth, Surrey

Mr J. B. Smith, Department of Pharmacology, Royal College of Surgeons, Lincoln's Inn Fields, London W.C.2

Dr A. R. Somerville, I.C.I. Ltd. (Pharmaceutical Division), Alderley Park, Macclesfield, Cheshire

Dr M. Stockham, Allen & Hanbury's Ltd., Ware, Herts.

Mr F. M. Sullivan, Department of Pharmacology, Guy's Hospital Medical School, London S.E.1

Mr G. Sunshine, Department of Biochemistry, University College London, Gower Street, London WC1E 6BT

Dr D. Szollosi, Animal Research Station, Huntingdon Road, Cambridge

Dr J. R. Tata, National Institute of Medical Research, Mill Hill, London NW7 1AA

Dr G. M. Tomkins, Department of Biochemistry, University of California Medical Center, San Francisco, California, U.S.A.

Dr Yale J. J. Topper, Department of Health, Education and Welfare, Public Health Service, National Institute of Health, Bethesda, Maryland 20014, U.S.A.

Dr M. Weller, Department of Biochemistry, Institute of Psychiatry, De Crespigny Park, London S.E.5

Dr D. J. Williams, Department of Biochemistry, University College London, Gower Street, London WC1E 6BT

Dr D. C. Wilton, Department of Physiology and Biochemistry, University of Southampton

'PLEIOTYPIC' AND 'SPECIFIC' HORMONAL CONTROL OF GENE EXPRESSION IN MAMMALIAN CELLS

G. M. Tomkins

Department of Biochemistry and Biophysics, University of California, San Francisco, California 94122

Pleiotypic Control

I should like to propose that regulation by a variety of hormones and other growth-stimulating substances is effected in two ways, which I shall refer to as the 'pleiotypic' [1] and 'specific' modes of regulation. The pleiotypic control system refers to a coordinated set of reactions which respond in a characteristic way when cellular growth is stimulated by a specific hormone. Some of the reactions under this type of general control are:

(1) the uptake of glucose and of various precursors for macro-molecular synthesis;
(2) RNA synthesis, particularly of ribosomal and transfer RNA;
(3) protein synthesis and the state of polysome assembly (probably determined by the initiation reaction);
(4) the degradation of intracellular proteins and other macro-molecules.

Responses in all of the above reactions follow the administration of the steroid hormones, thyroxin, insulin and growth hormone to animals (see [1] for references); similar reactions are regulated when lymphocytes are stimulated by phytohemagglutinin, erythroid cells by erythropoietin, and in other conditions where the growth of certain cells is stimulated by a specific humoral agent. Table 1 lists some of the reaction under pleiotypic control and how they are regulated in specific situations.

The near universality of such a response raises the question of whether the control of all of these reactions in a number of cell types

1

could be a manifestation of a common underlying mechanism. Since the discovery of the adenyl cyclase-cyclic AMP system we have become quite used to the idea that a single effector molecule can regulate a number of different processes in different cell types, but one of the strongest arguments that pleiotypic control is exerted in all cells by a common mechanism comes from a comparison of the reactions under pleiotypic control with those under 'stringent control' in bacteria deprived of an essential amino acid. In the latter case, a very similar set of reactions is affected which facilitate the adaptation of the organism to unfavourable growth conditions. These reactions include decreases in tRNA and rRNA synthesis (without

Table 1
**The Pleiotypic Response in Mammalian Cells and its Antagonism
by Serum and Insulin**

Process	Pleiotypic response	Antagonized by	
		Serum*	Insulin*
RNA synthesis	inhibition	+	+
Protein synthesis	inhibition	+	+
Polysome formation	inhibition	+	+
Protein degradation	stimulation	+	+
Nucleic acid			
precursor uptake	inhibition	+	+
Glucose uptake	inhibition	+	+

* For references see [1].

much effect on messenger production) an increase in the rates of intracellular protein degradation, and decreases in the permeation of nucleic acid precursors and of carbohydrates. These stringent responses in bacteria are strikingly similar to the pleiotypic responses in mammalian cells listed above. A mutation in the RC gene in bacteria prevents the organisms from responding in any of the above ways to amino acid deprivation suggesting a common control mechanism for all of these reactions. Furthermore, an unusual guanine-containing nucleotide ppGpp accumulates in stringently controlled bacteria deprived of an essential amino acid [2], and preliminary experiments suggest that this nucleotide may control directly at least some of the responses to amino acid deprivation [3].

These findings suggest that perhaps a similar common basic

control mechanism may operate in mammalian cells subject to growth regulation.

To attack this problem experimentally, my colleagues and I have carried out experiments in cultured cells deprived of serum [1]. Figure 1 (reprinted from [1]) illustrates the pleiotypic response in mouse fibroblasts deprived of serum and its reversal when dialysed serum is restored to the medium. Similar pleiotypic stimulation takes place when crystalline insulin is used instead of serum. Pleiotypic

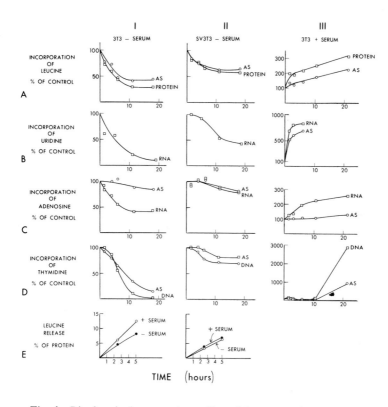

Fig. 1. Biochemical parameters affected by serum deprivation in 3T3 and SV 3T3 cells. *I-II, A-D*: The effect of serum deprivation on the incorporation of precursors into the acid-soluble (AS) and macromolecular components of 3T3 and SV 3T3 cells. *III, A-D*: Reversal of the effects of serum deprivation. *I-II, E*: Effect of serum deprivation on the degradation of intracellular protein. (Methods as described in Ref. [1]).

stimulation (measured with uridine uptake) does not require either concomitant protein or RNA synthesis and, in fact, certain of the effects of serum and insulin are mimicked when protein synthesis is inhibited by cycloheximide. These findings suggest that the reactions under pleiotypic control are coordinated in the same way as are those of bacteria subjected to amino acid starvation. Although a search for guanine nucleotides accumulating in these cells under step-down conditions has not revealed the presence of ppGpp [4], we imagine that a 'pleiotypic mediator' accumulates under these conditions and somehow coordinates all these responses.

An additional element in the pleiotypic control theory takes note of the fact (also illustrated in Fig. 1) that fibroblasts malignantly transformed by simian virus 40 are much less responsive to serum deprivation than are non-transformed cells. We therefore propose that the malignant phenotype derives, in part at least, from pleiotypic 'densensitization'. Sepharose-bound insulin is as effective as the crystalline product in reversing the pleiotypic response of serum-starved fibroblasts [1]. We argue, therefore, that interaction of 'pleiotypic activators' with the cell membrane relieves pleiotypic inhibition by decreasing the concentration of the mediator. Since malignant transformation of a number of cell lines is accompanied by changes in the cell membrane, the desensitization characteristic of the malignant state may be the result of these changes which would decrease the synthesis of the mediator. Malignant cells would therefore be constantly activated.

Specific Control

In addition to the pleiotypic response many hormones also stimulate the production of specific enzymes. Since these proteins are both hormone- and tissue-specific, it is unlikely that the pleiotypic mediator can account for these specific inductions. Furthermore, under certain special circumstances the hormones can elicit a specific response without the usual pleiotypic stimulation. For example, in cultured hepatoma cells (HTC) the adrenal steroids stimulate the rate of synthesis of tyrosine aminotransferase without altering the cell growth, overall rates of RNA or protein synthesis [5], or the rates of intracellular protein degradation [6]. Therefore, hormone-'specific' responses need not always be accompanied by a corresponding pleiotypic response and must therefore have a separate mechanism.

A number of studies using both synchronized and randomly growing populations of HTC cells have led us to the mechanism of 'specific' control illustrated in Fig. 2 [7]. In essence, the model states that the expression of a specific gene may be controlled in at least two ways: one determined by the position of the cell in the generation cycle, and the other determined by the specific inducer.

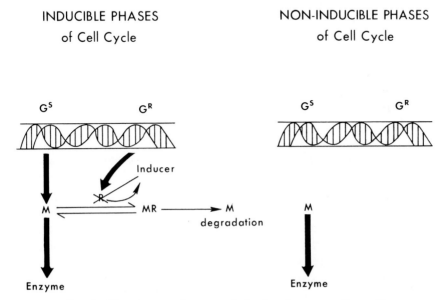

INDUCIBLE PHASES
of Cell Cycle

NON-INDUCIBLE PHASES
of Cell Cycle

Fig. 2. The theory of enzyme induction in mammalian cells. The configuration shown on the left is assumed to exist during the inducible phases of the cell cycle, while that on the right, during the non-inducible phases. The G^S refers to the structural gene for the inducible enzyme, while G^R refers to the regulatory gene. During the inducible periods, G^S is transcribed and the resulting messenger, M, can be translated to form the enzyme. The G^R is likewise transcribed and its messenger translated to produce the protein R. The R combines reversibly with M to produce the inactive complex MR which leads to M degradation. The R itself is labile as shown by the thin arrow leading away from R. The inducer is indicated to inactivate R by an unknown mechanism. During the non-inducible phases of the cycle, neither G^S nor G^R is transcribed, but M can be translated. Although for the case of tyrosine aminotransferase the degradation of the enzyme might also be depicted, we have not done so because its concentration is not regulated by changing the rate of its inactivation under constant cultural conditions. Reprinted from [7].

As illustrated, we consider that cell-cycle control is due to the fact that the structural gene is transcribed only during a limited portion of the cycle. In the case of tyrosine aminotransferase, this period of gene transcription occurs during the latter two-thirds of G1 and the entire S period [8]. Similar cell-cycle limited periods of gene expression have been reported in a number of other eukaryotic systems [9], but the nature of this transcription control is unknown. Preliminary studies in our laboratory [10] have not revealed gross differences between histone acetylation or phosphorylation during the periods of gene expression and repression.

When transcription control is lifted (i.e. during the periods of gene transcription) expression is modulated at the level of mRNA translation by a specific labile post-transcriptional repressor which has two functions. One action of the repressor is to inhibit the translation of the structural gene messenger, and its second function is to promote the degradation of the messenger. We assume that the gene coding for the repressor, i.e. the regulatory gene, is cyclically repressed and transcribed at the same times as the TAT structural gene. The experimental observations on which these conclusions are based have been presented in detail elsewhere [7]. Since the steroid induction of tyrosine aminotransferase takes place only during the periods of the cycle when the translational repressor is present, we propose that the steroids in some way antagonize the repressor.

We have begun studies in cell-free systems to attempt to localize the sites of hormone action in HTC cells [11]. Our experiments indicate that each cell contains about 10^5 specific cytoplasmic 'receptor' molecules which combine reversibly with both inducing and anti-inducing steroids. Quantitative studies of the kinetics of association and dissociation of the steroid from these receptor molecules, and a consideration of their affinity for a variety of steroids with different biological action in the HTC cells leads us to the conclusions that the interaction of the steroid inducers with the cytoplasmic receptors are the first step in the cell-hormone reaction leading to modulation of the expression of the TAT gene [11]. Other work carried out in intact cells [12] and in cell-free extracts has shown that once the steroid is bound to the cytoplasmic receptor, it can then associate with some component or components of the nucleus.

We investigated whether the steroid receptor molecules themselves might be the postulated translational repressor shown in Fig. 2.

However, cells freed of repressor (either by being trapped in repressor-free periods of the cell cycle, or by treatment with actinomycin D which allows the labile molecules to decay) have a constant concentration of cytoplasmic steroid receptor. Thus, the repressor and the receptor are not the same. If the site of repressor action is on the messenger RNA, the intra-nuclear localization of the inducing steroid indicates that the inducer-repressor interaction must be indirect.

This is the state of the art at present. It is obvious that what is needed is a cell-free system in which steroids stimulate the expression of the TAT gene. Although this seems at the moment like a distant dream we are encouraged by our microbiological colleagues who can easily study the induced synthesis of specific enzymes in bacterial extracts.

Conclusion

In summary, I should like to propose that many hormones have two distinct modes of action: 'pleiotypic' and 'specific'. The pleiotypic action of all the hormones may have an identical basis, derived from their ability to antagonize the action of a hypothetical, universal, 'pleiotypic mediator'. The latter is a negative regulator which maintains cells in the resting state similar to the way that ppGpp induces the resting state in bacteria deprived of an essential amino acid. In both mammalian and bacterial cells, a remarkably similar set of reactions is under pleiotypic control; these include RNA synthesis, polysome aggregation and protein synthesis, protein degradation and nucleic acid precursor and glucose penetration. In many hormone-stimulated tissues, these reactions are coordinately affected, presumably by pleiotypic activation.

In addition, hormone-specific responses take place so that different hormones may induce the synthesis of different proteins in the same cell. I propose that these specific inductions are controlled by indirect hormone antagonism of specific labile repressors of messenger RNA translation.

Discussion

Tata (Mill Hill)

You mentioned that pleiotypic responses are not elicited by malignant cells. Would you say that the induction of tyrosine transaminase by corticosteroids in hepatoma cells is brought about via a different route from that operating in normal rat liver?

Tomkins (San Francisco)

All indications are that the mechanism of tyrosine aminotransferase induction in malignant cells by the glucocorticoids is the same as in normal liver. Certainly, there are differences in control mechanisms beyond the particular induction, since a number of normal enzymes are missing in hepatoma cells. Therefore, the consequences of TAT induction in culture must be quite different from those *in vivo*, but the molecular mechanism of steroid action is very likely the same.

Lasnitzki (Cambridge)

What serum concentration did you use and how long were the cells deprived of it?

Did you also use lower and higher serum concentrations and if so, did you obtain a dose-response curve as regards the inhibition in the non-serum controls?

Tomkins (San Francisco)

Normally the cells were grown with 15% serum. Various times of deprivation were used up to 20 hours. We have not yet done a dose response curve, however.

King (London)

Serum contains several serum factors each having different effects. How do you account for these effects by your scheme?

Tomkins (San Francisco)

I know there are several growth promoting substances in serum. However, all or most of them can be substituted for by insulin so apparently a single effector can bring about reversal of the pleiotypic response although with a complex substance like serum, several effectors may be required to carry out the same reaction.

Grant (Glasgow)

Would you comment on the huge doses of insulin you have used?

Tomkins (San Francisco)

The dose of insulin we use, although large by physiological standards, is the same as that used by most other investigators for *in vitro* work. It has been suggested that the extensive binding of insulin to glass (see discussion by Y. J. Topper below) may account for the large insulin requirement.

Olson (Middlesex)

Can your pleiotypic effect be explained entirely from a coordinated response of the cellular membrane to a stimulus, or are intracellular controls also involved?

Tomkins (San Francisco)

We do not yet know whether the pleiotypic response is entirely a membrane-mediated affair, or whether intracellular controls are also involved.

Wilton (Southampton)

Assuming that all cells have a basal (resting) level of c-AMP, could the serum/insulin response be explained by a reduction of this c-AMP level to sub-basal levels?

Tomkins (San Francisco)

It is possible that insulin or serum lower the cyclic AMP level of the cells, but it appears from other studies that the cyclic nucleotide is not the pleiotypic mediator, since whatever effects c-AMP has on transformed and untransformed cells are too slow to account for the response itself.

References

1. Hershko, A., Mamont, P., Shields, R. and Tomkins, G. M.; *Nature New Biol.* **232**, (1971) 206.
2. Cashel, M.; *J. Biol. Chem.*; **244**, (1969) 3133.
3. Travers, A., Kamen, R. and Cashel, M.; *Cold Spring Harbor Symp. Quant. Biol.*; **35**, (1970) 415.
4. Mamont, P., Hershko, A. and Tomkins, G. M.; *private communication.*
5. Tomkins, G. M., Thompson, E. B., Hayashi, S., Gelehrter, T., Granner, D. and Peterkofsky, B., *Cold Spring Harbor Symp. Quant. Biol.*; **35**, (1966) 349.
6. Hershko, A. and Tomkins, G. M., *J. Biol. Chem.*; **246**, (1971) 710.
7. Tomkins, G. M., Gelehrter, T. D., Granner, D. K., Martin, D. W., Jr., Samuels, H. H. and Thompson, E. B.; *Science*; **166**, (1969) 1474.
8. Martin, D. W., Tomkins, G. M. and Bresler, M.; *Proc. Nat. Acad. Sci.*; **63**, (1969) 842.
9. Mitchison, J. M., *Science*; **165**, (1969) 657.
10. Tomkins, G. M., Martin, D. W., Jr., Stellwagen, R. H., Baxter, J. D., Mamont, P. and Levinson, B. B.; *Cold Spring Harbor Symp. Quant. Biol.*; **35**, (1970) 635.
11. Baxter, J. D. and Tomkins, G. M.; *Proc. Nat. Acad. Sci.*; **68**, (1971) 932.
12. Baxter, J. D. and Tomkins, G. M.; *Proc. Nat. Acad. Sci.*; **65**, (1970) 709.

CONTROL OF OESTROGEN ACTION BY SPECIFIC OESTROGEN-PROTEIN INTERACTION

R. J. B. King

Department of Hormone Biochemistry, Imperial Cancer Research Fund

Abbreviations: Oestradiol refers to the 17β-isomer.

Oestrogens have a wide range of physiological effects varying from the promotion of cell division in the vagina to the induction of specific enzymes in rat kidney (Table 1). At the pharmacological

Table 1
Effect of Oestrogens on Different Tissues

Species	Tissue	Effect	Reference
Rat	Vagina	Cell division, keratinisation	1
	Kidney	Induction of two enzymes	2,3
Chicken	Oviduct	Ovalbumen production	4
	Liver	Phosphoprotein production	5
Hamster	Kidney	Carcinogenic	6

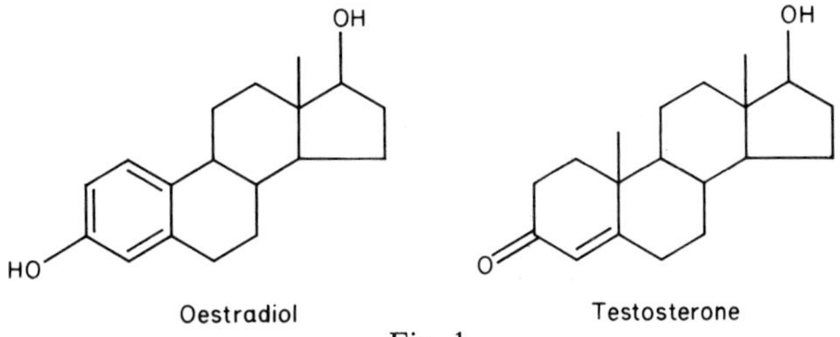

level, they have been used for the treatment of prostatic cancer [7] and the induction of kidney tumours [6]. Any explanation of how oestrogens exert their biological effects must answer two basic questions. How can a relatively simple molecule like oestradiol (Fig. 1) produce such a wide range of effects, and why are its effects very

Oestradiol   Testosterone

Fig. 1.

11

different from those of related androgenic molecules such as testosterone (Fig. 1)? Both types of molecule are relatively flat with oxygen functions at the 3 and 17 positions, the main distinguishing feature being the phenolic A ring and absence of the C_{19}-methyl group in the oestrogens.

This article will present some of the evidence implying that, at least part of the answer to the two questions just posed, is that oestrogen-responsive cells contain a specific receptor protein(s) that binds oestrogens but not androgens. Steroids have been described as 'low information molecules' in that they do not possess the complexity necessary for specific information transfer, but the 'information-content' could be markedly increased by association of the steroid with specific proteins. This mechanism exists in a wide range of steroid-responsive cells [8] and also in auxin-responsive plant cells [9].

The experiments to be described have evolved from studies on the fate of labelled oestrogens in responsive and unresponsive tissues. Several groups recognised the necessity for high specific-activity steroids [10, 11, 12] in order that specific interactions could be studied, but much of the credit for the developments in this field belongs to E. V. Jensen and his co-workers.

Oestrogen-binding and Transport Mechanism in Responsive Cells

The early experiments indicated that the naturally occurring oestrogen, oestradiol-17β, was attached non-covalently to a receptor without metabolic conversion of the steroid [11, 13]. The data at

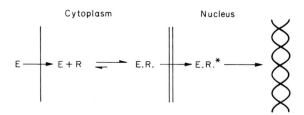

Fig. 2. E = oestrogen; R = receptor protein.

present available are summarised in Fig. 2, each step of which will be discussed below. For more detailed discussion the reader is referred to articles in reference [8].

Entry of oestradiol into the cell

There is no evidence of a permeability barrier to oestradiol at the cell membrane. The experiments of Martin [14] on the local application of steroids to mouse vagina indicate the rapidity with which such molecules can migrate through tissues. Erdos, Bessada and Fries [15] have pointed out that uterus has a high concentration of the so-called 'non-specific' binding proteins ($K_D - 10^{-5}$ M) and have suggested that they may provide the driving force for pulling oestradiol into the cell prior to its attachment to the specific receptor protein(s) ($K_D - 10^{-10}$ M).

Attachment to receptor protein

This is a non-enzymic, physico-chemical interaction which, because of the low-rate constant for dissociation has a K_D of about 10^{-10} M. Some of the factors that influence the oestradiol-receptor

Table 2
Factors affecting Oestradiol-Receptor Interaction

Factor	Effect	Reference
Proteolytic enzymes	Modify and destroy binding	16, 17
Divalent metal ions	Modify and precipitate receptor	18, 19
KCl	Reversibly converts receptor to 4 S form	20, 21
Polycations	Precipitate receptor	22
Urea, acid	Destroy binding	23
—SH reagents	Destroy binding	24
Iodination of tyrosine residues	Destroy binding	25
Oxidation of tryptophan residues	Destroy binding	22

interaction are shown in Table 2. As the receptor has not yet been purified, information about its properties is limited; even the size of the 'physiological' receptor as it exists in a responsive cell is not known for certain. Sedimentation coefficients varying from 10 S to 4 S have been reported, depending on the isolation conditions and age of animals used. Much of this confusion is due to the oligomeric nature of the receptor and its sensitivity to aggregating factors such as other proteins and divalent metal ions.

The isolated receptor is a protein, but because of its impurity, it is not known if other components are also present. Its specificity with respect to the steroids is high (Table 3); of the naturally occurring steroidal oestrogens, only oestradiol is bound to an appreciable extent, although potent synthetic compounds such as diethylstilboestrol and 17α-ethinyl oestradiol bind well. These data were obtained by adding these latter compounds to uterine cytosol in the presence of [6,7-³H] oestradiol and measuring the binding of the latter compound. In this closed system, oestrone is an effective competitor

Table 3
Competition of Steroids for [6,7-³H] Oestradiol-Binding Sites in Uterine Cytosol

Compound	Relative potency
Oestradiol-17β	100
Diethylstilboestrol	246
17α-Ethinyl oestradiol-17β	191
Oestrone	66
Oestriol	16
16-Oxooestradiol-17β	14
Oestradiol-17β diacetate	11
Oestradiol-17β—3-methyl ether	3

This data is taken from the work of S. G. Korenman [26]. The relative potency is the potency of the test compound relative to that of cold oestradiol to inhibit the binding of [6,7-³H] oestradiol.

for binding sites but, *in vivo*, oestrone does not appear to bind to receptors [27].

Entry into the nucleus

Whatever the true size of the cytoplasmic receptor, it changes its properties on passing into the nucleus; its size is no longer affected by ionic strength and the accessibility of the oestradiol is decreased [28]. As isolated in crude preparations it has a sedimentation coefficient of 5 S but on purification it may decrease to 4.5 S [29]. It is not certain if the change in properties of the cytoplasmic receptor occurs before or after its entry into the nucleus. The conversion is blocked by sulphydryl reagents and cannot occur at temperatures below 37° [16]. The scheme outlined in Fig. 2 proposes a net transfer of protein from cytoplasm to nucleus and the evidence for this is summarised in Table 4. As mentioned above, the nuclear and cytoplasmic receptors are not identical but many properties such as pK_I [29, 30] and polycation precipitability [22] are similar, which indicates that at least part of the protein from each locus is the same.

As the amount of nuclear receptor builds up, so that in the cytoplasm decreases [28]. This decrease continues for 4 hr after a single injection of oestradiol but then the number of binding sites increases due, in part, to the synthesis of new protein [31].

The third piece of evidence concerns the immunological properties of the various receptor preparations. Antibody to the cytoplasmic receptor cross reacts with the natural nuclear receptor but not with a

Table 4
Evidence that Protein is Transferred from Cytoplasm to Nucleus

1. Many properties of the 2 receptors are similar.
2. When oestradiol is transported into nucleus, the number of cytoplasmic binding sites decreases.
3. Antibody to cytoplasmic receptor cross reacts with nuclear receptor.

similar extract from endometrium that had not been treated with oestradiol [28].

Intranuclear attachment of receptor

Within the nucleus, the receptor is associated with the chromatin [32, 33] but two essential questions about this have not yet been fully answered; what is the chromatin acceptor molecule for the receptor, and does the acceptor have any specificity with respect to receptor recognition?

Acceptor   The receptor is an acidic protein that has an avidity for a range of polycations, including histones, and it was thought that the acceptor was a histone. This now seems unlikely as histones from a number of non-target cells effectively precipitate the receptor and it is difficult to envisage a cell-specific reaction between receptor and histone [34].

The receptor can attach to DNA and experiments are now in progress to test the idea that DNA is the acceptor [35, 36]. Oestradiol on its own does not bind to the DNA under these conditions (Table 5) although it does if milder equilibration procedures are used [37, 38]. It seems that the protein part of the receptor complex is essential for oestradiol attachment to the DNA, but it appears that the converse is not true; receptor, free of oestradiol, can compete with the oestradiol-receptor complex (Table 5). If these competition experiments can be substantiated by more direct means, an explanation must be found as to why receptor cannot be isolated from nuclei in the absence of oestradiol.

Table 5
Attachment of Uterine [6,7-^{3}H] Oestradiol-labelled Nuclear Receptor to Denatured Calf Thymus DNA

Treatment of receptor	Binding*
Intact [6,7-^{3}H] oestradiol-receptor	100
Heated 60°/5 min	10
[6,7-^{3}H] Oestradiol added to unlabelled nuclear extract	24
No receptor. [6,7-^{3}H] Oestradiol + serum albumen	1
Intact [6,7-^{3}H] oestradiol-receptor + unlabelled cytoplasmic receptor from ovariectomised uteri	43

*Expressed as a % of the binding of the intact complex.
The various preparations were equilibrated (final vol. 0.2 ml) for 1 hr at 4° with 45 μg denatured calf thymus DNA attached to filter paper discs. The discs were then washed with 20 ml cold 15 mM NaCl/0.1 mM sodium citrate pH 7.
Data from [35].

There is no specificity about the type of DNA required for receptor binding and single-stranded DNA is more effective than native DNA. The DNA-receptor interaction has a $K_D - 10^{-10}$ M which is strong enough to explain the prolonged nuclear retention of oestradiol and about one oestradiol molecule (as the receptor complex) is bound per 10^8 nucleotides. This agrees surprisingly well with the nuclear attachment obtained under either *in vivo* or *in vitro* conditions (Table 6). The table also indicates that, in the presence of physiological amounts of oestradiol, there are several thousand molecules of hormone per nucleus, which raises the question of whether there are several sites of action within the nucleus.

Receptor attachment is not confined to polydeoxyribonucleotides (Fig. 3). As far as one can tell from these experiments, guanine

Table 6
**Comparison of Uterine Nuclear Binding of [6,7-³H]Oestradiol under
Different Labelling Conditions**

Type of experiment	Molecules oestradiol bound/ 10^8 DNA nucleotide units	Reference
In vivo injection	20	39
In vitro incubation Nuclei + oestradiol receptor	4	35
In vitro incubation Chromatin + oestradiol receptor	4	35
In vitro incubation DNA + oestradiol receptor	25	35

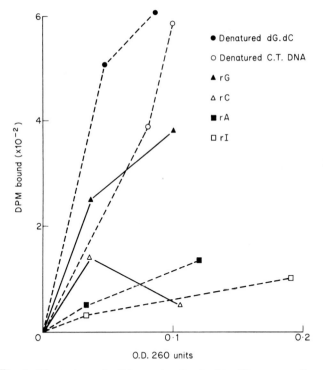

Fig. 3. The polynucleotides were attached to filter paper discs, equilibrated with [6,7-³H]oestradiol-nuclear receptor (15 × 10^3 disintegrations/min) washed and counted as described in Table 5. The amount of polynucleotide attached to the disc was determined by hydrolysis in 0.5 N PCA for 15 min at 70°C and measurement of the O.D. at 260 nm.

appears to be the most important base and the importance of the 2-amino group is illustrated by the comparison of polyguanylic with polyinosinic acid. This would agree with the observation that hydroxymethylation of the exocyclic amino groups of DNA by formaldehyde decreased receptor binding by 58%. Nothing is known about the influence of other nucleotides adjacent to the binding regions but the present data are compatible with the view that specific base sequences are required for receptor attachment. These experiments indicate that either DNA or RNA could be the acceptor. Hydrolysis of chromatin RNA with either $ZnNO_3$ or ribonuclease in

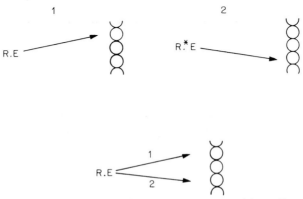

Fig. 4. 1 and 2 refers to different oestrogen-sensitive cell types. The suggestion in the top line is that the receptors (R and R*) are different in different cells. The bottom line represents the view that the oestrogen-receptor complex (RE) goes to different regions of the chromatin in different cells.

2 M NaCl/5 M urea [40] provided no evidence on this point. In both the treated and control (incubated in the absence of $ZnNO_3$ or ribonuclease) samples there was a general five-fold increase in acceptor property of spleen and uterine chromatins. This is probably due to the artifactual exposure of new acceptor sites. As these new sites are also available in dehistoned chromatin, they cannot be explained by receptor interaction with histones.

Uterine chromatin preparations, with DNA : RNA ratios of 1 : 0.02, bind the receptor complex which would tend to support the view that DNA and not RNA is the acceptor.

No tight binding of ^{3}H-guanosine to uterine cytoplasmic receptor was detected by chromatography of these two components through a Sephadex G50 column.

Specificity of the acceptor   One of the questions presented at the beginning of this article was, how do oestrogens exert their different effects on cells of various kinds? Is it due to the presence of different receptors (R and R* in Fig. 4) in different oestrogen-responsive cells or does the receptor go to one chromatin site in cell type 1 but to a different one in cell type 2? No evidence has been found that the receptors in different responsive cells are different but the methods

Table 7
Attachment of Uterine [6,7-^{3}H] Oestradiol-Cytoplasmic Receptor to Nuclei and Chromatin

Acceptor prepared from	Binding to*	
	Nuclei	Chromatin
Uterus	100	100
Liver	86 (97–69)	83 (98–57)
Spleen	53 (81–32)	29 (47–19)

*DPM/mg DNA expressed as a % of that bound to either nuclei or chromatin from uterus. The results are expressed as the mean and the range of three separate experiments.

Receptor complex was equilibrated at 4°C for 1 hr with either nuclei or chromatin (containing 40 μg DNA). Nuclei were reisolated, washed once with 0.01 M tris pH 7.4 and counted. Chromatin was filtered onto filter paper discs, washed with 10 ml 1.5 mM NaCl/0.1 mM sodium citrate pH 7 and counted. The amount of DNA per disc was determined by hydrolysis with 0.5 N PCA at 70°C for 15 min and the O.D. at 260 nm measurement.

that have been used are far too crude to permit any conclusion on this point. There is however some specificity at the acceptor level; uterine nuclei or chromatin will accept more uterine oestradiol-receptor than similar preparations from liver or spleen (Table 7). This difference cannot be due to their DNA and the most likely reason is the different composition of the chromatin proteins. If DNA is the acceptor, the chromatin proteins may determine if the correct region of the DNA is available for binding.

Relationship of Receptor Binding to Biological Activity of Oestrogens

The evidence that attachment of oestrogen to receptor is the initiating event in a sequence resulting in the biological effect of the hormone is circumstantial and can be divided into four parts.

Kinetics of binding and biological effect

The data available at present suggest that the speed with which oestradiol attaches to the receptor is compatible with the earliest known effects of oestradiol. The caution contained in this statement is due to the fact that parallel experiments measuring binding and biological effect (chromatin activation) have only been carried out by one group [41]. In this one case, binding and effect were concomitant. On the other hand, an effect on uterine RNA synthesis can be detected 2 min after intraperitoneal injection of oestradiol [42] as compared with the earliest time at which bound oestradiol has been measured of a few minutes. Szego and Davis [43] have reported that uterine cyclic 3'5'-AMP increases within 15 sec of oestradiol application: no comparable studies have been made with oestradiol binding although bound oestradiol can be detected 7 sec after local application of [6,7-^{3}H] oestradiol to mouse vagina [14].

Occurrence of receptor in different cells

Of the tissues thus far studied, receptors have been found in those that respond to oestrogen but not in the so-called unresponsive tissues such as liver, spleen, lung or muscle [8]. This does not mean that they are not present in small but undetected amounts. This is especially intriguing in respect to liver which responds to oestrogen, albeit in a small way [41, 44]. No one has demonstrated the presence of the classical 8-10 S receptor in rat liver cytoplasm but it does contain protamine-precitable material which is absent in mouse liver [22 and unpublished results].

Another possible exception is the hamster kidney in which oestrogen-responsive tumours develop under the prolonged influence of pharmacologic amounts of oestrogen [6]. No receptors were detected prior to the appearance of the tumours [45]. The number of oestrogen-sensitive cells in the hamster kidney is very small which may explain the apparent lack of receptors but it is possible that this carcinogenic effect of oestrogen is mediated via a 'non-receptor mechanism'.

Structure-function relationship

With the reservations mentioned below, there is a good structure-function relationship between the oestrogens that will attach to the receptor and their biological activity. This extends from the naturally occurring steroid oestradiol to the synthetic, non-steroid, diethyl-stilboestrol. This topic has been described in a number of publications [26, 27, 46, 47] and will not be discussed here apart from three points that, at first glance, indicate that there are exceptions to the above statements but for which rational explanations can be found.

Tissues such as liver can demethylate methyl ethers so that 3 methyl ethers of potent oestrogens are inactive when applied directly to the vagina both as oestrogens and for attachment to receptors. They are however active if given systemically [27, 48].

The second proviso concerns the duration of attachment of oestrogen to the receptor. It appears that the longer the oestrogen is attached to the receptor, the more potent it is in biological terms. Thus oestriol binds less tightly to the uterine receptor than does oestradiol [16, 49] and is a weaker oestrogen in this organ [50]. The situation with regard to oestriol and the vagina is less clear. Martin [47] has reported that, in vagina [15^{-3} H] oestriol is retained to the same extent as oestradiol but is less efficient at competing with oestradiol for receptor sites. Obviously one cannot entirely extrapolate the results obtained with one oestrogen-sensitive tissue to another one.

The duration of attachment to receptor can explain the action of some antioestrogens. Some antioestrogens exert their effect by blocking the attachment of potent oestrogens such as oestradiol and the evidence for this provides good evidence for a causal relationship between binding and biological effect. This is illustrated in Fig. 5, the data for which are taken from the work of Martin [47]. He compared the effect of increasing amounts of the synthetic anti-oestrogen, dimethylstilboestrol, given either simultaneously or 15 min prior to the injection of [$6,7-^3$H] oestradiol, on biological potency and binding. The parallelism between the two parameters is very evident. When the antioestrogen was given concomitantly with the oestrogen, both effects were depressed to an extent dependent on the dose. When the antioestrogen was given 15 min after the oestrogen, the dimethylstilboestrol only had a marginal effect.

Conclusive proof that receptor attachment is a prerequisite of biological effect can only be obtained by *in vitro* experiments showing that the oestrogen-receptor complex will mimic the early *in vivo* effect of oestrogen. One such example has been reported: Raynaud-Jammet and Baulieu [51] have shown that uterine nuclei isolated under conditions such that they would contain the oestradiol-receptor complex produce more RNA than those that contain

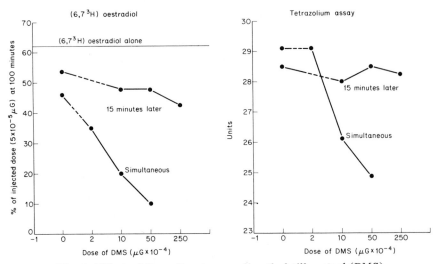

Fig. 5. Effect of the antioestrogen, dimethylstilboestrol (DMS) on [6,7-³H] oestradiol binding and biological activity of oestradiol binding and biological activity of oestradiol in mouse vagina. Data from [47].

oestradiol but no receptor. Beziat, Guilleux and Mousseron-Canet [52] have reported similar results but other workers have had difficulty in repeating these experiments.

Conclusions

This paper outlines a mechanism that can provide some of the answers to how oestrogens exert their biological effect but this does not mean that it is the only way by which these hormones can be effective. The following article by Rabin *et al.* [53] illustrates another potential effect and there is nothing to suggest that the physiological and pharmacological effects are mediated by the same route. It is also possible that one of the numerous reports of inhibition of enzymes by very high concentrations of steroids [54] may play some part in the pharmacological effects of steroids.

Discussion

Tomkins (San Francisco)

1. Is the early increase in RNA labelling in the uterus due to changes in nucleoside phosphorylation? If so, is it inhibited by AMP?

2. Does the receptor bind guanosine monomers like GTP?

King (London)

1. To the best of my knowledge this is not known.

2. No detectable binding of ^{3}H guanosine to uterine cytoplasmic receptor could be detected by Sephadex G25 chromatography. We have reported that GTP will interact with receptor [55], but I am no longer certain about those particular experiments as the pH of the medium was not accurately controlled.

Olson (Middlesex)

Are the cytoplasmic receptors for oestrogen and the analogous nuclear receptor the same or different?

King (London)

The current view is that at least part of the nuclear receptor is similar to the cytoplasmic one. This is discussed in the articles in ref. 8.

Jenkins (St George's Hospital)

Do non-steroid oestrogens such as diethyl stilboestrol bind specifically to receptor protein in the same way as natural steroid oestrogen?

King (London)

Yes.

Grant (Glasgow)

Would you not agree that the very lack of similarity in chemical structure provides evidence for your view that what goes in to the nucleus is the receptor protein and it is this which provides the biological specificity?

King (London)

Yes.

Jaitly (Delft)

If the role of the oestrogens is only the enhancement of passage of the receptor protein into the nucleus, and this protein is then responsible for the further oestrogenic effects of the oestrogen-protein complex, how do you explain the effect of the anti-oestrogens.

King (London)

I think the combined oestrogen-receptor complex is needed within the nucleus. One can picture the action of anti-oestrogens at a number of places after they have attached to the receptor. (These remarks are confined to those anti-oestrogens that exert their effect by receptor attachment.) Attachment of an anti-oestrogen to receptor in place of oestradiol could make nuclear transfer or chromatin binding less efficient or the anti-oestrogen receptor complex could remain for a shorter time in the chromatin.

As far as I know, no one has shown that anti-oestrogens actually get into the nucleus. One possible exception to this is the work of Brecher and Wotiz [49]. I personally think they do because all of the anti-oestrogens have some oestrogenic properties if you look hard enough.

Heald (Strathclyde)

1. Would Dr. King indicate the purity of the receptor preparations he discussed and how these are evaluated?

2. Since they are so impure would he comment on the validity of the immunological experiments?

King (London)

1. The purest preparations available contain less than 5% of the receptor [see ref. 8]. Most of the receptor preparations used thus far have been even less pure than this. The purity is evaluated on the basis of the molecular weight of the particular receptor protein and the assumption that 1 molecule of receptor binds 1 molecule of oestradiol.

2. It is not really possible to comment on the purity of the receptor used in the immunological work. It was prepared by adsorption of calf uterine cytosol on a column of oestradiol-cellulose and elution with sodium deoxycholate which destroys the binding of [6,7-^{3}H] oestradiol [28]. It is certainly not 100% pure and therefore the immunological experiments are not absolutely conclusive.

References

1. Biggers, J. D. and Claringbold, P. J.; *J. Anat.*; **89**, (1955) 124.
2. Herzfeld, A. and Knox, W. E.; *J. biol. Chem.;* **243**, (1968) 3327.
3. Ryan, K. J., Meigs, R. A., Petro, Z. and Morrison, G., *Science*; **142**, (1963) 243.
4. O'Malley, B. W., McGuire, W. L., Kohler, P. O. and Korenman, S. G.; *Recent Prog. Horm. Res.*; **25**, (1969) 105.
5. Heald, P. J. and McLachlan, P. M.; *Biochem. J.*; **94**, (1965) 32.
6. Kirkman, H.; *Nat. Cancer Inst. Monogr.*; **1**, (1959) 1.
7. Huggins, C. and Hodges, C. V.; *Cancer Res.*; **1**, (1941) 293.
8. *'Advances in the Biosciences'*; Vol. 7. Pergamon Press, Vieweg, W. Germany, (1971).
9. Matthyse, A. G. and Abrams, M.; *Biochim. Biophys. Acta*; **199**, (1970) 511.
10. Glasscock, R. F. and Hoeckstra, W. G.; *Biochem. J.*; **72**, (1959) 673.
11. Jensen, E. V. and Jacobsen, H. I.; *Recent Prog. Horm. Res.*; **18**, (1962) 387.
12. Pearlman, W. H. and Pearlman, M. R. J.; *J. Biol. Chem.;* **236**, (1961) 700.
13. King, R. J. B., Gordon, J. and Inman, D. R.; *J. Endocr.*; **32**, (1965) 9.
14. Martin, L.; *J. Endocr.*; **30**, (1964) 337.
15. Erdos, T., Bessada, R. and Fries, J.; *FEBS Letters*; **5**, (1969) 161.
16. Gorski, J., Toft, D., Shyamala, G., Smith, D. and Notides, A.; *Recent Prog. Horm. Res.*; **24**, (1968) 45.
17. Erdos, T.; In: 'Hormonal Steroids'; Excerpta Medica International Congress Series 210, (1971) in press.
18. Brecher, P., Pasquini, A. and Wotiz, H. W.; *Endocrinology*; **85**, (1969) 3.
19. DeSombre, E. R., Chabaud, J. P., Puca, G. A. and Jensen, E. V.; In: 'Hormonal Steroids'; Excerpta Medica International Congress Series 210, (1971) in press.
20. Erdos, T., Gospodarowicz, D., Bessada, R. and Fries, J.; *C.R. Acad. Sci. Paris*; **266**, (1968) 2164.
21. Korenman, S. G. and Rao, B. R.; *Proc. Natn. Acad. Sci. U.S.A.*; **61**, (1968) 1028.
22. Steggles, A. W. and King, R. J. B.; *Biochem. J.*; **118**, (1970) 695.
23. King, R. J. B., Gordon, J., Cowan, D. M. and Inman, D. R.; *J. Endocr.;* **36**, (1966) 139.
24. Jensen, E. V., Hurst, D. J., DeSombre, E. R. and Jungblut, P. W.; *Science*; **158**, (1967) 385.
25. Puca, G. A. and Bresciana, F.; *Research on Steroids,* **4**, (1970) 247.
26. Korenman, S. G.; *Steroids*; **13**, (1969) 163.
27. Jensen, E. V., Jacobsen, H. I., Flesher, J. W., Saha, N. N., Gupta, G. N., Smith, S., Colucci, V., Shiplacoff, D., Neumann, H. G., DeSombre, E. R. and Jungblut, P. W.; In: 'Steroid Dynamics'; Eds G. Pincus, T. Nakao and J. T. Tait. Academic Press, New York, (1966) p. 133.
28. Jungblut, P.W., McCann, S., Gorlich, L., Rosenfeld, G. C. and Wagner, R.; *Research on Steroids*; **4**, (1970) 213.
29. Puca, G. A., Nola, E., Sica, V. and Bresciani, F.; In: 'Advances in the Biosciences'; Vol. 7. Pergamon Press, Vieweg, W. Germany, (1971) p. 97.
30. Brecher, P. O., Chabaud, J. P., Colucci, V., DeSombre, E. R., Flesher, J. W., Gupta, G. N., Hurst, D. J., Ikeda, M., Jacobsen, H. I., Jensen, E. V., Jungblut, P. W., Kawashima, T., Kyser, K. A., Neumann, H. G., Numata, M., Puca, G. A., Saha, N., Smith and Suzuki, T.; In: 'Advances in the Biosciences; Vol. 7. Pergamon Press, Vieweg, W. Germany, (1971) p. 75.

31. Gorski, J., Sarff, M. and Clark, J.; In: 'Advances in the Biosciences.; Vol. 7. Pergamon Press, Vieweg, W. Germany, (1971) p. 5.
32. King, R. J. B.; *Archs. Anat. microsc. Morph. exp.*; **56**, (1967) 570.
33. Maurer, H. R. and Chalkley, R. G.; *J. mol. Biol.*; **27**, (1967) 431.
34. King, R. J. B., Gordon, J. and Steggles, A. W.; In: 'Hormonal Steroids.: Excerpta Medica International Congress Series 210, (1971) in press.
35. King, R. J. B., Beard, V., Gordon, J., Pooley, A. S., Smith, J. A., Steggles, A. W. and Vertes, M.; In: 'Advances in the Biosciences'; Vol. 7. Pergamon Press, Vieweg, W. Germany, (1971) p.21.
36. King, R. J. B. and Gordon, J.; Submitted for publication.
37. Ts'o, P. O. P. and Lu, P.; *Proc. Natn. Acad. Sci. U.S.A.*; **51**, (1964) 17.
38. Cohen, P., Chin, R.-C. and Kidson, C.; *Biochemistry*; **8**, (1969) 3603.
39. King, R. J. B. and Gordon, J.; *J. Endocr.;* **34**, (1966) 43.
40. Bekhor, I., Kung, G. M. and Bonner, J.; *J. Mol. Biol.*; **39**, (1969) 351.
41. Hamilton, T. H.; *Science*; **161**, (1968) 649.
42. Means, A. R. and Hamilton, T. H.; *Proc. Natn. Acad. Sci. U.S.A.*; **56**, (1966) 1594.
43. Szego, C. M. and Davis, J. S.; *Proc. Natn. Acad. Sci. U.S.A.*; **58**, (1967) 1711.
44. Church, R. H. and McCarthy, B. J.; *Biochim. Biophys. Acta*; **199**, (1970) 103.
45. King, R. J. B., Smith, J. A. and Steggles, A. W.; *Steroidologia*; **1**, (1970) 73.
46. Terenius, L.; *Mol. Pharmacol.*; **4**, (1968) 301.
47. Martin, L.; Proc. second inter. congr. hormonal steroids. Excerpta Medica International Congress Series 132, (1967) p. 608.
48. Emmens, C. W.; *J. Endocr.*; **2**, (1941) 444.
49. Brecher, P. I. and Wotiz, H. H.; *Steroids*; **9**, (1967) 431.
50. Merrill, R. C.; *Physiol. Rev.*; **38**, (1958) 463.
51. Raynaud-Jammet, C. and Baulieu, E. E.; *C.R. Acad. Sci. Paris*; **268**, (1969) 3211.
52. Beziat, Y., Guilleux, J. C. and Mousseron-Canet, M.; *C.R. Acad. Sci. Paris*; **270**, (1970) 1620.
53. Rabin, B. R. *et al.* This volume.
54. Tomkins, G. M. and Yielding, K. L.; In: 'Actions of Hormones on Molecular Processes'; Eds G. Litwack and D. Kritchevsky. J. Wiley & Son, New York (1964) p. 209.
55. King, R. J. B., Gordon, J., Marx, J. and Steggles, A. W.; In 'Basic Actions of Steroid Hormones on Target Organs'; Eds P. O. Hubinont, F. Leroy & P. Laland. Karger; Basle, (1971) p. 21.

THE EFFECTS OF STEROID HORMONES AND CARCINOGENS ON THE INTERACTION OF MEMBRANES WITH POLYSOMES

B. R. Rabin, Carol A. Blyth, Delma Doherty,
R. B. Freedman, Anne Roobol,
G. Sunshine and D. J. Williams

*Department of Biochemistry, University College London,
Gower Street, London, WC1E 6BT*

Protein synthesis in the cell, involves particulate elements called ribosomes which translate the information coded as specific nucleotide sequences in messenger RNA molecules into amino-acid sequences of proteins [1]. Ribosomes are frequently found in the cell in the form of aggregates called polysomes. The ribosomes in a polysome are believed to be attached to a single messenger RNA molecule and simultaneously to translate the encoded information to give polypeptides with a specific amino-acid sequence [2]. The basic mechanisms of the control of protein synthesis at the level of translation are not well understood.

Polysomes can be observed by electron microscopy to exist in the cell in two distinctive forms—free polysomes, unattached to membranes, and membrane-bound polysomes [3, 4]. The membrane-polysome complex constitutes the 'rough' membranes of the endoplasmic reticulum. A variety of other membranes also occur in the cell, including 'smooth' endoplasmic reticulum, which is characterised by the absence of bound polysomes.

Accumulating evidence indicates that free and bound polysomes are probably involved in the biosynthesis of different classes of proteins [5, 6]. For example, it is probable that proteins exported from the cell are biosynthesised by membrane-bound polysomes [5] and this may also be true of other important classes of protein such as those whose biosynthesis is induced by steroid hormones [7]. Clearly the control of the interaction of polysomes with membranes could be of profound importance in dictating the tissue-specific pattern of protein biosynthesis which characterises the processes of differentiation and development. Indeed there are indications that the ratio of free to bound polysomes is a function of the hormonal status of the organism [7, 8, 8a, 8b]. If chemical carcinogenesis is viewed as essentially an aberrant form of the processes of differentiation, it is obviously important to investigate the effects of carcinogens on the interaction of membranes with polysomes.

The problem of investigating membrane-polysome interactions is considerably simplified by the fact that an enzyme present in the reticular membranes—which we shall call the disulphide rearranging enzyme (or rearrangease)—has its activity masked when polysomes are bound to the membranes and its activity is only fully exposed when the polysomes are removed. Thus the activity of rearrangease provides a relatively simple means of measuring quantitatively polysome attachment to membranes *in vitro*. The enzyme is present in both 'rough' and 'smooth' membrane fractions, but the activity in rough membranes is zero and only appears when the polysomes are removed [9]. Rearrangease catalyses a complex reaction of disulphide exchange and is probably involved in the terminal stages of protein biosynthesis [10].

Native bovine pancreatic ribonuclease contains 4 disulphide bonds. By reduction and reoxidation of the enzyme under denaturing conditions, it is possible to produce a protein in which the disulphide bonds are 'wrongly' paired and which is devoid of any catalytic action. If this 'randomly oxidised' material is used as substrate, the activity of rearrangease can be measured by following the appearance of ribonuclease activity, since the membrane-bound rearrangease catalyses the 're-shuffling' of the sulphurs of the wrongly folded protein to give the native structure [10].

In Fig. 1, the specific activity of rearrangease is plotted against the RNA/protein ratio of various membrane sub-fractions prepared by differential centrifugation techniques from male rat liver. Similar and parallel plots are obtained from other tissues of the rat [11]. The RNA/protein ratio is a measure of the number of ribosomes bound per unit weight of the membrane. The linear relationship is not surprising, since the various sub-fractions are composed of rough and smooth membrane components but in different ratio. Notice that the 'roughest' components are totally devoid of enzymic activity. If those fractions with a high RNA/protein ratio are dialysed against EDTA, which causes polysome dissociation from the membranes, and the specific activity of the separated membranes determined, the values obtained approach that corresponding to the intersection of the line in Fig. 1 with the ordinate axis. The degranulated rough

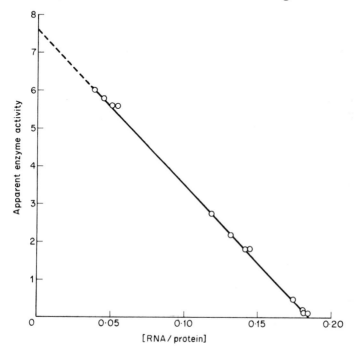

Fig. 1. The relationship between apparent disulphide inter-change activity (arbitrary units) and the RNA : protein ratio, for microsomal fractions derived from rat liver by differential centrifugation. Assay methods as in ref. [9].

membranes have approximately the same specific activity as smooth membranes: the 'enzyme density' is the same for all membranes from a given tissue and the enzyme is uniquely coupled to the loci of polysome binding. It may indeed be located in the vicinity of the ribosome binding site which would be a favourable location for the enzyme to operate in the terminal stages of protein biosynthesis using the newly formed nascent protein as substrate.

Figure 2 illustrates an experiment in which liver membranes were stripped of polysomes by EDTA treatment so as to uncover nearly all latent rearrangease activity and the resultant degranulated membranes were incubated with fresh polysomes in the presence of magnesium ions. The rearrangease activity falls to the initial low value of the original, mainly rough membranes as the polysomes reattach themselves to the membranes. Notice that the experimental curve does not cross below that of the control of the unstripped

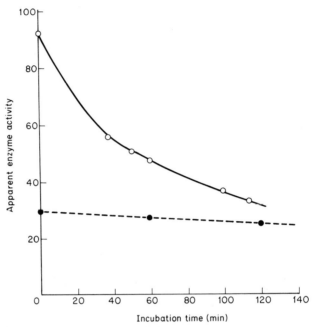

Fig. 2. The binding of polysomes to 'polysome-depleted' membranes, monitored by the masking of disulphide interchange activity. Rough microsomal membranes were degranulated by EDTA [9, 11], isolated, and then incubated (~4 mg/ml protein) with excess free polysomes (~1 mg/ml RNA) at 25°C. (—o—). Untreated rough membranes were also incubated with free polysomes as a control (—●—).

membranes incubated with polysomes. Now the activity present in these unstripped membranes is due to the presence of smooth membranes and it is clear that although degranulated, rough membranes will rebind polysomes, smooth membranes will not. This lack of interaction has been confirmed by using purified smooth membrane preparations. The reattachment of polysomes to stripped-rough membranes has also been confirmed by measuring directly RNA bound to the membranes after separation of unbound polysomes by centrifugation [11]. Clearly smooth membranes are operationally different from degranulated rough membranes: the difference seems to be due to a component present in rough but absent in smooth reticulum as we shall see later.

The reattachment of polysomes to degranulated rough membranes is remarkably sex-specific as illustrated in Fig. 3. It can be seen that degranulated rough membranes will re-bind polysomes

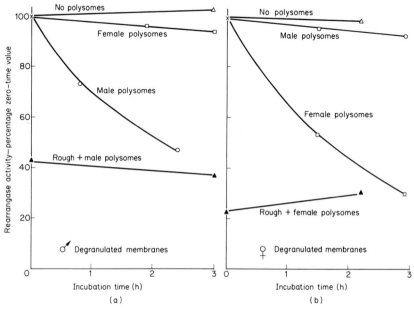

Fig. 3. The sex-specificity of association *in vitro* between free polysomes and degranulated rough membranes from rat liver. Conditions as described in legend of Fig. 2.

from the same, but not the opposite, sex. Before discussing the sex-specificity in detail, we shall consider the nature of the differences between smooth and degranulated rough membranes. It is possible to prepare an ethyl acetate extract of male rough membranes which will activate both male and female smooth membranes to bind polysomes of either sex. A similar extract from male polysomes will promote the binding of female polysomes to female smooth membranes but not male polysomes to male smooth membranes. Analogous extracts from female polysomes promote the attachment of male polysomes to male membranes. The data are summarised in Table 1. Although the presentation is qualitative, experimental determinations are actually very clear-cut and, binding in the experimental systems seems to be almost an all-or-none phenomenon. The male polysomes contain a material which will activate the female but not the male system and vice versa. Male rough reticulum contains the components required to activate both

Table 1
Interaction of Polysomes with Smooth Membranes as Measured by Disulphide Rearranging Enzyme

Smooth membrane	Polysomes	Ethyl acetate extract	Formation of membrane-polysome complex
male	male	none	—
male	male	male polysomes	—
male	male	female polysomes	+
male	male	male rough membranes	+
male	female	none	—
female	female	none	—
female	female	female polysomes	—
female	female	male polysomes	+
female	female	male rough membranes	+
female	male	none	—
female	male + female	none	+
male	male + female	none	+

Membranes (5-7 mg protein/ml) were incubated with polysomes (2-5 mg RNA/ml) in the presence and absence of various ethyl acetate extracts. The extracts were prepared by suspending the polysomes or rough membranes in water (3 ml) and extracting 3 times with 6 ml portions of ice-cold ethyl acetate. The pooled extracts were evaporated to dryness, dissolved in 0.05 ml dimethyl formamide and diluted with 0.15 ml of 0.25 M sucrose in 50 mM Tris-chloride containing 25 mM KCl and 5 mM $MgCl_2$ (TKM).

the male and female systems. These unknown substances can be provided by the polysomes without extraction since a mixture of male plus female polysomes, but not the separate components, will bind to either male or female smooth membranes.

The above experiments strongly suggest that in male rat liver, smooth membranes will not bind polysomes because there is a deficiency of a material which is soluble in organic solvents and present in female polysomes or male rough endoplasmic reticulum. In the female there would be an analogous deficiency, but of a different material which is present in male polysomes. One obvious possibility would be the involvement of the pair of sex hormones, with oestradiol being deficient in the male and testosterone deficient in the female. This would require that testosterone or oestradiol is present in male or female polysomes, respectively, as isolated. These hormones have, indeed, been previously implicated in the interaction

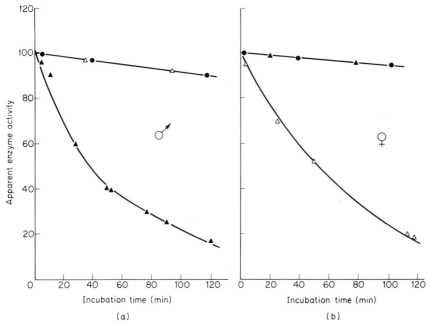

Fig. 4. The sex-specific effects of steroid hormones in promoting association of free polysomes and smooth micro-somal membranes *in vitro*. Incubations of steroids with male (a) and female (b) smooth microsomes and polysomes. No steroid present (—●—); in presence of 2 μg/ml oestradiol (—▲—); in presence of 2 μg/ml testosterone (—△—).

of smooth membranes with polysomes [12, 13] and some of the experimental evidence is presented in Figs 4a and 4b. It is clearly demonstrated in Fig. 4a that oestradiol promotes the binding of male polysomes to male smooth membranes. Testosterone is without any effect. The binding in the presence of oestradiol *in vitro* has been confirmed by electron microscopy [14] and it has been estimated, very approximately, that one molecule of steroid hormone is required per ribosome bound to the membrane. Figure 4b illustrates the situation in the female: the effects are totally opposite to the male. Testosterone promotes polysome binding, oestradiol is without effect. The concentrations of hormone required are again of the order of one molecule per bound ribosome. These experiments show very clear-cut differences between male and female animals, which could derive from sex specificity of steroid interactions with membranes and/or polysomes.

One, but by no means the only, possible explanation of the results is, (i) that in both sexes oestradiol and testosterone are required to be simultaneously present to activate the membranes for polysome binding and, (ii) that polysomes and/or membranes of the female already contain oestradiol, or an equivalent material, and those of

Table 2
**Steroid Hormone Requirements for the Interaction of
Polysomes with Female Smooth Membranes**

Polysome sex	Added steroid	Formation of membrane-polysome complex
female	none	—
female	oestradiol	—
female	testosterone	+
male	none	—
male	testosterone	—
male	oestradiol	+

Incubation of membranes and polysomes, and assay for complex formation as in Table 1.

the male, a substance with equivalent properties to testosterone. This explanation would, of course, be entirely consistent with the ability of the ethyl acetate extracts of polysomes to promote membrane-polysome interaction in the opposite sex. To shed further light on this problem some experiments were conducted to determine the steroid hormone requirements for the interaction of membranes with polysomes from the opposite sex. Some of these results are summarised in Tables 2 and 3. It can be seen that testosterone promotes the interaction of male membranes with female polysomes, and oestradiol a similar interaction of female membranes with male polysomes.

It seems clear, from the work described above, that steroid hormones (or equivalent materials extracted from polysomes *or* membranes) are required for membrane-polysome interactions to occur. The requirements are sex specific and are for oestradiol (or equivalent material extracted from female polysomes) in the male and testosterone (or equivalent material extracted from male polysomes) in the female. The crossed-sex experiments suggest there may also be a requirement for the other hormone, although this possibility cannot yet be tested experimentally in the interaction of membranes with polysomes from the same sex, because the male and female polysomes already contain, respectively, substances equivalent to testosterone and oestradiol. It is certainly true to say that, in all systems in which polysomes interact with membranes, both hormones (or equivalent materials) are present. We are at present

Table 3
Steroid Hormone Requirements for the Interaction of Polysome with Male Smooth Membranes

Polysome sex	Added steroid	Formation of membrane-polysome complex
male	none	−
male	testosterone	−
male	oestradiol	+
female	none	−
female	oestradiol	−
female	testosterone	+

Incubation of membranes and polysomes, and assay for complex formation as in Table 1.

attempting to deplete polysomes of their hormone content to test whether both hormones are involved in the binding process.

Further relevant information has been obtained by studies in the direct binding of steroid hormones to membranes [15]. Figure 5 shows the binding curves obtained for the interaction of oestradiol with male smooth and degranulated rough membranes. There are some quite profound differences between the two types of membranes. The smooth membranes have sites at which the hormone is bound very tightly (region A-B). We shall call these tight sites and these can be saturated; at higher hormone concentration (region B-C) there is an almost linear partitioning of the hormone between the membranes and solution. At still higher hormone concentration (region C-D) a further set of hormone binding sites come into operation. Degranulated rough membranes possess no sites in the regions A-B or C-D. We have evidence that binding in the region C-D involves the microsomal hydroxylase complex, which is mainly located in smooth membranes. We shall only consider binding in the region A-B. The binding curves of the tight sites only are shown in Figs 6 and 7. They show the same remarkable sex-specificity as the

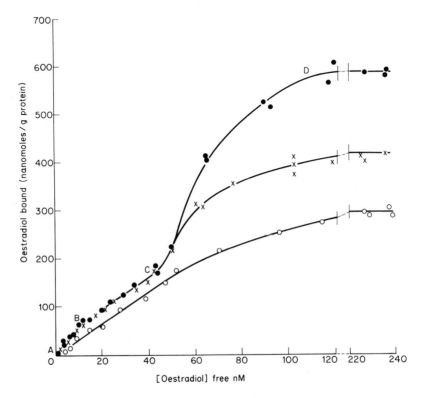

Fig. 5. Direct titration of ^{3}H-oestradiol with male rat liver microsomes. Methods as in ref. [15]. Smooth microsomes (—●—); EDTA-treated smooth microsomes (—x—); EDTA-degranulated rough microsomes (—○—).

interaction of smooth membranes with polysomes from the same sex. It can be seen that male smooth membranes possess tight sites for oestradiol and female membranes similar sites for testosterone. The sites are very specific since oestradiol and testosterone do not compete with each other for these tight sites. Degranulated membranes from either sex apparently possess no tight sites for either hormone.

Recent unpublished experiments in this laboratory by Dr Carol Blyth suggest that degranulated membranes do in fact possess tight sites for the binding of steroid hormones, but that these are already occupied. Ethyl acetate extracts of male degranulated rough membrane, block the tight oestradiol sites on male smooth membranes

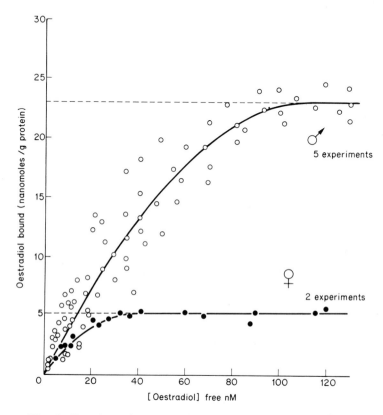

Fig. 6. Titration of the 'tight' binding sites [see ref. 15] for oestradiol in male (O) and female (●) rat liver smooth microsomes.

but have no effect on the tight testosterone sites on female smooth membrane. Similar extracts of female degranulated membrane block the tight testosterone sites on female smooth membranes and are without effect in the tight oestradiol sites of male smooth membrane.

We have also investigated the effects of a range of carcinogenic and other substances on the interaction of membranes with steroids and polysomes. Our earlier experiments showed that the hepatotoxin and carcinogen, Aflatoxin B_1, will directly degranulate the rough endoplasmic reticulum by irreversible interaction with the membranes [11]. Figures 8a and 8b show the degranulating effect for both male and female membranes as measured by assaying the

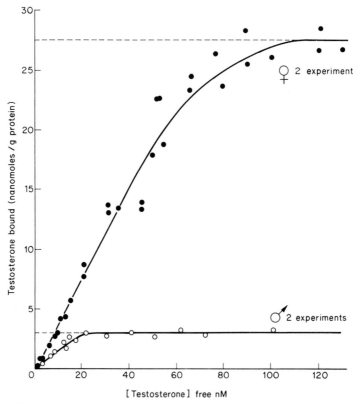

Fig. 7. Titration of the 'tight' binding sites [see ref. 15] for testosterone in male (○) and female (●) rat liver smooth microsomes.

'rearrangease' enzyme. The results have been confirmed by direct measurements of RNA attached to the membranes [11]. If the carcinogen is acting by interfering with a site on the membrane which binds steroid hormones, then it is to be expected that the appropriate hormone will protect the membrane against the degranulating effects of the carcinogen. This is indeed observed, as shown in Figs 8a and 8b and, again, the protection is sex-specific:

oestradiol protects male and, testosterone female membranes. Aflatoxin B_1 also destroys the ability of smooth membranes to interact with polysomes in the presence of the appropriate hormone. These effects of Aflatoxin B_1 are also observed by *in vivo* feeding experiments. The smooth membranes from male rats fed on a diet containing 5 ppm Aflatoxin B_1 totally lost their ability to bind polysomes in the presence of oestradiol in just two days. The

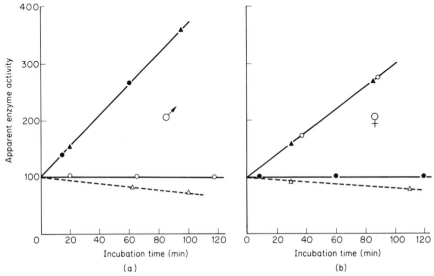

Fig. 8. The effects of steroid hormones on the reaction of aflatoxin B_1 with rough microsomes from male (a) and female (b) rat liver. Membranes at ~4 mg/ml protein. Control incubation (—△—); incubation with aflatoxin B_1 (40 μg/ml) alone (—▲—); incubation with aflatoxin B_1 and oestradiol (10 μg/ml) (—○—); incubation with aflatoxin B_1 and testosterone (10 μg/ml) (—●—).

carcinogen destroys the ability of smooth membranes to react with polysomes much more rapidly than it degranulates rough membranes.

Binding studies have demonstrated that Aflatoxin B_1 destroys the tight binding sites for steroid hormones on smooth membranes and some of the relevant experiments are illustrated in Figs 9a and 9b. It can be seen that oestradiol, but not testosterone protects the tight oestradiol sites on male smooth membranes. Similarly, testosterone, but not oestradiol, protects the sites for this hormone on female membranes.

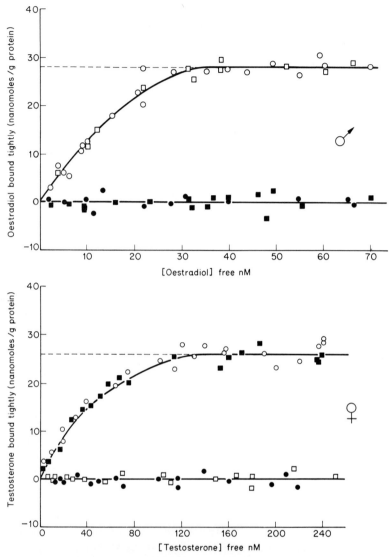

Fig. 9. The effect of aflatoxin B_1 on the 'tight' steroid binding sites [see ref. 15] of smooth microsomes from rat liver. (a) Titration of male microsomes with ^{3}H-oestradiol. (b) Titration of female microsomes with ^{14}C-testosterone. For both graphs: untreated membranes (—○—); membranes (3 mg/ml protein) incubated at 25°C with aflatoxin B_1 (3 μM) for 20 hours before titration (—●—); membranes incubated with aflatoxin, as above, in presence of oestradiol (375 nM) (—□—); membranes incubated with aflatoxin, as above, in presence of testosterone (375 nM) (—■—).

To summarise, the data presented show that oestradiol and testosterone respectively activate male and female smooth membranes to bind polysomes. There are specific tight sites for oestradiol on male, and for testosterone on female smooth membranes. These sites are destroyed irreversibly by Aflatoxin B_1. These hormones, or equivalent substances, are already present in rough reticulum.

Table 4

The Rate of Increase of Apparent Disulphide Interchange Enzyme Activity of Microsomal Membranes from Rat Liver on Incubation with the Substances indicated in the Presence of NADPH

Substance tested*	Rate of enzyme activation†	Carcinogenicity
Naphthalene	0	Nil
2-Naphthylamine	0-3	±
Anthracene	0	Nil
2,7-Diaminofluorene	8	+
1,2-Benzanthracene	5	+
1,2-Benzanthraquinone	8	+
2-Aminochrysene	8	+
6-Aminochrysene	0	Nil
3-Aminopyrene	9	+
3,4-Benzpyrene	20	+
Benzo[b]chrysene	0	Nil
3,4,8,9-Dibenzpyrene	13	+
Carbon tetrachloride (15 μg/ml)	8	+
Aflatoxin B_1 ‡ (10 μg/ml)	10	+

* Incubated at 20°C with microsomal membranes (~ 10 mg protein/ml) at a concentration of 5 μg/ml (unless otherwise stated) in the presence of 1 mM NADPH, 50 mM tris, 25 mM KCl, 5 mM $MgCl_2$ and 250 mM sucrose, at pH 7.3. Post microsomal supernatant was added to 10% final volume.

† Percentage of total enzyme activity released per hour.

‡ Absence of NADPH.

Aflatoxin B_1 causes the irreversible displacement of polysomes from rough membranes and the evidence is consistent with the blocking of a specific hormone site. The steroid sites, on both rough and smooth membrane, can be specifically protected by the hormone involved, against destruction by the carcinogen.

A number of other carcinogenic substances have been shown to produce the same effects as Aflatoxin B_1. Table 4 shows the relative degranulation (measured as increase in rearrangease enzyme activity), caused by incubation of microsomal membranes, mainly rough but containing some smooth, with various carcinogenic compounds and some innocuous relatives, in the presence of 1 mM NADPH (and post-mitochondrial supernatant). Clearly some of the compounds do indeed cause degranulation and in this series correlation with carcinogenicity is complete. The NADPH is an absolute requirement in each case. The term 'carcinogenicity', as applied to the active compounds in the table, needs some definition. A compound is deemed 'carcinogenic' if it can cause tumour formation in any tissue

Table 5

The Degranulation of Rough-Surfaced Microsomal Membranes from Male Rat Liver caused by Incubation with the Substance indicated in the Presence of NADPH

Substance tested*	RNA removed from membrane (% control)		Carcinogenicity
	measured directly	calculated†	
Naphthalene	0	0	Nil
Anthracene	0	0	Nil
2,7-Diaminofluorene	30	30	+
2-Aminochryscne	30	30	+
6-Aminochrysene	0	0	Nil
3-Aminopyrene	27	35	+
3,4-Benzpyrene	28	40	+
Carbon Tetracholoride (15 μg/ml)	35	30	+

* Mixture of rough and smooth membranes incubated at 20°C for 2 hours as described in footnote to Table 4, and centrifuged over a layer of 2.0 M sucrose for 4 hours, 120,000 g, to remove unbound ribosomes.

† Corresponding values calculated from the data summarised in Table 4.

in the rat; clearly not all of the compounds listed in the table are hepatocarcinogens.

To confirm that the apparent enzyme activation was the result of degranulation, a selection of the compounds, listed in Table 4, were incubated with microsomal membranes in the presence of NADPH. The incubates were then centrifuged at 120,000 g for 4 hours over a layer of 2.0 M sucrose to separate membranes from unbound ribosomes. The difference in RNA/protein ratios of the membranes, floating on the 2.0 M sucrose layer, compared with that of untreated membrane gives a direct measure, in terms of RNA, of the degranulation. Table 5 summarises the results obtained which correlate well with the results obtained indirectly in Table 4. The carcinogen-pretreated membranes would not bind additional fresh ribosomes in the presence of oestradiol (1 μg/ml) even after extensive washing. Thus not only is the degranulation operationally irreversible, but all of the potential ribosome binding sites on the original smooth membrane are destroyed as well.

The mechanism of the carcinogen activation and subsequent degranulation is not yet clear, but studies with various modifiers of the microsomal hydroxylase complex, summarised in Table 6,

Table 6
The Effect of Various Substances on the Carcinogen-induced Degranulation of Microsomal Membranes from Male Rat Liver

Incubation*	Benzanthraquinone	Rates of Degranulation†	
		Dibenzpyrene	2-aminochrysene
Control	8	13	8
−NADPH	0	0	0
+Naphthalene (10 μg/ml)	2	2	2
+CO	0	0	not tested
+SKF 525A (1 mM)	0	0	0
+Oestradiol (1 μg/ml)	0.5	0	0.5
+Testosterone (1 μg/ml)	not tested	9	not tested

* Conditions exactly as described for Table 4 except additions where indicated.
† Measured as the rate of increase of apparent disulphide interchange enzyme activity.

suggest the involvement of the cytochrome P450-flavoprotein enzyme system present in microsomal membranes [16]. The absolute requirement for NADPH, the partial inhibition by alternative substrates, and the complete inhibition by CO and the P450 specific inhibitor—SKF 525A—all point to this conclusion. Similarly the complete inhibition of the overall degranulation by low concentrations of oestradiol, strongly suggest that it is the steroid specific site, responsible for maintaining membrane-polysome complex integrity, that is attacked by the activated 'carcinogen'.

The importance of this type of interaction in the transformation of tissues *in vivo* is clearly impossible to evaluate at the present time. However such an initial interaction *in vivo* is certainly consistent with the frequent reports of rough endoplasmic membrane degranulation [17, 18, 19] and the binding of carcinogens to cytoplasmic and microsomal protein [20, 21, 22] during chemical tumorigenesis.

Acknowledgements

We are grateful to the Cancer Research Campaign, Nuffield Foundation and Medical Research Council for grants in support of this work. We are also grateful to the Science Research Council and the Salters' Company for personal grants to C.A.B. and R.B.F.

Discussion

Schlessinger (St Louis)

How many tight-binding sites are present per ribosome in liver and how does the binding affinity compare to the oestradiol-binding protein described by Dr King and others?

Rabin (London)

It is possible to estimate the concentration of ribosome binding sites in the membrane by combining the known RNA:protein ratios of ribosomes and of very rough microsomes before and after degranulation. This suggests that there are between 10^{-7} and 10^{-8} mole of ribosome binding sites per gramme of membrane protein. The figures quoted above for the concentration of tight steroid sites are 2-3 x 10^{-8} mole per gramme and so the stoichiometry of steroid to ribosome binding sites in the membrane is approximately 1:1.

As for the affinity of these specific steroid sites, we do not feel that it is possible to establish a satisfactory dissociation constant because of the complication introduced by the non-specific association which we have mentioned. However the specific sites are certainly saturated at free steroid concentrations below 10^{-7} molar; the true dissociation constant is probably at least an order of magnitude lower. This compares with values of 10^{-9}–10^{-10} molar for the dissociation constant of the soluble uterine receptor protein for oestradiol [23, 24].

Tomkins (San Francisco)

  1. Have you tested dihydrotestosterone—the true androgen?
  2. Is the aflatoxin result related to its blocking effect on the cholesterol feedback inhibition?

Rabin (London)

1. Dihydrotestosterone has just been tested by Mr G. Sunshine. It promotes the binding of female polysomes to female membranes of rat liver at rather high concentrations. Lower concentrations have yet to be tested. Thus the preliminary work indicates that dihydrotestosterone acts like testosterone.

2. In the *in vitro* systems the effects of aflatoxin are due to direct interaction of the carcinogen with the membranes. Cholesterol itself causes dissociation of polysomes from membranes *in vitro*. Inhibition of the cholesterol feedback system should thus cause enhanced, and perhaps sustained, degranulation *in vivo*.

Clemens (Mill Hill)

1. Have you examined the effects of binding of polysomes to membranes *in vitro* on their protein synthetic activity *in vitro*.

2. A related point—in view of the evidence from several groups on the synthesis of different groups of proteins by free and bound ribosomes would you care to speculate on the biological significance of binding of free polysomes to membranes *in vitro*?

Rabin (London)

1. No.

2. The biological significance is at present unknown. It is certainly possible, however, to speculate. It could be that the rate of translation of some messengers is enhanced and others diminished by interaction with the membranes. Interaction with membranes could then act as a switch device for controlling the overall pattern of protein synthesis. Interaction with membranes could also affect the rate of messenger breakdown. It would be wise to await further experimental information before attempting to make any sweeping generalizations.

Kosterlitz (Aberdeen)

It would be very interesting to know whether castration affects the sex specificity of the responses of the polysomes. Did you include castrated rats in your experiments?

Rabin (London)

We are at present investigating the effects of castration and adrenalectomy.

Powis (Glasgow)

Could I ask what other enzyme activities you uncover when you transform rough endoplasmic reticulum to smooth endoplasmic reticulum? In particular I am thinking of drug metabolizing activities.

Rabin (London)

We have not found any other enzyme which is unmasked in the same way as rearrangease.

Cox (Chelsea)

The rat appears to be anomalous with regard to certain aspects of liver function in that there are quite marked differences in the rates of metabolism of certain compounds by male and female animals. These differences are not apparent in the mouse or guinea pig. I wonder whether the sex differences that you have reported can also be demonstrated in liver from other species?

Rabin (London)

We are investigating other tissues and species at the present time. Sheep parotids show similar sex differences to rat liver.

References

1. Lambourg, M. R. and Zamecnik, P. C.; *Biochim. Biophys. Acta*; **42**, (1960) 206.
2. Howell, R. R., Loeb, J. N. and Tomkins, G. M.; *Proc. Nat. Acad. Sci. U.S.A.*; **52**, (1964) 1241.
3. Palade, G. E.; *J. Biophys. Biochem. Cytol.*; **1**, (1955) 59.
4. Teng, C. S. and Hamilton, T. H.; *Biochem. J.*; **105**, (1967) 1091.
5. Siekevitz, P. and Palade, G. E.; *J. Biophys. Biochem. Cytol.*; **7**, (1960) 619.
6. Campbell, P. N.; *FEBS Letters*; **7**, (1970) 1.
7. Cox, R. F. and Mathias, A. P.; *Biochem. J.*; **115**, (1969) 777.
8. Rancourt, M. W. and Litwack, G.; *Exp. Cell Res.*; **51**, (1968) 413.
8a. Mills, E. S. and Topper, Y. J.; *Science*; **165**, (1969) 1127.
8b. Meggi, V., Steggles, A. W. and Gahan, P. B.; *Histochem. J.*; **2**, (1970) 381.
9. Williams, D. J., Gurari, D. and Rabin, B. R.; *FEBS Letters*; **2**, (1968) 133.
10. Goldberger, R. F., Epstein, C. J. and Anfinsen, C. B.; *J. Biol. Chem.*; **238**, (1963) 628.
11. Williams, D. J. and Rabin, B. R.; *FEBS Letters*; **4**, (1969) 103.
12. Sunshine, G. H., Williams, D. J., and Rabin, B. R.; *Nature Lond.*; **230**, (1971) 133.
13. Rabin, B. R., Sunshine, G. H. and Williams, D. J.; Biochemical Society Symposia No. 31 'Chemical Reactivity and Biological Role of Functional Groups in Enzymes'; Academic Press, (1970) p. 203.
14. James, D. W., Rabin, B. R. and Williams, D. J.; *Nature, Lond.*; **224**, (1969) 37.

15. Blyth, C. A., Freedman, R. B. and Rabin, B. R.; *Nature, Lond.*; **230**, (1971) 137.
16. Orrenius, S.; *J. Cell Biol.*; **26**, (1965) 713.
17. Svoboda, D. and Higginson, J.; *Cancer Res.*; **28**, (1968) 1703.
18. Flaks, B.; *Chem. Biol. Interactions*; **2**, (1970) 129.
19. Baglio, C. M. and Farber, E.; *J. Mol. Biol.*; **12**, (1965) 466.
20. Miller, E. C. and Miller, J. A.; *Cancer Res.*; **12**, (1952) 547.
21. Wiest, W. G. and Heidelberger, C.; *Cancer Res.*; **13**, (1953) 250.
22. Huttin, T.; *Exp. Cell Res.*; **10**, (1956) 697.
23. Steggles, A. W. and King, R. J. B.; *Biochem. J.*; **118**, (1970) 695.
24. Mester, J., Robertson, D. M., Feherty, P. and Kellie, A. E.; *Biochem. J.;* **120**, (1970) 831.

THE CONTROL OF LYSOSOMAL ENZYME SYNTHESIS AND EFFECTS OF STEROIDS

A. C. Allison and P. Davies

Clinical Research Centre, Harrow, Middlesex

Anti-inflammatory effects of adrenal cortical hormones have attracted a great deal of attention during the last decade, especially in connection with rheumatoid arthritis. The following points are well accepted:

1. Rheumatoid synovia contain large numbers of mononuclear cells: lymphocytes (including large pyroninophilic cells, which may be blasts or transformed cells) and macrophages [1, 2].

2. In cultures of chick embryonic cartilage, release of lysosomal hydrolases following exposure to anti-cellular antibody or other stressing agents brings about the breakdown of matrix. Studies with specific antibody show that cathepsin D plays a major role in this process [3]. It is likely that release of hydrolases from mononuclear cells is also an important cause of cartilage erosion in rheumatoid arthritis [2].

3. The spontaneous release of lysosomal hydrolases from cultured cells, and that induced by complement-sufficient antibody or ultraviolet light, is in large measure prevented by administration of hydrocortisone [4, 5].

4. Glucocorticoids diminish the release of hydrolases from isolated lysosomes *in vitro* under a variety of conditions [6]. These steroids also decrease the redistribution of lysosomal hydrolases which follows the administration of endotoxin [7]. The latter does not necessarily imply intracellular release of hydrolases after endotoxin administration, but the lysosomes may be more readily disrupted by homogenization.

These observations have been taken as evidence for an overall effect of glucocorticoids on the 'stabilization' of lysosomes in cells, and this has come to be regarded as an adequate explanation for the

49

anti-inflammatory effects of the steroids. However, more recent evidence suggests that steroids have many actions on cells, including enzyme induction [8], and alteration in the properties of cell membranes [9]. The complexity of the mechanisms controlling hydrolase formation and release are also becoming apparent, and it is already clear that the attribution of glucocorticoid effects entirely to lysosomal membrane stabilization is a considerable over-simplification. Some of the complexities will be discussed in this chapter, which outlines what is known about the control of hydrolase synthesis in lymphocytes and macrophages—the two cell types mainly involved in chronic inflammatory reactions—and effects of glucocorticoids on these processes.

Lysosomes and transformation of lymphocytes

Small lymphocytes in peripheral blood have few lysosomes and a low content of lysosomal enzymes. One of the prominent changes accompanying lymphocyte transformation, stimulated by phyto-haemagglutinin (PHA) or specific antigen, is an increase in the number of lysosomes and the content of hydrolases [10-12]. This is a remarkable example of selective activation of certain lymphocyte genes, and may play a role in graft and tumour rejection.

Several metabolic changes accompany lymphocyte transformation. One of the earliest, occurring within 30 minutes, is stimulation of $^{32}PO_4^{3-}$ incorporation into phosphatidyl inositol but not other phospholipids [13]. There is a very early increment in histone acetylation [14], followed by an increase in RNA synthesis, the latter beginning as early as 30 minutes after PHA addition [15]. There is next an increase in protein synthesis and then DNA replication and subsequent mitosis, beginning at 28 hours [16]. There is, however, no indiscriminate stimulation. Activities of several other enzymes remain unchanged during transformation [16]. The most recent enzyme to attract interest in transformed lymphocytes is RNA-dependent DNA polymerase [17], which may play some role in gene amplification.

It has long been known that continued administration of glucocorticoids leads to lysis of lymphocytes and a decrease in the weights of lymphoid organs, especially the thymus [18]. The cells mainly affected are short-lived lymphocytes rather than the long-lived recirculating lymphocytes that are transformed by PHA and participate in cell-mediated immune responses [19]. Nevertheless glucocorticoids, in concentrations that do not lyse lymphocytes, inhibit transformation by PHA and antigen [10, 20]. An example is given in Table 1, which shows that the responses of human peripheral blood cells to antigens (tuberculin or foreign cells) are almost abolished by hydrocortisone whereas the very strong stimulus following exposure to PHA is substantially, but not completely overcome. Steroids are most effective during the first 24 hours of a 72-hour culture, but significant depression is seen when they are added at 24 hours. This suggests that steroids do not only counteract the initial inductive effect of PHA or antigen, although this could be their major mode of action.

Table 1

Transformation of Human Peripheral Blood Leucocytes by Antigens (Tuberculin and Mitomycin-treated Allogeneic Cells and by Phytohaemagglutinin). Incorporation of ^{3}H-thymidine into DNA at 72 hours and Inhibition by Hydrocortisone

Exposure	Control	Hydrocortisone
None	346	310
Tuberculin	4138	679
Allogeneic cells	3229	488
Phytohaemagglutinin	20,372	5679

The mechanism by which lymphocyte transformation is triggered is still under debate. One suggestion is, that release of protease or some other constituent of lysosomes may itself initiate transformation [10, 11, 21]. Another theory is that alteration in the lymphocyte plasma membrane is the trigger, perhaps through formation of cyclic AMP [22]. In either case, membrane stabilization by glucocorticoids might contribute to inhibition of transformation. Some general and specific effects of steroids on membranes are discussed below, and analogous effects on lymphocyte membranes may well occur.

Relationship of endocytosis to lysosome formation in macrophages

Since the work of Lewis and Lewis [23], it has been known that in culture, peripheral blood monocytes survive with a marked increase in cytoplasmic mass and in the number of granules stainable by vital dyes. The cytoplasmic granules were found by Cohn and

Wiener [24] to have the properties of lysosomes. Cells washed out from the unstimulated peritoneal cavity rapidly attach to and spread on the surface of culture vessels. The unattached lymphocytes and other cells can readily be washed away, leaving a population of mononuclear phagocytes resembling peripheral blood monocytes. Moderate numbers of small granules, dense by phase-contrast microscopy, are seen around the nucleus. In a high-serum medium, phase-contrast cinemicroscopy shows the development of pseudo-podia with ruffled membrane activity and at the same site, formation of pinocytotic vacuoles. The vacuoles are phase-lucent, close to the limit of resolution of the microscope, and pass rapidly towards the centre of the cell; this movement is readily visible by direct observation. The pinocytic vacuoles pass to the lysosomes, which usually lie in a perinuclear position, and fusion with lysosomes takes place.

During the next few days, the phase-dense lysosomes increase greatly in number and size [25] and these morphological changes which occur during macrophage maturation *in vitro* are accompanied by marked changes in the enzyme content of the cells. No cell division was observed but the protein content of the cells was increased about threefold, as expected from the larger size of the mature cells. The content of three typical lysosomal hydrolases—acid phosphatase, β-glucuronidase and cathepsin—increased much more than the overall protein content: in the case of acid phosphatase a 40 to 50-fold increase was observed in 3 days.

The major environmental factor stimulating the formation of macrophage lysosomes was the level of serum in the medium. Cultures exposed to low serum formed few dense granules and little or no hydrolase, whereas high levels of serum resulted in marked pinocytosis and formation of lysosomes [26-28]. Inhibitors of protein synthesis prevent lysosome development.

Reviewing the electron microscopic evidence, Cohn [29] has concluded that newly synthesized proteins—and, presumably, hydro-lytic enzymes—are packaged within the Golgi vesicles and are carried to the pinosome. The primary lysosome of the macrophage is a small, smooth-surface Golgi vesicle, a package of hydrolase which has not yet come in contact with substrate. The secondary lysosome, containing both substrate and enzyme, is a demarcated cytoplasmic locus in which intracellular digestion is constantly taking place.

It is clear from these and other observations that environmental

factors which stimulate pinocytosis also stimulate hydrolase formation. This is indeed a remarkable adaptation in which the cell
responds to a particular need: for the production of hydrolases
which can digest material taken into the cell by endocytosis.

The stimulus to endocytosis

Several factors in serum increase endocytosis. The most potent is
anti-cellular antibody, including a macroglobulin in bovine serum
with the properties of an interspecies antibody [30]. This antibody
was found to be cytotoxic to mouse macrophages in the presence of
complement, but in the absence of complement it markedly
stimulated endocytosis and formation of lysosomes, as well as
increasing the content of hydrolases. In other systems, anti-cellular
antibody stimulates the synthesis and release of hydrolases [4]. It
has long been known that antigen-antibody complexes near equiva-
lence are rapidly endocytosed by macrophages and degraded within
these cells [31]. Immunoglobulins G and M are attached to specific
and independent sites on macrophages [32-35], but the attachment
of native immunoglobulins does not initiate endocytosis. In contrast,
when the configuration of immunoglobulin is altered so that it can
fix complement, it is rapidly taken into macrophages [36]. Complement is not necessary for this process.

It therefore seems likely that the natural factor which stimulates
endocytosis is immunoglobulin which has undergone a configura-
tional change in the course of interaction with antigen (which may
be on the cell membrane itself). This would have obvious advantages
as a trigger mechanism, since it would ensure that immunoglobulins
present in tissue fluids would not stimulate endocytosis unless they
had already reacted with antigen. Combination of antigen with
antibody can trigger other important events at the cell membrane.
Thus the attachment of IgE and related antibodies to leucocytes does
not by itself bring about release of histamine and other mediators of
acute hypersensitivity. Subsequent exposure to specific antigen,
however, acts as the trigger for mediator release.

Other serum factors inducing pinocytosis include bovine plasma
albumin and fetuin [37]. Removal of fatty acids from albumin or
sialic acid from fetuin abolished the stimulatory effect, which was
attributed to the high net negative charge of albumin. Other anionic
polymers had a similar effect, whereas cationic compounds did not.
This contrasts with the observations of Ryser [38] on stimulation of

pinocytosis in tumour cells by basic compounds. Possibly, acidic polymers interacted with immunoglobulin in the culture medium, so that the stimulus to pinocytosis is the same. Adenosine and its 5'-phosphates (including ATP) were also inducers of pinocytosis in mouse macrophages [39]; other nucleotides were much less effective.

The mechanism of pinocytosis

Cohn [40] has presented evidence that pinocytosis in macrophages is an energy-dependent phenomenon. It is prevented by inhibitors of respiration and oxidative phosphorylation, including anaerobiosis, cyanide, antimycin A, 2,4-dinitrophenol and oligomycin, which implies that ATP may be required. Inhibitors of protein synthesis, such as *p*-fluorophenylalanine and puromycin, prevented pinocytosis, suggesting that synthesis of new plasma membrane may be necessary for continuing membrane interiorization. There was a high-temperature coefficient for pinocytosis, and Cohn concluded that pinocytosis is a reaction dependent on temperature and energy and one in which outgoing protein synthesis is essential.

We have investigated the possibility that contraction of actomyosin-like filaments in the peripheral cytoplasm of the macrophage is required for pinocytosis and the directional movement of pinosomes towards the centre of the cell. Evidence is accumulating that many cells have filaments about 500 Å in diameter in their cytoplasm, which are quite distinct from microtubules (diameter about 2200 Å). The actin-like nature of some of these filaments has been demonstrated by the fact that they bind heavy meromyosin to form typical 'arrowhead-like' structures in electron micrographs [41]. Actomyosin-like fibrous proteins have been extracted from several different cell types, including slime moulds and blood platelets. In the presence of Ca^{2+} and ATP these contract *in vitro.* Our colleague S. de Petris has found that the peripheral cytoplasm of macrophages contains a dense network of microfilaments which bind heavy meromyosin. Some appear to be inserted into the cell membrane and some are observed encircling vacuoles which correspond in size to pinosomes. Analysis of the role of microfilamentous contractile systems in cell function has been greatly advanced by the demonstration [42, 43] that the antibiotic cytochalasin B selectively interferes with the function of such systems in a variety of cell types.

In dividing cells, for instance, cytochalasin does not interfere with the functioning of the mitotic spindle, so that the daughter nuclei separate, but the drug prevents the contraction of a band of microfilaments located just beneath the cleavage furrow that is thought to pinch the cell in two. As a result, a binucleate cell is formed. Binucleate cells and discharge of cell nuclei are two characteristic effects of cytochalasin. We believe that enucleation occurs because normally the nucleus is held away from the plasma membrane by a network of microfilaments in the peripheral cytoplasm; in cytochalasin-treated cells, the nucleus comes in close contact with, and is enveloped by, the cell membrane; often it is then discharged from the cell.

We have found that when mouse macrophages are exposed to cytochalasin B, in concentrations of 1 μg or 10 μg/ml of culture medium, movements of the cell, movements of the ruffled membrane, pinocytosis and movement of pinosomes are all strongly inhibited. In the higher concentration, the cells take on a remarkable 'spidery' appearance, apparently because of collapse of the cortical cytoplasm, the rigidity of which contributes to the maintenance of normal shape. These changes are fully reversible within a few minutes of replacement of fresh medium lacking cytochalasin.

We therefore conclude that the movement of the ruffled membrane and associated movements of the plasma membrane which result in pinocytosis, as well as the movement towards the lysosomal region of the cell, are brought about by contraction of suitably oriented microfilaments inserted into the plasma membrane itself. This system provides an opportunity for analysing whether pinocytosis itself is required for stimulation of hydrolase formation. If the signal were arising from the cell membrane, it might be possible after addition of an inducer to block pinocytosis and still observe an increase in hydrolase levels.

The stimulus to hydrolase formation

The results described in the previous section suggest that the process of pinocytosis is required to stimulate hydrolase synthesis. The question can therefore be asked whether the rate of pinocytosis or the rate of resolution of secondary lysosomes is the controlling factor? Here, the results of experiments with sucrose and other sugars that cannot be digested within the secondary lysosomes are relevant. As shown by Dingle *et al.* [44], using embryonic skeletal cells and by Cohn and Ehrenreich [45], for macrophages, addition of sucrose to culture media considerably increases the amount of hydrolase synthesized and (in the case of skeletal cells) released from the cells. Experiments with [^{14}C]-dextran on embryonic skeletal cells [44] and observations of pinocytotic vesicles by Cohn and Ehrenreich [45] and ourselves show that sucrose does not only increase the rate of endocytosis, but greatly prolongs the persistence of the vacuoles. As a result, the cells develop large numbers of secondary lysosomes. If invertase (which can split sucrose into glucose and fructose) is taken up into the same cells, the sucrose-containing lysosomes promptly shrink. From these and other experiments it is clear that the ability of small neutral carbohydrates to produce lysosomal swelling is dependent on their molecular weight and resistance to lysosomal hydrolases. Disaccharides cannot pass through the lysosomal membrane whereas monosaccharides can.

The stimulation of hydrolase synthesis brought about by sucrose therefore appears to be due to failure of resolution of secondary lysosomes. Whether the 'message' comes from the membrane or some other constituent of the secondary lysosome is not clear, nor is the mechanism by which hydrolase formation is de-repressed or potentiated.

A possible role of the products of lysosomal digestion in stimulation of hydrolase formation comes from experiments described by Cohn [46]. It was found that endocytosis of digestible particulates (including aldehyde-treated red cells, heat-aggregated gamma globulin and a coacervate of L-glutamic acid and L-poly-lysine) stimulated hydrolase synthesis whereas ingestion of non-digestible material (polystyrene spheres, starch and coacervates of D-glutamic acid and D-polylysine) had no effect on hydrolase levels. However, the fact that sucrose and other non-digestible sugars stimulate hydrolase synthesis shows that digestion is not required for stimulation. The nature of the stimulus is still unknown.

Some of the ways in which synthesis of hydrolases might be regulated are illustrated in Fig. 1. It is not known whether the control is exerted at the level of transcription, to form messenger RNA's coding for hydrolases, or at the translational level, but it is possible that the message for increased hydrolase synthesis comes from the plasma membrane itself. The role of membranes in control of contact-dependent phenomena such as mitosis is now widely accepted. Alternatively, the control could come from the secondary lysosomes: while these are unresolved, a message passes from their membrane or contents to signal the need for more hydrolases. When the contents of the secondary lysosome are digested and absorbed, the secondary lysosomes themselves will shrink and perhaps disappear, along with the stimulus for more hydrolase production.

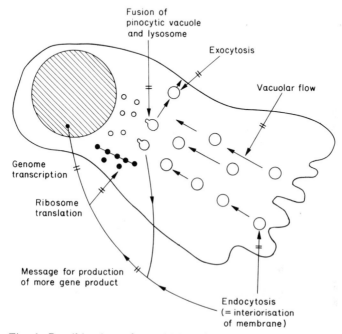

Fig. 1. Possible sites of steroid interference with macrophage function.

Inhibitors of the formation and release of lysosomal hydrolases in macrophages might then be able to act in several different ways, including:

1. Prevention of endocytosis or of the movement of endocytotic vacuoles from the periphery of the cell.

2. Prevention of the passage of a signal from the cell membrane or from the secondary lysosomes.

3. Prevention of the response to such a message.

4. Prevention of the release of preformed lysosomes.

In an attempt to throw some light on this interesting and practically important system of control, we have put together published evidence and our own experimental results.

Effects of steroids on hydrolase synthesis in macrophages

Dingle and his colleagues have found that hydrocortisone considerably reduces the release of acid protease from embryonic skeletal tissues in organ culture, induced by complement sufficient antiserum. Comparable observations have been made by Wiener and Marmary [47] who reported that hydrocortisone, added to cultures of mouse peritoneal monocyte cultures, retarded the rise of intracellular acid phosphatase and cathepsin following exposure to foreign serum. The depressant effect of hydrocortisone on hydrolase levels was dose-dependent, but statistically significant depression was observed at the lowest concentration of hydrocortisone used (1.4×10^{-7} M). No immediate effect of hydrocortisone on pinocytotic activity was noted.

We have investigated effects of hydrocortisone on mouse peritoneal exudate cells. Cells incubated in medium 199 with 10% foetal calf serum and 10^{-5} M hydrocortisone were more rounded than control cells. Although ruffled membrane movements were not abolished they were reduced, as was microscopically observable pinocytosis. When normal medium was replaced by medium containing 10^{-5} M hydrocortisone no immediate effect was observable, but after about 30 minutes cells began to withdraw their processes and pinocytosis was retarded.

Cortisone administration has long been known to diminish host resistance against infections [48]. However glucocorticoids have slight, if any, effects on intracellular killing or phagocytosis of bacteria [49-51]. It has been claimed that fusion of primary lysosomes with phagocytic vacuoles containing fungal spores is inhibited by cortisone [52], but this result has not been readily repeatable in other hands [53]. Thus the mechanism by which cortisone reduces resistance against infections is not yet understood.

Our results suggest that one of the factors by which glucocorticoids inhibit lysosome formation is depression of pinocytosis; the hormones probably also inhibit release of hydrolases from macrophages. Both of these effects may be related to membrane stabilization, so that it is necessary to review briefly what is known of the effects of corticosteroids on membranes.

Effects of steroids on natural and artificial membranes

The actions of steroids on membranes are rather complex, and reports of different authors reveal some apparent discrepancies. Bangham, Standish and Weissmann [54] concluded that steroids can be arranged on a linear scale relating their effects on isolated lysosomes to those on phospholipid-cholesterol liposomes (concentric spheres of lipid bilayers separated by an aqueous phase). At one extreme are glucocorticoids, such as cortisone and hydrocortisone, which diminish the release of enzymes from isolated lysosomes and of cations from liposomes. These have stabilizing effects on membranes promoting the release of enzymes from lysosomes and of marker ions from liposomes.

The group of steroids with labilizing effects includes etiocholanolane and related compounds with 5β-H atoms; in these the A:B junction is *cis* so that the A ring is at a sharp angle to the rest of the molecule. However, this configuration is not necessary for labilizing effects since these are also shown by progesterone which has the more conventional 5α- configuration in which the A:B ring junction is *trans.* In fact, the configuration of progesterone is rather like that of hydrocortisone although it lacks most of the hydroxyl groups of the latter and is correspondingly less soluble in an aqueous phase.

Weissmann and Keiser [55] have reported that as a general rule, steroids with the capacity to augment the release of hydrolases from isolated lysosomes are haemolytic when added to erythrocyte suspensions in isotonic media. However, Seeman [56], has questioned this interpretation in view of his observations that in hypotonic media all steroids tested in rather low concentrations, including 5β-H compounds, protect erythrocytes against the spontaneous haemolysis that occurs under these conditions. Higher steroid concentrations augmented the lysis due to hypotonicity alone. Seeman concluded that all compounds affecting membrane stability have a biphasic effect, being protective at low concentrations and lytic at high concentrations.

In view of this apparent discrepancy we have compared the effects of representative steroids on erythrocytes under isotonic and hypotonic conditions. The labilizing effect of progesterone (Fig. 2) occurs at the same concentration ($>10^{-4}$ M) under both sets of conditions, but at lower concentrations the steroid does indeed protect against hypotonic haemolysis.

It is not certain whether the protective effect occurs only under hypotonic conditions, when some increase of tension in the membrane might be expected. Seeman claims that it does not, and has replotted Weissmann's data in an attempt to show that so-called labilizing steroids may, in low concentrations, confer some measure

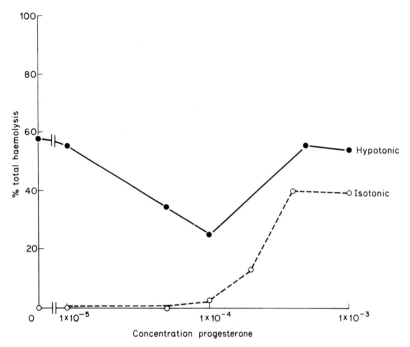

Fig. 2. Erythrocyte haemolysis by progesterone under isotonic and hypotonic conditions. Erythrocytes (2% v/v) were incubated at 37°C for 1 hour in either isotonic or 0.4 isotonic phosphate-buffered saline. Progesterone was included as an ethanolic solution of desired concentration. Haemolysis was estimated as haemoglobin release measured at 540 nm.

of protection against spontaneous release of lysosomal enzymes; but this is unconvincing [57].

The complexity of the situation is illustrated by observations of Weissmann and Keiser [55], which we have confirmed, that glucocorticoids, which usually stabilize membranes and help to counteract the effects of labilizing compounds (Fig. 3), actually *augment* the haemolysis produced by etiocholanolone under isotonic conditions (Fig. 4). The ability of hydrocortisone to protect against progesterone but not etiocholanolone may be due to the difference in configuration of the two labilizers discussed above.

Despite these difficulties, there is remarkable agreement between effects of steroids on natural membranes and on cholesterol : lecithin liposomes. The importance of cholesterol in these interactions is suggested by the finding of Heap *et al.* [58] that all steroids *increase* leakage of ^{42}K from lecithin liposomes, in contrast to the opposite effect of glucocorticoids on phospholipid: cholesterol liposomes and

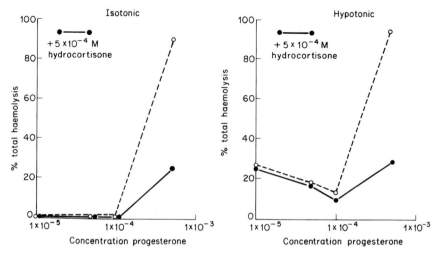

Fig. 3. The inhibition of progesterone induced erythrocyte haemolysis by hydrocortisone. Erythrocytes (2% v/v) were incubated at 37°C for 1 hour in either isotonic or 0.4 isotonic phosphate-buffered saline. Steroids were included as ethanolic solutions of desired concentration. Haemolysis was estimated as haemoglobin release measured at 540 nm.

natural membranes (except under unusual conditions). The importance of cholesterol in stiffening up and stabilizing membranes is well known [59].

Spin-label techniques also allow investigation of the mobility and availability of various membrane components. Butler *et al.* [60] have used the method to show the role of cholesterol in increasing the degree of order in membranes: the extent to which the long axes of lipids are oriented preferentially in a direction perpendicular to the lamellar plane. Hubbell *et al.* [61] have reported that in erythrocytes a spin-labelled steroid can gain access to previously inaccessible highly immobile protein sites in the presence of haemolytic

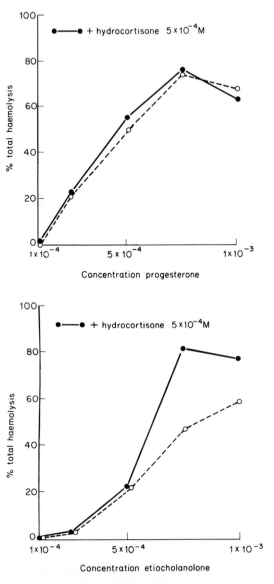

Fig. 4. The effect of hydrocortisone on progesterone and etiocholanolone induced erythrocyte haemolysis. Erythrocytes (2% v/v) were incubated at 37°C for 1 hour in phosphate-buffered saline. Steroids were included as ethanolic solutions of desired concentration. Haemolysis was estimated as haemoglobin release measured at 540 nm.

concentrations of benzyl alcohol. It is possible that similar binding occurs with lytic steroid concentrations. Lower concentrations of steroids may increase disorder of membrane lipids up to a critical level when they interfere with interactions between protein and lipid (mainly hydrophobic) so that haemolysis results. Effects of steroids on membrane proteins could be of major importance in control of lysosomal hydrolase synthesis and release, as well as many other processes.

The relatively high concentrations of steroids required for demonstrable effects on phospholipid : cholesterol liposomes, lysosomes and erythrocytes suggest that these could be major control mechanisms *in vivo* only if there is some selective mechanism increasing the concentrations of steroids in certain membranes. In view of the concentration of many drugs in lysosomes [62], some such effect may well occur. Selective effects on membranes are suggested by the observations of Ballard and Tomkins [9] on the promotion by corticosteroids in low concentrations of the attachment of hepatoma cells to culture vessels. The authors suggest that glucocorticoids induce the biosynthesis of a protein which either modifies the cell surface (an enzyme) or is incorporated into surface structures (structural protein). Steroids, with their hydrophilic and hydrophobic sites, complex three-dimensional configuration, hydrogen bonding and charge-transfer properties [63] are well constructed to become correctly oriented at the lipid-aqueous interface of membranes and specifically interact with membrane constituents.

Discussion

Jenkins (St George's Hospital)
One point against the physiological relevance of the experiments involving lysosome stabilisers is that you have shown cortisone to be comparable in activity to cortisol whereas in most biological systems cortisone has little or no activity until converted to cortisol.

Allison (Northwick Park)
As pointed out, extrapolation from *in vitro* experiments, especially with model systems such as liposomes, to *in vivo* effects of steroids must be made with caution. In many biological systems interconvertibility of cortisol and cortisone is known, and it would be of

interest to know whether this occurs in macrophages and lymphocytes.

Sullivan (Guy's Hospital Medical School)

What is the relationship between the endocytotic and pinocytotic
vesicles and lysosomes?

Allison (Northwick Park)

Endocytosis is a general term used to cover both pinocytosis (the
uptake of colloids into small vacuoles) and phagocytosis (the uptake
of particles into large vacuoles). The pinocytic vacuoles move
towards the centre of the cell and fuse with primary lysosomes
(organelles, packaged in the outer part of the Golgi system,
containing hydrolytic enzymes) to form secondary lysosomes, in
which digestion occurs.

Szollosi (Animal Research Station)

Would you tell us more details of the interaction between microfilaments and cytochalasin?

Allison (Northwick Park)

We suppose that cytochalasin combines rather firmly with either the
actin or the myosin component of the contractile system and so
prevents the interaction of the protein components which is required
for normal function. The actomyosin system of striated muscle is
resistant to cytochalasin. Actin or myosin from blood platelets will
combine with the complementary components from striated muscle
to form a functional system, and we are currently ascertaining
whether this recombination system can be used to establish whether
cytochalasin interacts with actin or myosin from platelets. We know
that the platelet actomyosin system, which is responsible for clot
retraction, is highly sensitive to cytochalasin, although platelet
aggregation is not.

Tata (Mill Hill)

Have you looked for qualitative differences in the lysosomal enzymes
that are inducible with antigens and phytohaemagglutinin and
inhibited by corticosteroids?

Allison (Northwick Park)

Some lysosomal enzymes are increased to a greater extent than
others in macrophages exposed to foreign serum, e.g. acid phos-

phatase is increased forty- to fifty-fold whereas others are increased five- to ten-fold. We have not yet looked for differential effects of corticosteroids, although this would be interesting to do.

Schofield (Bristol)

Dr Allison, do you observe pinocytotic vesicles bound to microfilaments under electron microscopy?

Allison (Northwick Park)

Some relatively large endocytic vacuoles (*ca.* 0.2-0.5 μm diameter) are seen in electron micrographs to be enveloped by concentric circles of micro-filaments. Other microfilaments appear to be inserted into the plasma membrane or the membrane surrounding pinocytic vesicles. These results suggest that the microfilaments are attached to the vesicles, but appearances could be deceptive since the cell has to be rather roughly handled in order to reveal the microfilaments which are normally obscured because their electron density is similar to that of the background cytoplasm.

Slater (Brunel)

1. I was most interested in your mention of the biological effects of the cytochalasins. Was it cytochalasin B that you used and does this substance not have very interesting effects in terms of nuclear extrusion when applied to cells in culture?

2. You mentioned that the addition of sucrose with serum increased pinocytotic activity in your *in vitro* system. Have you tried using Triton-WR-1339 in place of sucrose as this detergent is taken up into secondary lysosomes in liver and the particles so formed are relatively fragile?

Allison (Northwick Park)

1. We used cytochalasin B although other cytochalasins have rather similar effects. Our explanation of the nuclear extrusion phenomenon is that in normal cells the nucleus is held away from the cell membrane by a network of microfilaments. When this is dispersed by cytochalasin the nucleus can move to the cell membrane and is closely enveloped by it; indeed the nucleus is often seen bulging out of the side of the cell, which never happens in normal cells. Extrusion can easily follow. We suppose that this is what happens to developing normoblasts in the bone marrow, and intend to study that system shortly.

2. We have not yet looked at Triton-WR-1339 in macrophages, although this detergent would probably, like sucrose, stimulate hydrolase synthesis to a remarkable degree.

References

1. Lack, C. H.; In: 'Lysosomes in Biology and Pathology'; Eds J. T. Dingle and H. B. Fell. Amsterdam: North Holland Publishing Company. **1**, (1969) p. 493.
2. Page Thomas, D. P.; In: 'Lysosomes in Biology and Pathology'; Eds J. T. Dingle and H. B. Fell. Amsterdam: North Holland Publishing Company. **2**, (1969) p. 87.
3. Weston, P. D., Barrett, A. J. and Dingle, J. T.; *Nature, Lond.*; **222**, (1969) 285.
4. Dingle, J. T., Fell, H. B. and Coombs, R. R.; *Int. Arch. Allergy*; **31**, (1967) 283.
5. Weissmann, G. and Fell, H. B.; *J. exp. Med.*; **116**, (1962) 365.
6. Weissmann, G.; *Biochem. Pharm.*; **14**, (1965) 525.
7. Weissmann, G. and Thomas, L.; In: 'Bacterial Endotoxins'; Eds M. Landy and W. Braun. New Jersey: Rutgers University Press. (1964) p. 602.
8. Tomkins, G. M., Thompson, E. B., Hayashi, S., Gelehrter, T., Gronner, D. and Peterkofsky, B.; *Cold Spr. Harb. Symp. quant. Biol.*; **31**, (1966) 349.
9. Ballard, G. P. and Tomkins, G. M.; *J. Cell Biol.*; **47**, (1970) 222.
10. Allison, A. C. and Mallucci, L.; *Lancet*; **2**, (1964) 1371.
11. Hirschhorn, R., Kaplan, J. M., Goldberg, K., Hirschhorn, K. and Weissmann, G.; *Science*; **147**, (1965) 55.
12. Brittinger, G., Hirschhorn, R., Douglas, S. and Weissmann, G.; *J. Cell. Biol.*; **37**, (1968) 412.
13. Fisher, D. B. and Mueller, G. C.; *Proc. Nat. Acad. Sci.*; **60**, (1968) 1396.
14. Pogo, B. G. T., Allfrey, V. G. and Mirsky, A. E.; *Proc. Nat. Acad. Sci.* **55**, (1966) 805.
15. Kay, J. E. and Cooper, H. L.; *Biochim. biophys. Acta*; **186**, (1969) 62.
16. Loeb, L. A., Ewald, J. L. and Agarwal, S. S.; *Cancer Res.*; **30**, (1970) 2514.
17. Penner, P. E., Cohen, L. H. and Loeb, L. A. *Nature, Lond*; (1971) in press.
18. Dougherty, T. F.; In: 'The Lymphocyte and Lymphocyte Tissue'; Ed. J. W. Rebuck. New York: Hoeber. (1960) pp. 112-124.
19. Esteban, J. N.; *Anat. Rec.*; **162**, (1968) 349.
20. Nowell, P. C.; *Cancer Res.*; **21**, (1961) 1518.
21. Hirschhorn, R., Brittinger, G., Hirschhorn, K. and Weissmann, G.; *J. Cell Biol.*; **37**, (1968) 394.
22. Whitfield, J. F., McManus, J. P. and Gillan, D. J.; *J. cell Physiol.*; **76**, (1970) 65.
23. Lewis, M. R. and Lewis, W. H.; *J. Am. Med. Assoc.*; **84**, (1925) 798.
24. Cohn, Z. A. and Wiener, E.; *J. exp. Med.*; **118**, (1963) 991.
25. Cohn, Z. A., Hirsch, J. G. and Fedorko, M. E.; *J. exp. Med.*; **123**, (1966) 747.
26. Cohn, Z. A. and Benson, B.; *J. exp. Med.*; **121**, (1965) 153.
27. Cohn, Z. A. and Benson, B.; *J. exp. Med.*; **121**, (1965) 279.
28. Cohn, Z. A. and Benson, B.; *J. exp. Med.*; **121**, (1965) 835.
29. Cohn, Z. A.; *Adv. Immunol.*; **9**, (1968) 163.

30. Cohn, Z. A. and Parks, E.; *J. exp. Med.*; **125**, (1967) 213.
31. Sorkin, E. and Boyden, S. V.; *J. Immunol.*; **82**, (1959) 332.
32. Huber, H., Polley, M. J., Linscott, W. D., Fuderberg, H. H., Muller-Eberhard, H. J.; *Science*; **162**, (1968) 1281.
33. Lay, W. H. and Nussenzweig, V.; *J. exp. Med.*; **128**, (1968) 991.
34. Huber, H., Douglas, D. S., Nusbacher, J., Kochwa, S. and Rosenfeld, R. E.; *Nature Lond.*; **229**, (1971) 419.
35. Cohen, S.; (1971) Unpublished observations.
36. Hess, M. W. and Luscher, E. F.; *Exp. Cell Res.*; **59**, (1970) 193.
37. Cohn, Z. A. and Parks, E.; *J. exp. Med.*; **125**, (1967) 213.
38. Ryser, H. J.-P.; *Bull. Swiss Acad. Med. Sci.*; **24**, (1968) 363.
39. Cohn, Z. A. and Parks, E.; *J. exp. Med.*; **125**, (1967) 213.
40. Cohn, Z. A.; *J. exptl. Med.*; **124**, (1966) 557.
41. Ishikawa, H., Bischoff, R. and Holtzer, H.; *J. Cell Biol.*; **43**, (1969) 312.
42. Schroeder, T. E.; *Biol. Bull.*; **137**, (1969) 413.
43. Wessells, N. K., Spooner, B. S., Ash, J. F., Bradley, M. O., Luduenda, M. A., Taylor, E. L., Wrenn, J. T. and Yamada, K. M.; *Science*; **171**, (1971) 135.
44. Dingle, J. T., Fell, H. B. and Glauert, A. M.; *J. Cell Sci.*; **4**, (1969) 139.
45. Cohn, Z. A. and Ehrenreich, B. A.; *J. exp. Med.*; **129**, (1969) 201.
46. Cohn, Z. A.; In: 'Mononuclear Phagocytes'; Ed. R. van Furth. Oxford: Blackwell (1970) 121.
47. Wiener, E. and Marmary, Y., *Lab. Invest.*; **21**, (1969) 505.
48. Thomas, L.; *Ann. Rev. Med.*; **3**, (1952) 1.
49. Heller, J. H.; *Endocrinology*; **56**, (1955) 80.
50. Hirsch, J. G. and Church, A. B.; *J. clin. Invest.*; **40**, (1961) 794.
51. Berger, R. R. and Karnovsky, M. L.; *Fed. Proc.*; **25**, (1966) 840.
52. Merkow. L., Pardo, M., Epstein, S. M., Verney, E. and Sidransky, H.; *Science*; **160**, (1968) 79.
53. Remington, J. S.; (1971) Private communication.
54. Bangham, A. D., Standish, M. and Weissmann, G.; *J. Mol. Biol.*; **13**, (1965) 253.
55. Weissmann, G. and Keiser, H.; *Biochem. Pharm.*; **14**, (1965) 537.
56. Seeman, P. M.; *Internat. Rev. Neurobiol.*; **9**, (1966) 145.
57. Weismann, G.; In: 'The Interactions of Drugs and Subcellular Components of Animal Cells'; Ed. P. N. Campbell. London: J. & A. Churchill. (1968) p. 203.
58. Heap, R. B., Symons, A. M. S. and Watkins, J. C.; *Biochim. biophys. Acta*; **218**, (1970) 482.
59. Chapman, D. and Wallach, D. F. H.; In: 'Biological Membranes'; Ed. D. Chapman. New York: Academic Press. (1968) p. 125.
60. Butler, K. W., Smith, I. C. P. and Schneider, M.; *Biochim. biophys. Acta*; **219**, (1970) 514.
61. Hubbell, W. L., Metcalfe, J. C., Metcalfe, S. M. and McConnell, H. M.; *Biochim. biophys. Acta*; **219**, (1970) 415.
62. Allison, A. C. and Young, M. R.; In: 'Lysosomes in Biology and Pathology'; Eds J. T. Dingle and H. B. Fell. Amsterdam: North Holland Publishing Company. **2**, (1969) 600.
63. Allison, A. C., Peover, M. E. and Gough, T. A.; *Life Sciences*; **12**, (1962) 729.

THE EFFECTS OF DRUGS AND STEROID HORMONES ON THE ENZYMES OF THE ENDOPLASMIC RETICULUM

D. V. Parke

Department of Biochemistry, University of Surrey, Guildford, Surrey, U.K.

The endoplasmic reticulum is the intracellular location of many diverse enzyme activities including several concerned with carbohydrate metabolism, e.g. glucose-6-phosphatase and glucuronyl transferase, and with protein synthesis. This subcellular structure is, however, more widely associated with the activities of the mixed function oxidases, enzyme(s) requiring reduced nicotinamide adenine dinucleotide phosphate ($NADPH_2$) and molecular oxygen for activity, and concerned with the oxidative metabolism of drugs, steroids and other hormones, with the biosynthesis of cholesterol [1, 2] and its catabolism to the bile acids [3, 4], the ω-oxidation of fatty acids [5, 6], and the oxidation of prostaglandins [7].

Much of the current knowledge on the control mechanisms governing enzymes of the endoplasmic reticulum has been derived from the stimulus provided by the study of the hepatic metabolism of drugs and other foreign compounds [8, 9]. I propose therefore, to confine this paper to considerations of the regulation of the activities of the mixed function oxygenases of the endoplasmic reticulum of mammalian liver, and to consider the effects of drugs and steroids upon these enzymes.

The enzymes of the hepatic endoplasmic reticulum, which metabolize drugs and steroids, are often referred to as the 'microsomal drug-metabolizing enzymes' and are responsible for the oxidation, reduction and conjugation of drugs and other foreign compounds (xenobiotics) such as pesticides, food additives, and industrial chemicals. These enzymes have proved exceptionally difficult to solubilize and purify so that 'microsomal suspensions' consisting of the 10,000 x *g* supernatant fraction, or the re-suspended 100,000 x *g* deposit, fortified with the necessary co-enzyme requirements, have been most frequently used in studies of these enzymes. This has considerably hindered the study of the mechanisms of these reactions, and in particular the identification of the components of the intermediate electron transport chain and elucidation of the nature of the terminal oxygen-activating/oxygen-transferring enzyme. Furthermore, it suggests that these enzyme activities are integral components of the membranes of the endoplasmic reticulum.

The mixed-function oxygenase system of the hepatic endoplasmic reticulum although similar, in its 'hydroxylating' activity, to the oxygenase system of the adrenal mitochondria responsible for steroidogenesis, differs in its component structure. The system of the hepatic endoplasmic reticulum is believed to consist of $NADPH_2$, a phospholipid-protohaeme-sulphide-protein complex known as cytochrome P450, and a linking electron transport system containing cytochrome P450 reductase and probably $NADPH_2$-cytochrome *c* reductase. The mechanism of oxygenation (hydroxylation) of a drug or steroid is postulated to be as follows:

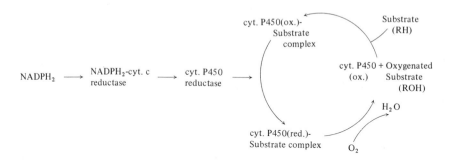

It has been suggested that one single enzyme system, is responsible for all the differing types of hepatic microsomal hydroxylation, which may include the following:

Aliphatic oxygenation $-RCH_3 \xrightarrow{[O]} -RCH_2OH$

Alicyclic oxygenation   ⬡ $\xrightarrow{[O]}$ ⬡$-OH$

Aromatic oxygenation

$$\text{(benzene ring)} \xrightarrow{[O]} \text{(benzene ring)}-OH$$

Epoxidation

$$\text{C=C} \xrightarrow{[O]} \text{epoxide}$$

O- and *N*-Dealkylation

$$>\!NCH_3 \xrightarrow{[O]} >\!NCH_2OH \longrightarrow$$

$$>\!NH + HCHO$$

N-oxidation

$$>\!NR \xrightarrow{[O]} >\!\overset{\text{O}}{\underset{\uparrow}{N}}R$$

Sulphoxidation

$$>\!SR \xrightarrow{[O]} >\!\overset{\text{O}}{\underset{\uparrow}{S}}R$$

Desulphuration

$$>\!C\!=\!S \xrightarrow{[O]} >\!C\!=\!O$$

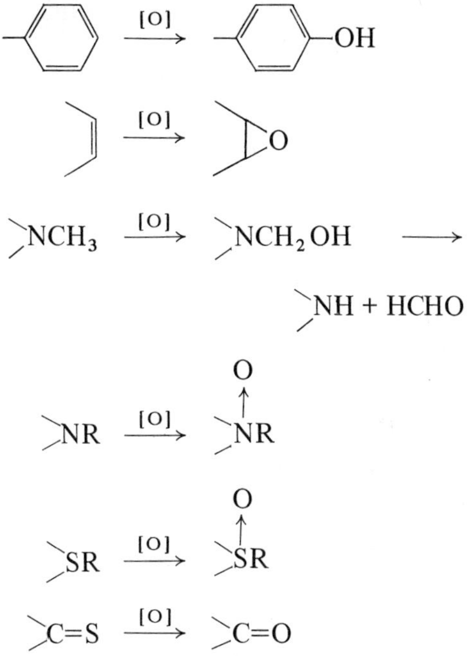

Furthermore, it is considered that this one enzyme system is responsible for the oxygenation of all the different substrates, including drugs and other foreign chemicals, steroids, and fatty acids. In support of this hypothesis, it is known that drugs and steroids may competitively inhibit each other in this hepatic microsomal oxygenation or alternatively, may inhibit the microsomal peroxidation of lipids, but this could merely imply a common electron transport system with different terminal oxygen transferases for each substrate. Evidence for the existence of only one terminal oxygenase, namely cytochrome P450, is provided by ultraviolet absorption spectral data [10]. Most drugs, including phenobarbital and the mixed function oxygenase inhibitor SKF-525A (β-diethylaminoethyl-diphenylpropylacetate hydrochloride) react with hepatic microsomal preparations to produce the same characteristic difference spectrum with an absorption minimum at 419-425 nm, and an absorption maximum at 385-390 nm (type I spectrum). Other drugs and chemicals, usually those containing a nitrogen or sulphur atom that could directly ligand with the haeme moiety of cytochrome P450, and which include aniline and the inhibitor DPEA (2,4-dichloro-6-

phenylphenoxyethylamine), produce a second type of difference spectrum with an absorption minimum at 390-405 nm, and an absorption maximum at 426-435 nm (type 2 spectrum).

This spectral evidence has been interpreted to imply that the diverse substrates studied may react with cytochrome P450 in two different ways, namely by interaction with the lipoprotein moiety of the cytochrome (type 1 spectrum), or by forming a ligand complex with the haeme moiety (type 2 spectrum). The first mode of reaction, and possibly also the second, could of course involve interactions of the substrates with different areas of the apoenzyme and yet still produce the same spectral shift. This would explain the apparent anomaly of a single enzyme protein catalysing many differing chemical reactions with a multitude of substrates, yet manifestly preserving a high degree of both substrate and reaction specificity. If this hypothesis eventually becomes substantiated it will create a new and more sophisticated concept of enzyme action.

Cytochrome P450 is reputed to be the most abundant cytochrome of the liver, and in addition to being a component of the hepatic endoplasmic reticulum and the adrenal mitochondria is found also in many other tissues which hydroxylate xenobiotics. In its reduced form cytochrome P450 forms a ligand complex with carbon monoxide which shows a characteristic absorption maximum at 450 nm, hence its name cytochrome P450 and its earlier synonym of 'carbon monoxide-binding pigment'. This cytochrome requires $NADPH_2$ and molecular oxygen for activity, it is inactivated by the presence of carbon monoxide, and is induced by pretreatment of animals with phenobarbital and a number of other drugs and foreign chemicals. Consequently, the accepted criteria for the involvement of cytochrome P450 as the catalyst of a given biochemical reaction are: (a) the requirement for $NADPH_2$ (and O_2); (b) inhibition by carbon monoxide; and (c) induction by phenobarbital. Induction of the hepatic microsomal enzymes by certain carcinogenic polycyclic hydrocarbons, such as methylcholanthrene, produces a cytochrome with a characteristic carbon monoxide difference absorption spectrum at 448 nm, instead of the usual 450 nm, from which it may be inferred that perhaps more than one distinct form exists, only one of which is produced by the methylcholanthrene pretreatment [11]. In addition to cytochrome P450 the hepatic endoplasmic reticulum contains another cytochrome, cytochrome b_5, whose biological function is, as yet, largely unknown, but which may also be increased by the inductive pretreatment with phenobarbital and other foreign chemicals.

In addition to the mixed function oxygenase activities the hepatic endoplasmic reticulum also contains a number of reductases, certain of which may be mediated through cytochrome P450, e.g. nitroreductase [12]. The pesticide, DDT, is reductively dechlorinated into DDD by a hepatic microsomal system, which requires $NADPH_2$, is inhibited by CO but is also anaerobic. As the reductive dechlorination of DDT is also catalysed by reduced porphyrin the microsomal reaction may involve a non-enzymic reduction by reduced cytochrome P450 or reduced cytochrome b_5 [13].

The biological function of the hepatic microsomal drug-metabolizing enzymes

The metabolic transformations which drugs and other foreign compounds undergo in the endoplasmic reticulum of the mammalian liver result in their conversion from predominantly lipid-soluble molecules into more polar substances, that are consequently more readily eliminated from the hepatocyte and more readily excreted from the body. In this way, compounds which are of little or no nutritive value to the living organism (anutrients or xenobiotics) are prevented from accumulating in the cells and impeding vital processes. Anutrients naturally present in the diet far outnumber the essential nutrients so it is not surprising that, in the course of biological development, living organisms have developed a versatile defence system for the comprehensive metabolism of anutrient molecules which leads to their rapid deactivation and elimination. It is probably only fortuitous that drugs, pesticides, food additives and other synthetic chemicals are detoxicated by these biochemical mechanisms which were developed for the protection of the organism against natural foreign compounds.

A second, and equally fundamental, role for these enzymes of the hepatic endoplasmic reticulum is the metabolism by oxygenation, reduction and conjugation of endogenous steroids and other hormones. As with drugs, this similarly leads to deactivation of these steroid hormones and facilitation of their excretion in the bile and urine. The low Michaelis constants which characterize the hydroxylation of testosterone, progesterone and oestradiol by hepatic microsomal enzymes support the concept that the endogenous steroids are the normal physiological substrates, and indeed preferential substrates, of the oxidative drug-metabolizing enzymes [14].

The effect of drugs and foreign compounds on the hepatic drug-metabolizing enzymes

The increased activities of the hepatic microsomal drug-metabolizing enzymes following the treatment of animals with a wide variety of drugs, pesticides, food additives, polycyclic hydrocarbons and other foreign compounds is now well known and extensively documented [15, 16]. Stimulation of these enzymes occurs only when the inducing compounds are administered to the living animal or are perfused through isolated liver [17], and addition to preparations of the microsomal enzymes *in vitro* produces no stimulatory effect. Microsomal enzyme induction has also been shown to occur in mammalian cell cultures and a sensitive model system to study the induction of aryl hydroxylase in foetal tissue culture has been devised [18].

The drugs and foreign compounds which produce stimulation of these enzymes have widely differing pharmacological activities and the only factors which they would all seem to have in common are that they are lipid soluble and hence become localized in the endoplasmic reticulum of the liver, and are substrates of the microsomal mixed-function oxygenases. It is moreover, significant that all the compounds studied show initial inhibition of these enzymes which is followed by the increase in enzyme activity some 12-24 hours later. This phenomenon would thus appear to be an example of substrate induction where, because of the unique, multifunctional nature of the enzyme system involved, one substrate is able to increase not only the enzymic activity required for its own metabolism but also that for many others.

The drug-metabolizing enzymes are largely absent or latent in the neonate but develop to normal levels during the first few weeks of life. They may readily be induced in the neonatal animal, or in the foetus and indeed may be induced at any age although the extent of induction falls off with advancing maturity [19]. The postnatal development of the mixed-function oxygenases might therefore be the result of substrate-induced derepression initiated by the greatly increased level of anutrient compounds entering the animal system from the diet and from the metabolic activity of the newly acquired intestinal microflora.

A number of naturally occurring anutrients have now been shown to be inhibitors and stimulators of the hepatic drug-metabolizing enzyme system, thus confirming the fundamental nature of anutrients as natural substrates for these enzymes. Rats pretreated with caffeine have an increased drug-metabolizing activity, an increased $NADPH_2$-cytochrome P450 reductase and a slight increase of cytochrome P450 [20]. Similar increases of these enzymes have been produced by pretreatment of animals with coumarin derivatives [21], the terpenoids eucalyptol, [22] β-ionone [23], cedrol and cedrene present in cedarwood chips [24], the flavones, β-naphtho-flavone, quercetin pentamethyl ether, and rutin [25] and with the aromatic ethers safrole and isosafrole [26]. The administration of nicotine to rats [27] and cigarette smoking in man also increase these drug-metabolizing enzymes [28]. The hepatic endoplasmic reticulum has recently been found to oxidize ethanol, quite independently of the alcohol dehydrogenase of the cytoplasm. This enzyme activity has a requirement for $NADPH_2$ and O_2, is inhibited by carbon monoxide, and would appear to be another of the mixed function oxidase activities [29]. Feeding of ethanol increases the activities of hepatic microsomal drug-metabolizing enzymes, in both man and rat, and like phenobarbital and other inducing agents also give rise to proliferation of the endoplasmic reticulum, and to increase in microsomal protein and cytochrome P450 [30]. It exhibits a biphasic effect on the *in vivo* metabolism of aminopyrine in rats, first inhibiting and later stimulating the metabolism [31]. Conversely, the pretreatment of rats with phenobarbital, butylated hydroxytoluene (BHT) or 3-methylcholanthrene enhances the microsomal metabolism of ethanol [32]. These findings would explain the observation that alcoholics are more resistant to drugs, such as barbiturates when sober, whereas inebriated individuals are more sensitive.

Alternative pathways for the metabolism of a drug are not necessarily all equally stimulated by inducing agents, and even within the same class of substrate, the relative extents of induction of alternative paths may differ from one compound to another and with different inducing agents and animal species. In the metabolism of anilines by rabbits induced with phenobarbital or chlorophenothane, the *N*-hydroxylation of aniline was markedly stimulated with little or no increase of *p*-hydroxylation, whereas the *p*-hydroxylation of *N*-ethylaniline was markedly stimulated with no increase in *N*-

hydroxylation; moreover, the *N*-dealkylation of *N*-ethylaniline was stimulated by phenobarbital but not by chlorophenothane [33]. Similarly, whereas the 2- and 4-hydroxylation of biphenyl is stimulated by pretreatment of rats with carcinogenic polycyclic hydrocarbons, only the 4-hydroxylation is stimulated by non-carcinogenic hydrocarbons and by drugs [34]. Another model system of these microsomal enzymes that is induced by carcinogens but not by drugs, is the 5-hydroxylation of oxindole [35].

Similarly, the extent of ^{3}H-migration in the *in vitro* 4-hydroxylation of [4-^{3}H]acetanilide (the NIH effect), which is dependent on species, strain and sex, also varies on pretreatment with drugs and, furthermore, with the nature of the inducing agent. With phenobarbital, isotope retention is greater than normal, but with methylcholanthrene or 3,4-benzpryrene it is less, thus confirming many previous findings that inductions produced by these two classes of substance are different in nature [36]. The shift of the pH optimum for the 4-hydroxylation of aniline from pH 7.0 to 8.1 by the treatment of rats with benzpyrene also incidates that polycyclic hydrocarbons may result in a change, or at least a modification, of the enzymes involved in hepatic microsomal hydroxylation [37]. Several examples of stereospecific hydroxylations of drugs are known, one such reaction being the oxidation of ethylbenzene into methylphenylcarbinol which, in the rat yields a mixture of 90% D(+) and 10% L(−) isomers. After treatment with phenobarbital the stereospecificity is reduced to 77% D(+), from which it may be inferred that the proliferation of the endoplasmic reticulum may be accompanied by a structural change in the membrane [38].

Inducers of the microsomal enzymes, such as phenobarbital, 3-methylcoumarin, butylated hydroxytoluene (BHT) or 4-methylcoumarin, administered to rats for several days, increased the activities of the hepatic drug-metabolizing enzyme system but generally had no effect on other enzymes, such as the phosphatases (glucose-6-phosphatase, pyrophosphatase, inosine diphosphatase, guanosine diphosphatase, or uridine diphosphatase) of the endoplasmic reticulum, whereas hepatotoxic compounds such as carbon tetrachloride, ethionine, thioacetamide and coumarin, which had little or no effect on the drug-metabolizing enzymes produced a marked reduction of the microsomal phosphatases [39]. Other workers have shown that although the available glucose-6-phosphatase is reduced by phenobarbital pretreatment, the latent enzyme manifested by high pH or deoxycholate treatment of the microsomal membranes, is markedly increased, resulting in an overall increase of the enzyme activity of 50%. The phenobarbital therefore results in an induction of this enzyme which is accompanied by a change in conformation of the membrane which masks the increased activity [40].

This induction phenomena has found useful therapeutic application and phenobarbital treatment has been used successfully to induce the hepatic glucuronyl transferase, and thus reduce serum bilirubin levels, in cases of congenital, non-haemolytic, unconjugated hyperbilirubinaemia [41], and in neonatal jaundice due to ABO incompatability, glucose-6-phosphate dehydrogenase deficiency, and other various causes [42]. Treatment of pregnant women with phenobarbital or DDT shortly before birth considerably reduces the incidence of neonatal hyperbilirubinaemia [43]. However, a non-hypnotic, barbiturate, enzyme inducer such as *N*-phenylbarbital, might be more acceptable to patients than either the hypnotic phenobarbital or DDT.

With regard to inhibitors of these enzymes, the alkylating agents, cyclophosphamide (cytoxan), mechlorethamine HCl and pipobroman show no effect on the hepatic drug-metabolizing enzymes *in vitro*, but *in vivo* produce prolonged inhibition and consequently alter the rates of metabolism and toxicity of many drugs [44]. It is therefore important to be aware of the possible potentiation of drugs by simultaneous cytotoxic chemotherapy.

Mechanisms of induction of hepatic drug-metabolizing enzymes by drugs and polycyclic hydrocarbons

The molecular basis for the phenomenon of microsomal enzyme induction has not been fully elucidated, but Conney and Gilman [45] showed that the increased enzyme activity was inhibited by puromycin and actinomycin D and therefore probably involved the synthesis of new enzyme protein. This was confirmed by Kato, and his co-workers [46] who found that phenobarbital increased the incorporation, *in vitro* and *in vivo*, of labelled amino acids into liver microsomal protein. As the phenobarbital-induced enzyme activity is inhibited by actinomycin D, induction may be due to an enhanced DNA-RNA polymerase activity due to genomal derepression [47], and both phenobarbital and methylcholanthrene administered to rats have been shown to stimulate hepatic RNA-polymerase activity [48], giving rise to nuclear chromatin which is a more effective template for RNA synthesis than that isolated from control animals. These differences in template activity are abolished when basic proteins are removed from the chromatin [49]. It has also been shown that phenobarbital administration to rats induces the synthesis of a specific class of acidic, hepatic, nuclear protein, which may play a role in the increased transcription [50]. Other workers have suggested that phenobarbital primarily affects the transcription of ribosomal RNA whereas 3-methylcholanthrene produces an increase in the transcription of RNA resembling messenger RNA [51]. In the induction of aryl hydrocarbon hydroxylase activity by benz[a]-anthracene in hamster foetal cell culture, there is an accumulation of the inducer within the cells, with the major concentration of covalently-bound inducer associated with the nuclear fraction [52]. The consequent enzyme induction has been shown to consist of two phases, namely an initial phase of synthesis of an induction-specific RNA which is translation-independent (cycloheximide insensitive) followed by a second phase of protein synthesis related to the induction-specific RNA, which is transcription-independent (actino-mycin D insensitive) [53].

Alternatively, the increased synthesis of enzymic protein could be the result of an increase in the translation process due to a reduced rate of turnover of messenger- and other RNA, since phenobarbital pretreatment of rats results in inhibition of ribonuclease activity in the hepatic microsomal and post-microsomal fractions which parallels an increase in the hepatic microsomal oxidative demethylation of aminopyrine [54, 55].

In addition to the increase in protein synthesis, treatment with phenobarbital also leads to an increase in hepatic microsomal phospholipid which Orrenius and his colleagues [47] attributed to an increased synthesis since at 3-24 hours after phenobarbital treatment of fasted male rats there was an increased rate of incorporation of ^{32}P into the microsomal phospholipid. Holtzman and Gillette [56] however, subsequently found that no increase in phospholipid occurred until 24 hours after dosage with phenobarbital, and that this was due to inhibition of the catabolism of phospholipid and not to its increased synthesis.

It has also been suggested that chronic phenobarbital pretreatment had no effect on the rate of degradation of total microsomal protein and that the increase of this protein must therefore be due, almost entirely, to increased synthesis [57]. Other workers, however, have shown that a single dose of phenobarbital induced the synthesis of rat hepatic $NADPH_2$-cytochrome c reductase with no similar increase in cytochrome b_5, whereas, repeated dosage produced a large increase in $NADPH_2$-cytochrome c reductase with a moderate increase of cytochrome b_5, resulting from a drastic reduction in the rates of degradation of these enzymes [58]. In the induction of these microsomal enzymes, the increases in microsomal phospholipid and microsomal proteins, including the cytochromes, are accompanied by a proliferation of the endoplasmic reticulum. The herbicide, 3-amino-1,2,4-triazole, an inhibitor of haeme synthesis, when administered to rats inhibits the phenobarbital induction of cytochrome P450 but does not affect the proliferation of the endoplasmic reticulum, indicating that the induced increases of cytochrome P450 and membrane lipoprotein are regulated by separate mechanisms [59].

Induction of the hepatic drug-metabolizing enzymes by phenobarbital follows a similar pattern to that produced by other drugs, pesticides (DDT) and steroids, but differs in many respects from the pattern of enzyme induction resulting from treatment with 3-methylcholanthrene and other carcinogenic polycyclic hydrocarbons. Phenobarbital induces an increase in hepatic microsomal cytochrome P450 which shows u.v. spectral absorption maxima at 450 nm with carbon monoxide as ligand, and at 430 and 455 nm with ethyl isocyanide. In contrast, methylcholanthrene induces an hepatic microsomal haemoprotein with maxima at 448 nm (with carbon monoxide as ligand) and at 455 but not 430 nm with ethyl isocyanide [60, 61, 11]. Furthermore, in the hydroxylation of 3,4-benzpyrene by rat liver microsomes, methylcholanthrene pre-treatment reduced the K_m value to 0.2×10^{-5} M from 1.4×10^{-5} M for normal microsomes, indicating that the induced cytochrome has a greater affinity than the normal liver enzyme for the substrate [62]. On the other hand, phenobarbital resulted in an increase of the normal enzyme since for the oxidation of 3,4-benzpyrene there was an increase of $V_{max.}$ with no decrease of K_m. Similar increases of $V_{max.}$ with no change of K_m have also been observed for the O-demethylation of p-nitroanisole [63] and the N-demethylation of ethylmorphine [64] by hepatic microsomal preparations from phenobarbital-stimulated animals. These findings may, in some part, be explained by the finding that the RNA formed in the presence of chromatin, which has been isolated from the liver of rats treated with methylcholanthrene, differs from that made in the presence of chromatin from control rats, suggesting that methylcholanthrene activates a new region(s) of the genome [65].

Although the induced increases in hepatic microsomal enzyme activity are not always directly related to an increase in cytochrome P450, and indeed cytochrome P450 reductase may often be the rate-limiting factor in hydroxylation reactions, the microsomal CO-binding haemoprotein is nevertheless a major determinant. Studies of the reaction or binding spectra of hepatic microsomal cytochrome P450 with hexobarbital (type 1) and aniline (type 2) show that whereas the hexobarbital reaction spectrum was increased by phenobarbital pretreatment, it was reduced by methylcholanthrene, but the aniline reaction spectrum was increased by both. These changes in the binding spectra were reflected in the *in vitro* oxidations of aniline and hexobarbital, for after methylcholanthrene pretreatment the microsomes gradually increased their ability to oxidize aniline and lost their ability to oxidize hexobarbital, though both activities increased after phenobarbital. These results suggest that phenobarbital increases the content of cytochrome P450 and its affinity for both type 1 and 2 substrates, whereas methylcholanthrene results in an increase of a haemoprotein which has increased affinity for type 2 substrates but decreased affinity for type 1 substrates. This could be either cytochrome P450 with a modified conformation, or a new, related haemoprotein-cytochrome $P_1 450$ [66, 67].

The 'CO-binding particles' (steapsin-treated microsomes, free from cytochrome b_5) of rat liver, normally contain two haemoprotein fractions (cytochrome P450) with different stabilities, of $t_{0.5}$ of 8 hours and 48 hours, present in the ratio of 4:1. Pretreatment with phenobarbital or chlordane increased the amounts of both components similarly, but methylcholanthrene only increased the concentration of the more stable component so that the ratio of the two components became 1 : 1 [68]. Methylcholanthrene and phenobarbital also differently affect the distribution of the haemoprotein within the microsomal vesicles, as subfractionation of the hepatic microsomes by rate-zonal centrifugation showed that phenobarbital resulted in an increase in cytochrome P450 in the lighter fraction, in contrast to the fact that methylcholanthrene resulted in an increase in both this fraction and the fraction of heavier particles [69]. All these facts would seem to indicate the inhomogeneity of cytochrome

P450, with both forms of the haemoprotein being equally increased by phenobarbital, but only one form or conformation increased by methylcholanthrene.

Induction of the rat hepatic drug-metabolizing enzymes by the naturally-occurring anutrients safrole and isoSafrole increases both the 2- and the 4-hydroxylation of biphenyl [26]; the increase of the former enzymic activity being characteristic of carcinogenic inducing agents [34]. We have further shown that simultaneous administration of thioacetamide, to inhibit nuclear-directed protein synthesis, or of 3-amino-1,2,4-triazole, to inhibit the synthesis of haeme, results in the abolition of the increase in cytochrome P450 and of the parallel increase in biphenyl-4-hydroxylase activity, but the increased activity of biphenyl-2-hydroxylase is only partially abolished by these two inhibitors (see Table 1). Further studies with these inhibitors and with actinomycin D, have shown that whereas the increases of cytochrome P450 and the 4-hydroxylation of biphenyl are the result of increased enzyme synthesis and decreased enzyme breakdown, the increase in biphenyl-2-hydroxylase activity is the result of an initial change of conformation of the microsomal enzyme, followed later by an increase in enzyme protein.

The microsomal enzyme-inducing agents such as phenobarbital and 3-methylcholanthrene also result in an increase in the content of the hepatic microsomal cytochrome b_5. Pretreatment of rats with safrole or isoSafrole similarly results in an increase of cytochrome b_5 but also gives rise to a new redox difference absorption spectrum with a maximum at 455 nm (cytochrome b_5 has 425 nm; cytochrome P450 has 445 nm), which is indicative of the formation of a new microsomal haemoprotein [70]. The appearance of this new cytochrome is abolished by simultaneous administration of thioacetamide or aminotriazole. Like cytochrome P450 it is not readily solubilized but unlike cytochrome P450 it is reduced by both NADH and NADPH. The increase in the 2-hydroxylation of biphenyl, induced by safrole and isoSafrole, is not necessarily related to the appearance of this new cytochrome since 3-methylcholanthrene, which also gives rise to a considerable increase of biphenyl-2-hydroxylase activity, does not result in the appearance of the new cytochrome. Like the cytochrome P448 resulting from pretreatment of animals with methylcholanthrene, this new cytochrome may be further evidence for the existence of a family of microsomal haemoproteins of the hepatic endoplasmic reticulum.

Table 1

Changes in Hepatic Microsomal Enzymes and Cytochromes Following Pretreatment with Safrole and isoSafrole

Pretreatment	Percentage of Normal Activity						New Cytochrome (as % normal cyt. b_5)
	Glucuronyl transferase	Nitro reductase	Biphenyl-2-hydroxylase	Biphenyl-4-hydroxylase	Cytochrome P450	Cytochrome b_5	
Safrole	150	200	475	145	160	160	160
Safrole + Thioacetamide	120	200	350	70	100	70	30
Safrole + Aminotriazole	150	200	350	110	120	130	40
isoSafrole	160	200	575	140	150	135	150
isoSafrole + Thioacetamide	120	200	175	70	100	70	30
isoSafrole + Aminotriazole	150	200	250	70	100	120	40
Aminotriazole	100	100	70	70	100	100	0
Thioacetamide	90	100	25	70	70	80	0

The metabolism of steroids by the endoplasmic reticulum

Many tissues other than the liver, for example, the adrenal cortex, the testicular interstitial tissue, the corpus luteum and the placenta, which are concerned with the biogenesis of the steroid hormones, have been shown to contain well-developed endoplasmic reticula and microsomal enzymes, which are involved in metabolic pathways of cholesterol and the steroid hormones. The endoplasmic reticulum of the liver is known to be concerned in the biosynthesis of cholesterol, which requires $NADPH_2$ for the conversion of squalene into lanosterol and the saturation of the $\Delta 7$- and $\Delta 24$-bonds, and NAD for the C-4 demethylations [2]. The transformation of 2,3-oxido-squalene to lanosterol is also catalysed by an hepatic microsomal enzyme (2,3-oxidosqualene sterol cyclase) which has been obtained in a soluble and partially purified form by treatment of the microsomes with deoxycholate [71]. The $NADPH_2$-dependent C-4 demethylation of cholesterol precursors, using 4,4-dimethyl-Δ^7-cholesterol as substrate, is inhibited by cyanide but not by carbon monoxide; furthermore, purification of the methylsterol demethyl-ase has separated cytochrome P450 from this activity [72].

A number of enzymes concerned in corticoidogenesis, including the 17α- and 21-hydroxylases and the Δ^5-3β-hydroxysteroid dehydrogenase, have been shown to occur in the endoplasmic reticulum of the adrenal cortex, and other tissues. Moreover, it has been suggested that cytochrome P450 is the terminal oxygenase for both the 17α- and 21-hydroxylases of the adrenal microsomes [73, 74] as it is for the adrenal mitochondrial steroid 11-hydroxylase, and possibly also for the 18-, 20- and 22-hydroxylases and for the side-chain cleavage enzymes [75, 76]. Other workers, however, found no cytochrome P450 in a soluble preparation of the adrenal 21-hydroxylase and claimed that cytochrome P450 particles actually inhibited this enzyme [77, 78]. The adrenal also contains enzymes that further hydroxylate cortisol into 2α- and 6β-hydroxycortisol and studies in different strains of guinea pig have revealed that different rates of hydroxylation of cortisol were paralleled by different levels of cytochrome P450 in the adrenal cortex [79].

The endoplasmic reticulum of the liver contains a number of enzymes which further metabolize and deactivate the steroid hormones, and these include the 2β-, 6α-, 6β-, 7α-, 16α- and 18α-hydroxylases, and the 4,5α-Δ^4-oxidoreductase [80, 81]. Also located in the hepatic endoplasmic reticulum are the enzymes concerned in the conversion of cholesterol into the bile acids, including cholesterol 7α-hydroxylase and chenodeoxycholate 6β-hydroxylase. The former enzyme probably catalyses the first step of the conversion, and has been shown to require $NADPH_2$ and O_2 and to be inhibited by CO and an antibody to NADPH-cytochrome *c* reductase [3, 4]. This enzyme, although an hepatic microsomal oxygenase mediated probably through cytochrome P450, is not identical with the drug-metabolizing enzymes since it is competitively inhibited *in vitro* by cortisol (50% at 0.5 mM) but is unaffected by aniline (5 mM) or aminopyrine (5 mM) [4]. The

Table 2

Similarities between the Hepatic Microsomal Enzymes which Hydroxylate Drugs and Steroids (after Conney *et al.* [16])

(i)	both require $NADPH_2$ and O_2 for activity
(ii)	activity is higher in male than female rats, with little or no difference in mice
(iii)	activity is high in mammalian liver but low in fish liver
(iv)	activity is increased by pretreatment with drugs, pesticides and steroids
(v)	activity is inhibited by *in vitro* addition of SKF 525-A or chlorthion
(vi)	drugs and steroids exhibit competitive inhibition with each other *in vitro*
(vii)	activity shows a diurnal variation with minimal drug-metabolizing activity coincident with maximum plasma levels of corticosteroid

6β-hydroxylase is also inhibited by CO and is considered to be mediated through cytochrome P450 [82]. Bile acids probably undergo further oxidative metabolism in the liver since they react with hepatic microsomes to give a type 1 reaction spectrum and competitively inhibit the oxidation of type 1, but not type 2, substrates. Longer exposure to bile acids results in irreversible inhibition of type 1 substrates, and increased concentration (1.2 mM) causes degradation of cytochrome P450 with a parallel decrease in metabolism of type 2 substrates [83].

The microsomal fraction of human placenta extensively converts C_{19} steroids into the C_{18} phenolic female sex hormones [84, 85], and further converts oestradiol into 2-hydroxyoestrone [86]. Apart from this 2-hydroxylase the only other oestrogen-metabolizing enzyme present in the placental microsomes is the ubiquitous 7β-dehydrogenase. Various workers [87, 88] have shown that the placenta contains cytochrome P450 and have claimed that certain drugs may be metabolized *in vitro*. A comprehensive survey of the drug-metabolizing activity of human placental tissue carried out in our laboratories has failed to reveal the presence of any significant level of these enzymes. This may be explained by a high degree of substrate specificity of the placental steroid hydroxylases or by a high level of competitive inhibition due to the high concentration of steroids present [89].

The similarities between the enzymes that metabolize steroids and those which metabolize drugs are well known [16] and a list of the similarities between these enzyme activities present in the liver is given in Table 2.

Regulation of hepatic steroid metabolism

Both the biosynthesis of cholesterol from acetate and its subsequent metabolism into bile acids are affected by inhibitors and inducers of the hepatic microsomal enzymes. Certain inhibiting drugs such as SKF 525-A and triparanol inhibit both the synthesis of cholesterol and the activities of the drug-metabolizing enzymes [90] whereas phenobarbital, the classic inducer of the hepatic drug-metabolizing enzymes, similarly induces the synthesis of cholesterol, substantially increasing the incorporation rate of labelled acetate, and probably also mevalonate, into this sterol [91, 92, 93]. The rate of turnover of labelled serum cholesterol in rats was unaltered by phenobarbitone [92] and chlorcyclizine [94], whereas in mice, triglycerides, phospholipids and cholesterol were reduced by continuous treatment with phenobarbital, and even more markedly reduced by chlorcyclizine [94]. In contrast, the increased serum cholesterol and phospholipid and the development of atheromata, that are produced by feeding cholesterol to rabbits, are inhibited by phenobarbital but not by chlorcyclizine [95]. It is interesting to note that the development of atheromata in cholesterol-fed rabbits is enhanced by exposing the animals to carbon monoxide, a potent inhibitor of cytochrome P450 and of the hydroxylation of cholesterol and testosterone [96].

The breakdown of cholesterol by rat liver microsomes was shown to be significantly increased by phenobarbital treatment [93] and although the 7α-hydroxylation of cholesterol, an early step in the formation of bile acids, was found by some authors [97] also to be stimulated, others did not confirm this [98]. Phenobarbital has also been shown to stimulate the hydroxylations involved in the interconversions of the bile acids, namely, the 6β-hydroxylation of taurochenodeoxycholate and lithocholate and the 7α-hydroxylation of taurochenodeoxycholate [99].

The polycyclic hydrocarbon inducer, 3,4-benzpyrene, had no effect on the incorporation of either labelled acetate or mevalonate into cholesterol, but consistently raised the plasma cholesterol level [91]. It is suggested by these authors that whereas phenobarbital stimulates the overall turnover of cholesterol, 3,4-benzpyrene may act by inhibiting the conversion of cholesterol into bile acids. Methylcholanthrene treatment of rats certainly produces a moderate inhibition of the 6β-hydroxylations of taurochenodeoxycholate and lithocholate, and results in no stimulation of any of the reactions involved in the biosynthesis of the bile acids [100].

The hepatic microsomal enzyme activities involved in the synthesis of cholesterol would appear to be more sensitive to inhibitors than are the drug-metabolizing enzymes, as administration to rats of hypocholesteremic agents, such as AY-9944 (*trans*-1,4-*bis*[2-chloro-benzylaminomethyl]*cyclo*hexane dihydrochloride), in doses sufficient to lower the plasma cholesterol, had no effect on a number of drug-metabolizing enzymes [91]. Moreover, though hypocholesteremic drugs, and certain insecticide synergists such as piperonyl butoxide, inhibited the synthesis of cholesterol *in vitro*, they had no appreciable inhibitory effect on the drug-metabolizing enzymes [91] (see Table 3).

It is well known that endogenous oestrogens have a hypolipaemic effect. Merola and co-workers [101, 102] have shown that in rats given oestrone orally, cholesterol biosynthesis is inhibited and there is a redistribution of cholesterol from the blood into the liver. The hepatic mitochondrial oxidation of cholesterol is increased by oestrogens [103] and in perfused male rat livers added estrone, and probably oestradiol, increase the rate of biliary excretion of neutral sterols and bile acids, without increasing the rate of bile production [104]. The overall effect of oestrogens on cholesterol metabolism would therefore appear to be inhibition of synthesis and stimulation of catabolism and excretion.

The metabolism of the steroid hormones may be similarly affected by the simultaneous administration of drugs and other foreign compounds which inhibit or stimulate the hepatic microsomal enzymes. Treatment of humans with phenobarbital, diphenyl-

Table 3

The Effects of Some Enzyme Inhibitors and Inducers on Hepatic Cholesterol Synthesis and Drug Metabolism (from Mitoma et al. [91])

Compound	Cholesterol synthesis in vitro (% control)	Plasma cholesterol (mg/100 ml)	Drug metabolized in vitro (% controls) Hexobarbital	o-Nitroanisole	Aminopyrine	Hexobarbital sleeping time (% control)
In vivo						
None	100	58				
Phenobarbital	1100	53		225	380	90*
Benzpyrene	80	70		230	70	80*
In vitro						
AY-9944 (10^{-5} M)	3		100	100	95	220†
Piperonyl butoxide (10^{-4} M)	11		79	100	73	
SKF 525-A (10^{-4} M)	11		23	74	54	

* 100 μmole/kg dose of inhibitor.
† 15 μmole/kg dose of inhibitor.

hydantoin or phenylbutazone markedly stimulates the metabolism of cortisol into 6β-hydroxycortisol which is excreted in the urine [16]. A more detailed study of the effect of phenobarbital in humans showed that the adrenal secretion of 6β-hydroxycortisol is increased by 50%, the peripheral production by 300%, and the urinary excretion by 200%, while the urinary excretion of tetrahydro-cortisone is reduced by 50% and the cortisol production is unaffected [105]. The authors infer that these findings may result either from an induction of the hepatic cortisol 6β-hydroxylase or from an inhibition of the alternative pathway for cortisol deactivation, namely reduction of ring A. The potentiation of corticosteroids, such as cortisol or prednisolone, by menadione has been shown to be due to inhibition of the deactivation of cortisol by ring A reduction, probably by oxidative depletion of $NADPH_2$ the coenzyme for the hepatic microsomal enzyme, cortisol-5α-Δ^4-reductase [106]. Other workers [107, 108] have shown that, in the rat and the guinea pig, phenobarbital induces the hepatic microsomal 6β-hydroxylase. This increase in the 6β-hydroxylation of cortisol appears to be of therapeutic benefit in Cushing's syndrome, possibly because the enhanced levels of 6β-hydroxycortisol may inhibit the action of cortisol [109]. The non-hypnotic barbiturate inducer, N-phenylbarbital (Phetharbital), administered chronically to man gives rise to a marked increase in 6β-hydroxycortisol excretion, with no increased adrenal output, and with no undesirable hypnotic effects and is therapeutically preferable to hypnotic barbiturates in the treatment of Cushing's syndrome [110]. The metabolism of cortisol to 6β-hydroxycortisol is also stimulated by administration of o,p'-DDD(2,2-[o-chlorophenyl, p-chlorophenyl] 1,1-dichloroethane) to man [111] guinea pigs or rats [112]. Moreover, phenobarbital pretreatment of guinea pigs has been shown to increase also the 2-hydroxylation of cortisol [108].

Pretreatment of experimental animals with phenobarbital and many other drugs also increases the hepatic microsomal metabolism of the endogenous sex hormones, including testosterone, Δ^4-andro-stene-3,17-dione, androsterone, oestradiol-17β, oestrone and pro-gesterone, but in contrast methylcholanthrene has little or no stimulatory effect on these hydroxylations [15]. Phenobarbital, chlorcyclizine [113] chlordane and DDT [16] markedly stimulate the 2β-, 6β-, 7α- and 16α-hydroxylations of testosterone and androstenedione by rat liver microsomes, the greatest effect being with the 16α-hydroxylation of testosterone; methylcholanthrene however, stimulates only the 7α-hydroxylation [114] (see Table 4). On the other hand, the insecticide chlorthion inhibits the 16α-hydroxylation but not the 7α-hydroxylation of testosterone [115]. These variations in the extent of induction in the testosterone hydroxylations by phenobarbital and methylcholanthrene, plus the facts that they are affected by carbon monoxide to different extents and that their rates of neonatal development differ, provide further evidence for the existence of different enzymic entities and different

Table 4
Characteristics of Hepatic Microsomal Testosterone Hydroxylases
(from Kuntzman *et al.*[114])

	Hepatic testosterone hydroxylase		
	6β-	7α-	16α-
Neonatal development:			
Ratio of: $\dfrac{\text{activity at age 1 week}}{\text{activity at age 10 weeks}}$	0.4	2.5	0.01
Phenobarbital induction:			
In adult male (% controls)	230	220	150
In immature male (% controls)	290	140	1900
Methylcholanthrene induction:			
In adult male (% controls)	70	170	25
In immature male (% controls)	140	190	100
Carbon monoxide inhibition:			
(% CO required for 50% inhibition)	60	70	45

regulating mechanisms of these enzymes [116]. The 7α-, 7β-, and 16α-hydroxylations of 3β-hydroxyandrost-5-en-17-one (DHEA) are similarly stimulated by phenobarbital in the female rat, whereas only the 7-hydroxylations are increased in the male, another instance of the individuality and independent regulation of the hepatic steroid hydroxylases [117]. In the hepatic microsomal metabolism of 4-androstene-3,17-dione the various hydroxylases, but not the 5α-reductase, are carbon monoxide-sensitive and are probably mediated through cytochrome P450, but both of these alternative pathways of hydroxylation and ring A reduction are stimulated by phenobarbital [118].

Pretreatments with drugs and pesticides have a similar stimulatory effect on the hepatic metabolism and deactivation of the oestrogens, oestradiol-17β and oestrone [119]. On the other hand, the 17α-ethinyl-19-norsteroids may initially inhibit this metabolism, and norethindrone, norethynodrel and ethynodiol diacetate, when added to liver microsomal preparations, have been shown to inhibit markedly the *in vitro* metabolism of oestradiol into more polar metabolites [120], although it might be anticipated that administered *in vivo* they might subsequently lead to the induction of the same enzymes. This increased rate of metabolic deactivation of the sex hormones *in vitro* is accompanied by the expected physiological effects *in vivo*. The anaesthetic action of progesterone and other steroids is reduced, as is also the uterotropic activity of oestrone and oestradiol, and studies have further indicated that the enzymic stimulatory effects of the pesticides, DDT, chlordane and aldrin, may finally result in decreased fertility [16].

The effects of steroids on hepatic drug metabolism

Steroids of all kinds, the endogenous corticosteroids, androgens, oestrogens and progestogens, and various synthetic steroids, have been shown to effect the metabolism of drugs by altering the activity of the drug-metabolizing enzymes of the liver [15]. Since drugs and steroids would appear to be alternative substrates for the same hepatic microsomal mixed-function oxygenase system, they might be expected to exhibit competitive inhibition of the enzyme system *in vitro* and within a short period after administration *in vivo*, though after a longer interval should give rise to an increase in the enzymic activity. These speculations have now been largely substantiated by experiment.

Adrenalectomy decreases the rates of metabolism of hexobarbital and many other drugs in the male rat but possibly not the female [15]. The activities may be restored by administration of prednisolone, cortisol or phenobarbital [121]. Application of short-term stress, such as exposure to cold or hind-limb ligation, increases the rate of drug metabolism [122]. Restoration of enzyme activity in adrenalectomized rats by repeated treatment with phenobarbital, cortisol or exposure to cold produces different effects according to the drug metabolized and suggests that both phenobarbitone and stress can bring about changes in drug metabolism independent of the adrenal and independent of each other [121]. More recent work has shown that adrenalectomy of male rats decreases hepatic O-demethylase activity, NADPH-cytochrome c reductase and cytochrome P450 reductase much more than it reduces the cytochrome P450 content of the liver, and it is inferred that the effect of adrenal function is more concerned with the reductases of the microsomal hydroxylating system than with cytochrome P450, the supposed terminal oxygenase [123]. Hepatic drug metabolism is restored by corticosterone (but not ACTH) in adrenalectomized rats, and by both corticosterone and ACTH in hypophysectomized animals. This suggests that the pituitary-adrenal system exerts a regulatory function on the drug-metabolizing enzymes. This was substantiated by the work of Radzialowski and Bousquet [124] who have shown that the rates of metabolism of aminopyrine, p-nitroanisole, hexobarbital and 4-dimethylaminoazobenzene by microsomal preparations of rat liver follow a circadian rhythm which matches a circadian rhythm of plasma corticosterone concentration, with the maximum level of microsomal drug-metabolizing enzyme activity coinciding with the minimum level of plasma corticosteroid and vice versa. Adrenalectomy removes this circadian variation of activity of the hydroxylating enzymes but does not similarly affect hepatic azo reductase. Pretreatment with phenobarbitone, or supplementation of corticosterone, also remove this variation in enzyme activity.

The effect of corticosteroid hormones on intermediary metabolism is believed to be due to increases in the activities of the particular enzymes concerned, possibly resulting from an increased synthesis of enzyme protein. The rates of synthesis of enzyme protein are dependent on, among other factors, the stability of the polysomes which in turn is related to the stability of the ribonucleic acid, which is controlled by ribonuclease activity. Administration of the synthetic steroid triamcinolone diacetate to rats has been shown to result in a gradual, but marked, decrease in liver ribonuclease activity, maximal at 72 hours after dosage and returning to normal at 96 hours, which is paralleled by increases in liver RNA and liver aminotransferase activity [125]. This is comparable with the discovery that phenobarbital pretreatment suppresses liver ribonuclease which is paralleled by an increase in drug metabolizing activity [55]. The increased drug metabolism produced by stress is blocked by inhibitors of protein synthesis, such as actinomycin D [122], and in view of the possible role of histones in regulating gene activity in the eucaryotic cell it is perhaps interesting to note that the acetylation of liver histones is stimulated by cortisol which is bound to the F3 histones of the liver when administered to rats [126]. Another possible role of steroid hormones in regulating the pattern of hepatic enzyme synthesis is their ability to cause the 'smooth' membranes of the liver endoplasmic reticulum to react with polysomes to form 'rough' membranes [127].

It has long been known that in the rat, the duration and intensity of drug action is greater in the adult female than in the male. This difference of activity is due to an enhanced level of the hepatic microsomal drug-metabolizing enzymes in the adult male rat and must be produced by the male sex hormones for it only appears at puberty and may be abolished by castration. This sex difference has not been observed to the same extent in other animals. Testosterone administered to female rats increases the rates of metabolism of many drugs and conversely the opposite effect is produced by the administration of oestrogens to male animals [15]. Mice behave somewhat differently and a single dose of testosterone to female mice produces a biphasic effect, initially prolonging the action of hexobarbital and after 4 days reducing this. Long-term pretreatment of female mice with testosterone reduces the pharmacological activities of hexobarbital and chlorzoxazone by increasing their metabolism [128]. Various anabolic 19-nortestosterone derivatives such as norethandrolone and 19-nortestosterone increase the metabolism of hexobarbital and zoxazolamine within 6-12 hours after a single dose in mice, though prolonged treatment is required to produce this effect in rats [129].

Certain synthetic anabolic and anti-mineralocorticoid steroids have been shown to inhibit the action of various drugs and toxic compounds, e.g. digitoxin and picrotoxin, by increasing the activity of the hepatic drug-metabolizing enzymes—the so-called 'cataxoxic' effect. The diuretic spironolactone, administered to male mice, increased the microsomal metabolism of hexobarbital, aniline and ethylmorphine [130] and pretreatment of rats with spironolactone, norbolethone, or ethylestrenol increased the microsomal hydroxylation of hexobarbital and aminopyrine [131]. That this induction involved the synthesis of new enzyme protein was shown by the complete inhibition of the stimulatory effects of spironolactone or ethylestrenol on the metabolism of pentobarbital in rats by the simultaneous administration of actinomycin D, puromycin aminonucleoside and cycloheximide, known inhibitors of RNA- and protein-synthesis [132].

Cortisol, progesterone, testosterone, androsterone and estradiol-17β all competitively inhibit the *in vitro* hydroxylation of hexobarbital and the *N*-demethylation of ethylmorphine by rat liver microsomes, consistent with the view that steroids and drugs are alternative substrates for the hepatic microsomal mixed-function oxygenase system [133]. Cortisol and prednisolone also competitively inhibit the *in vitro* activities of the microsomal drug-metabolizing enzymes (e.g. aniline hydroxylase and aminopyrine demethylase, of mouse liver) but do not inhibit other hepatic microsomal enzymes (e.g. ATP-ase, glucose-6-phosphatase, esterase, NADH-diaphorase or NADPH-diaphorase) [134]. Metapyrone (2-methyl-1,2-*bis*[3-pyridyl]-1-propanone), a potent inhibitor of adrenal mitochondrial 11-hydroxylase (a cytochrome P450 mediated enzyme), and of several other steroid hydroxylases, also inhibits the metabolism of hexobarbital and aminopyrine by rat liver microsomes; but in the hydroxylation of acetanilide only high concentrations of metapyrone inhibit, lower concentrations ($10^{-2}-10^{-4}$ M) enhancing the reaction [135]. The activation of the latent alkylating agent, cyclophosphamide, is inhibited *in vitro* by addition of prednisolone, and *in vivo* by simultaneous administration to rats [136] but pretreatment with phenobarbital enhances the rate of activation [137]. In view of the simultaneous usage of cytotoxic drugs and immunosuppressive steroids in the management of transplantation surgery, or in the treatment of malignancy, particularly leukaemia, these particular types of drug-steroid interactions merit further investigation.

The effect of pregnancy on the metabolism of drugs

There has been a growing opinion among clinicians that pregancy in humans imposes an inhibition of the ability to metabolize and deactivate drugs [138]. During pregnancy there is a considerable increase in the formation and circulation of the female sex steroid hormones, both progestogens and oestrogens [139, 140] and, since these steroid hormones may be metabolized by the same hepatic microsomal enzymes which metabolize drugs it is possible that they may competitively inhibit the metabolism of drugs.

Cessi [141] showed that the glucuronide conjugation of *o*-amino-phenol in pregnant guinea pigs was only half that of non-pregnant female animals, and it was later shown that the glucuronide conjugation of bilirubin by rat liver slices was inhibited by the addition of serum from pregnant women and new-born infants, and also by progesterone, pregnanediol and pregnanolone [142]. It was concluded that the inhibitor present in the serum of pregnant women was pregnane-3α,20α-diol and that this steroid hormone was likely to be a contributory factor in the hyperbilirubinaemia of new-born infants [143]. Later workers showed that administration of oestriol and cortisone increased the plasma level of unconjugated bilirubin in infants [144], as did pregnanediol present in the mothers' milk [145]. Creaven and Parke [146] showed that in both pregnant rats and rabbits, and in animals pretreated with progesterone, the glucuronide conjugation of a number of substrates was markedly inhibited. Sulphate conjugation is also inhibited during pregnancy and it has been suggested that this is due to the high levels of oestrogens [147].

A more recent survey of the effects of pregnancy on the hepatic microsomal drug-metabolizing enzymes [148] has shown that at full-term, pregnant rats exhibit reductions of the order of 30-50% in the concentration of liver microsomal protein and cytochrome P450, and in the specific activities of biphenyl-4-hydroxylase and 4-methylumbelliferone glucuronyl transferase. However, due to the greatly increased size of the liver these deficiencies are fully compensated for, and the total contents of the microsomal drug-metabolizing enzyme activities of the liver in the pregnant rat are the same or even greater than in the non-pregnant animal. This is somewhat different from the picture in the pregnant rabbit, where there is only minor liver enlargement with no change in the contents of microsomal protein or cytochrome P450; biphenyl-4-hydroxylase is unaffected but glucuronyl transferase activity is decreased by some 20% and coumarin-7-hydroxylase activity is inhibited to an extent of 70% [148].

These findings are confirmed by the kinetic studies of Guarino and his co-workers [149] who showed that with hepatic microsomal preparations from 20-day pregnant rats, the K_m values for the metabolism of aniline and ethylmorphine are the same as for non-pregnant animals, but that the V_{max} values were significantly decreased, suggesting that a reduced concentration of enzyme is responsible for the diminished rate of metabolism, possibly as a result of the high circulating levels of oestrogenic and progestational steroids during pregnancy.

The effects of oral contraceptive steroids

Since endogenous steroid hormones may act as competitively inhibiting substrates for the hepatic drug-metabolizing enzymes [133, 150], and both natural oestrogens and progestogens of pregnancy have been shown to be associated with the inhibition of these enzymes, it may follow that oral contraceptive steroids could also have an inhibiting effect, which in view of the extensive and prolonged usage of these compounds, might be highly undesirable. Juchau and Fouts [150] showed that 1 hour after administration of norethynodrel to rats the *in vitro* metabolism of both hexobarbitone (a type I substrate of cytochrome P450) and of zoxazolamine (a type II substrate) were inhibited, whereas 24 hours later the metabolism of both compounds was increased. The oestrogen mestranol administered to mice daily for 4 days inhibited the metabolism of hexobarbital and pentobarbital and increased the sleeping times produced by these barbiturates; on the other hand lynestrenol, a progestogen similarly administered, enhanced the metabolism of these barbiturates [151] and also that of phenobarbital and phenytoin [152]. With acute treatment (2 hours after dosage) norethynodrel and ethinyl oestradiol (though not medroxyprogesterone or mestranol) inhibited the *in vivo* metabolism of pentobarbital in rats, whereas after chronic treatment (30 days) this *in vivo* metabolism was significantly increased [153].

A study of the *in vitro* inhibitory effects of a number of oral contraceptive steroids by Neale and Parke [154] showed that there was inhibition of the 4-hydroxylation of biphenyl and of the demethylation of 4-methoxybiphenyl at concentrations of $10^{-3}-10^{-4}$ M progesterone, norethynodrel, norethisterone, and ethynodiol diacetate, which are considerably higher concentrations than were found necessary by other workers for the inhibition of the side-chain hydroxylation of hexobarbital and the aromatic-ring hydroxylation of zoxazolamine by norethynodrel and progesterone [150]. Both groups of workers, however, found little or no reduction in inhibition of *p*-nitrobenzoate at concentrations of 10^{-4} M of the steroids.

The prolonged pretreatment of rats (18 days) by intraperitoneal injection of the contraceptive steroids mestranol, plus ethynodiol

Oestrogens

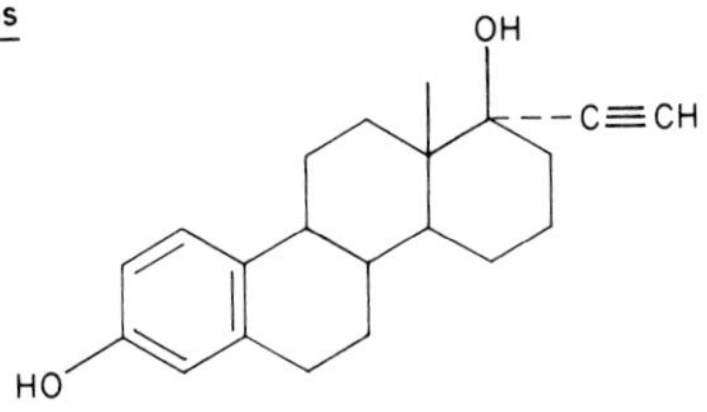

Ethinyl oestradiol

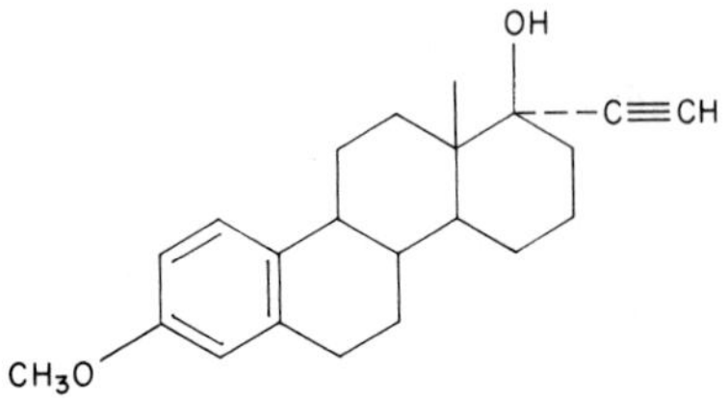

Mestranol

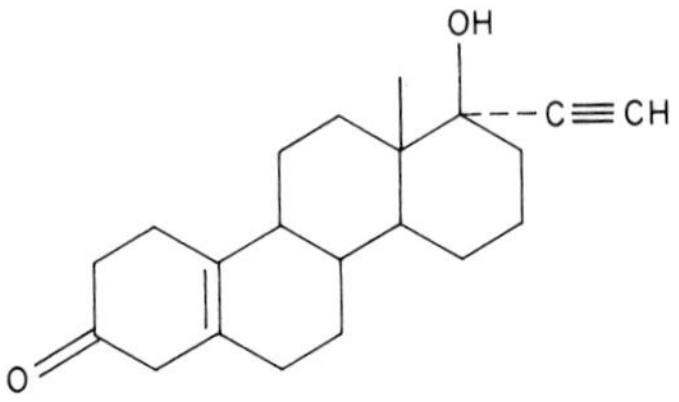

Norethynodrel

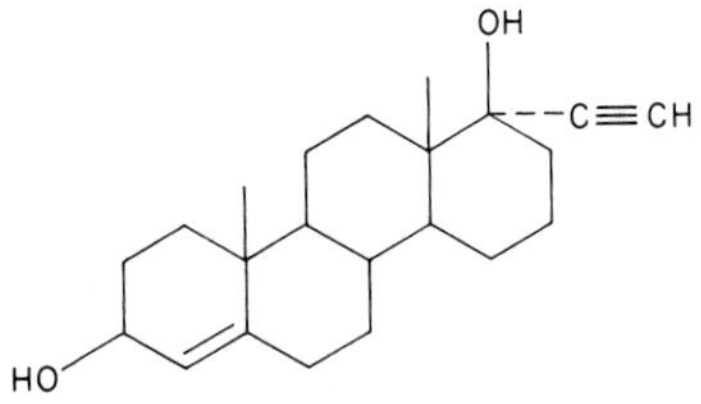

Ethynodiol

Progestogens

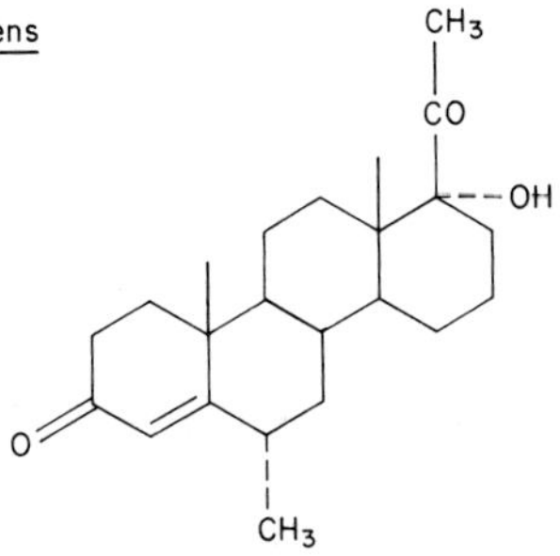

Medroxyprogesterone

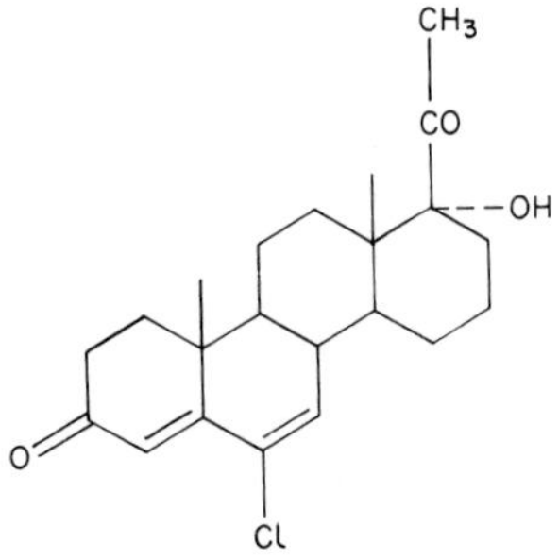

Chlormadinone

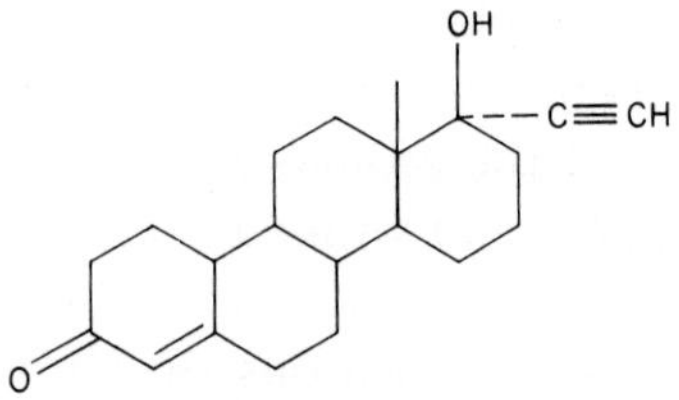

Norethisterone

diacetate, results in a significant increase in the aromatic hydroxylation of biphenyl (30%), which is not shown by the same doses of mestranol or ethynodiol acetate alone; but neither cytochrome P450 nor glucuronyl transferase was similarly stimulated [154]. This is comparable with the work of Jori, and his co-workers [153] who showed that pretreatment of rats for 30 days with mestranol, norethynodrel, medroxyprogesterone acetate or ethinyl oestradiol, alone and in combination, frequently lead to the induction of drug metabolism as measured by the *O*-demethylation of 4-nitroanisole,

Table 5
Effect of †Chronic Oral Pretreatment with Contraceptive Steroids on some Microsomal Drug-Metabolizing Enzymes of Rat Liver

Liver Parameter:	Steroid Pretreatment			
	None	Ethynodiol diacetate	Norethynodrel	Chlormadinone acetate
Liver weight (g)	8.5	8.5	8.5	7.5*
Microsomal protein (mg/g)	29	27	28	32*
Cytochrome P450 (mμmol/g)	0.74	0.73	0.73	0.70*
Biphenyl-4-hydroxylase (μmol product/g/hr)	4.8	3.7*	4.6	4.0*
4-Nitrobenzoate reductase (μmol product/g/hr)	2.7	2.6	2.7	2.8
4-Methylumbelliferone glucuronyl transferase (μmol product/g/hr)	61		65	71

* Significant difference from control.
† 120 days at 5 mg/kg for all three steroids.

the *N*-demethylation of aminopyrine and the aromatic hydroxylation of aniline. On the other hand, Juchau and Fouts [150] found that prolonged pretreatment of rats with norethynodrel and mestranol decreased the rate of hydroxylation of hexobarbital. In our laboratories, chronic oral treatment for 120 days with ethynodiol diacetate, norethynodrel or chlormadinone acetate showed only minor changes; with a moderate reduction of biphenyl-4-hydroxylase activity after ethynodiol diacetate and chlormadinone acetate, and a similar reduction of cytochrome P450 and liver weight in the case of the latter. None of the other enzymes examined were changed, and norethynodrel produced no abnormalities whatsoever [154] (see Table 5). In summary it would appear that many of these contraceptive steroids are acceptable substrates for the hepatic microsomal drug-metabolizing enzymes, giving rise to modest inhibition of drug metabolism *in vitro*, and variable extents of induction of the various microsomal drug-metabolizing enzymic activities *in vivo*, which on prolonged treatment finally return to approximately normal levels. The long-term use of these oral-contraceptive steroids thus appears unlikely to result in any major changes in the levels of the hepatic drug-metabolizing enzymes, and hence is unlikely to result in any marked changes in the activity of drugs or the toxicity of environmental chemicals.

Acknowledgements

The work carried out in the author's laboratories was supported by The Sir Halley-Stewart Trust, Glaxo Laboratories Limited and Schering Chemicals Limited.

Discussion

Powis (Glasgow)

Would you care to qualify the remarks you made concerning latency in the Cotton-tail rabbit and also as you suggested, in humans. Do you think this may have any possible relationship to the uncovering of latent enzyme activity in the rough endoplasmic reticulum as discussed by Professor Rabin in an earlier paper?

Parke (Surrey)

Several examples of latency of enzymes of the endoplasmic reticulum are now known. The latent activity is manifested following the action of certain surface-active, detergent compounds *in vitro* and certain lipophilic compounds, such as safrole, *in vivo*. It would appear that conformational changes of the membrane may occur, or that the inter-relationships of the protein and lipid components, the membrane environment, are altered, so that more active sites of the particular enzyme become available. The characteristics of the enzyme itself do not appear to be changed.

I do not think that these are the same enzyme sites as previously discussed by Professor Rabin, though, of course, the mechanisms may be similar.

Marshall (King's College Hospital)

It seems to me that there are many similarities between the induction of microsomal enzymes that you have been discussing, and the growth-promoting effects of hormones about which we heard from Dr Tomkins this morning. In both cases a variety of chemically and physically different compounds gives rise to broadly similar effects. Dr Tomkins has proposed that a pleiotypic effector mediates the growth-promoting effects of hormones. Might there not be an analogous substance involved in microsomal enzyme induction?

Parke (Surrey)

There would certainly seem to be a case for one or two common effector substances, through which the multitude of different inducing substances would act. Because of the basic differences in mechanisms between drugs and carcinogens, and to some extent also steroids, in the induction of the microsomal enzymes, one would expect these to be mediated through different intermediary effectors, so more than one such substance is likely to be involved.

Hughes (Beecham)

You showed a sex difference in the rat in the action of drug metabolizing enzymes. Bearing in mind the circadian variation in the female which you illustrated, how significant is this sex difference? What would the comparison be like if estimates were taken at a different time of day?

Parke (Surrey)

This work has not been done, but certainly the sex differences in rats have been studied at the same time of day, and to my knowledge at almost every different hour—and they do persist despite variation in the plasma corticosteroids. I would not think that these phenomena are very interdependent.

Cohen (Open University)

Are there synergistic effects of drugs on drug-metabolizing enzymes?

Parke (Surrey)

Yes, and many examples of these have been published.

Slater (Brunel)

You showed a slide in which drug metabolizing activity in several different strains of rabbit was contrasted. The activity in Cotton-tail rabbits seemed particularly low but was induced by phenobarbital to the same maximal activity found in the other strains. This reminds me of some work by Stevenson in Dundee with Gunn rats. The activity of glucuronyl transferase in the microsomes from Gunn rats is normally very low but treatment *in vitro* with diethylnitrosamine produced a rise in activity to within the normal range. Do you think that the drug metabolizing enzymes in Cotton-tail rabbits are similarly latent and would respond to diethylnitrosamine treatment?

Parke (Surrey)

I believe that this may be a similar phenomenon, involving changes of membrane conformation or changes in membrane environment.

References

1. Bloch, K.; *Science, N.Y.*; **150**, (1965) 19.
2. Scallen, T. J., Dean, W. J. and Schuster, M. W.; *J. biol. Chem.*; **234**, (1968) 5502.
3. Danielsson, H., Einarsson, K. and Johansson, G.; *Eur. J. Biochem.*; **2**, (1967) 44.
4. Wada, F., Hirata, K., Nakao, K. and Sakamoto, Y.; *J. Biochem., Tokyo*; **66**, (1969) 699.
5. Preiss, B. and Bloch, K.; *J. biol. Chem.*; **239**, (1964) 85.
6. Bjorkhem, I. and Danielsson, H.; *Eur. J. Biochem.*; **14**, (1970) 473.
7. Israelsson, U., Hamberg, M. and Samuelsson, B.; *Eur. J. Biochem.*; **11**, (1969) 390.
8. Parke, D. V.; *The Biochemistry of Foreign Compounds*; International series of Monographs in Pure and Applied Biology. Oxford: Pergamon Press, (1968).
9. Parke, D. V.; The metabolism of drugs; In: 'Recent Advances in Pharmacology'; Eds J. M. Robson and R. S. Stacey. Churchill, London. 4th ed. (1968) p. 29.
10. Remmer, H., Schenkman, J., Estabrook, R. W., Sasame, H., Gillette, J., Narasimhulu, S., Cooper, D. Y. and Rosenthal, O.; *Molec. Pharmac.*; **2**, (1966) 187.
11. Sladek, N. E. and Mannering, G. J.; *Biochem. biophys. Res. Commun.*; **24**, (1966) 668.
12. Gillette, J. R., Kamm, J. J. and Sasame, H. A.; *Molec. Pharmac.*; **4**, (1968) 541.
13. Walker, C. H.; *Life Sci.*; **8**, (1969) 1111.
14. Kuntzman, R., Lawrence, D. and Conney, A. H.; *Molec. Pharmac.*; **1**, (1965) 163.
15. Conney, A. H.; *Pharmac. Rev.*; **19**, (1967) 317.
16. Conney, A. H., Welch, R. M., Kuntzman, R. and Burns, J. J.; *Clin. Pharmac. Ther.*; **8**, (1967) 2.
17. Juchau, M. R., Cram, R. L., Plaa, G. L. and Fouts, J. R.; *Biochem. Pharmac.*; **14**, (1965) 473.
18. Nebert, D. W. and Gelboin, H. V.; *J. biol. Chem.*; **243**, (1968) 6242 and 6250.

19. Kato, R. and Takanaka, A.; *J. Biochem., Tokyo*; **63**, (1968) 406.
20. Leon, L. and Mitoma, C.; *Biochem. Pharmac.*; **19**, (1970) 2317.
21. Feuer, G.; *Can. J. Physiol. Pharmac.*; **48**, (1970) 232.
22. Jori, A., Bianchetti, A., Prestini, P. E. and Gorathini, S.; *Eur. J. Pharmac.*; **9**, (1970) 362.
23. Parke, D. V. and Rahman, H.; *Biochem. J.*; **113**, (1969) 12P.
24. Wade, A. E., Holl, J. E., Hilliard, C. C., Molton, E. and Greene, F. E.; *Pharmacology*; **1**, (1968) 317.
25. Wattenberg, L. W. and Leong, J. L.; *Cancer Res.*; **30**, (1970) 1922.
26. Parke, D. V. and Rahman, H.; *Biochem. J.*; **119**, (1970) 53P.
27. Ruddon, R. W. and Cohen, A. M.; *Toxicol. Appl. Pharmac.*; **16**, (1970) 613.
28. Beckett, A. H. and Triggs, E. J.; *Nature, Lond.*; **216**, (1967) 587.
29. Lieber, C. S. and DeCarli, L. M.; *Science, N.Y.*; **162**, (1968) 417.
30. Rubin, E., Bacchin, P., Gang, H. and Lieber, C. S.; *Lab. Invest.*; **22**, (1970) 569.
31. Schuppel, R.; *Naunyn-Schmiedebergs, Arch. exp. Path. Pharmak.*; **265**, (1969) 156.
32. Lieber, C. S. and DeCarli, L. M.; *Life Sci.*; **9**, (1970) 267.
33. Lange, G.; *Naunyn-Schmiedebergs Arch. exp. Path. Pharmak.*; **257**, (1967) 230.
34. Creaven, P. J. and Parke, D. V.; *Fed. Eur. Biochem. Soc. Second Meeting Absts.*; **128**, (1965) 88.
35. King, L. J., Parke, D. V., Turbert, H. and Wynne, D.; *Fed. Eur. Biochem. Soc. Fifth Meeting Absts.*; (1968) 39.
36. Daly, J., Jerina, D., Farnsworth, J. and Guroff, G.; *Arch. Biochem. Biophys.*; **131**, (1969) 238.
37. Rickert, D. E. and Fouts, J. R.; *Biochem. Pharmac.*; **19**, (1970) 381.
38. McMahon, R. E. and Sullivan, H. R.; *Life Sci.*; **5**, (1966) 921.
39. Feuer, G. and Granda, V.; *Toxicol. Appl. Pharm.*; **16**, (1970) 626.
40. Pandhi, P. N. and Baum, H.; *Life Sci.*; **9**, (1970) 87.
41. Crigler, J. F. Jr., and Gold, N. I.; *J. clin. Invest.*; **48**, (1966) 42.
42. Yeung, C. Y. and Field, C. E.; *Lancet*; **2**, (1969) 135.
43. Maurer, H. M., Wolff, J. A., Finster, M., Poppers, P. J., Pantuck, E., Kuntzman, R. and Conney, A.; *Lancet*; **2**, (1968) 122.
44. Tardiff, R. G. and Dubois, K. R.; *Archs. int. Pharmacodyn. Ther.*; **177**, (1969) 445.
45. Conney, A. H. and Gilman, A. G.; *J. biol. Chem.*; **238**, (1963) 3682.
46. Kato, R., Loeb, L. and Gelboin, H. V.; *Biochem. Pharmac.*; **14**, (1965) 1164.
47. Orrenius, S., Ericson, J. E. and Ernster, L.; *J. cell Biol.*; **25**, (1965) 627.
48. Gelboin, H. V., Wortham, J. S. and Wilson, R. G.; *Nature, Lond.*; **214**, (1967) 281.
49. Piper, W. N. and Bousquet, W. F.; *Biochem. biophys. Res. Commun.*; **33**, (1968) 602.
50. Ruddon, R. W. and Rainey, C. H.; *Biochem. biophys. Res. Commun.*; **40**, (1970) 152.
51. Wold, J. W. and Steele, W. J.; *Fed. Proc. Fedn. Am. Socs. exp. Biol.*; **28**, (1969) 484.
52. Nebert, D. W. and Bausserman, L. L.; *Molec. Pharmac.*; **6**, (1970) 293.
53. Nebert, D. W. and Gelboin, H. V.; *J. biol. Chem.*; **245**, (1970) 160.
54. Stolman, S. and Lou, H. H.; *J. Pharm. Pharmac.*; **22**, (1970) 713.

55. Louis-Ferdinand, R. T. and Fuller, G. C.; *Biochem. biophys. Res. Commun.*; **38**, (1970) 811.
56. Holtzman, J. L. and Gillette, J. R.; *Biochem. biophys. Res. Commun.*; **24**, (1966) 639.
57. Holtzman, J. L.; *Biochem. Pharmac.*; **18**, (1969) 2573.
58. Kuriyama, Y., Omura, T., Siekevitz, P. and Palade, G. E.; *J. biol. Chem.*; **244**, (1969) 2017.
59. Raisfeld, I. H., Bacchin, P., Hutterer, F. and Schaffner, F.; *Molec. Pharmac.*; **6**, (1970) 231.
60. Alvares, A. P., Schilling, G. R., Levin, W. and Kuntzman, R.; *Biochem. biophys. Res. Commun.*; **29**, (1967) 521.
61. Alvares, A. P. and Mannering, G. J.; *Fed. Proc.*; **26**, (1967) 462.
62. Alvares, A. P., Shilling, G. R. and Kuntzman, R.; *Biochem. biophys. Res. Commun.*; **30**, (1968) 588.
63. Netter, K. J. and Seidel, G.; *J. Pharmac. exp. Ther.*; **146**, (1964) 61.
64. Rubin, A., Tephly, T. R. and Mannering, G. J.; *Biochem. Pharmac.*; **13**, (1964) 1007.
65. Bresnick, E. and Mosse, H.; *Molec. Pharmac.*; **5**, (1969) 219.
66. Kato, R. and Takanaka, A.; *Jap. J. Pharmac.*; **19**, (1969) 171.
67. Shoeman, D. W., Chaplin, M. D. and Mannering, G. J.; *Molec. Pharmac.*; **5**, (1969) 412.
68. Levin, W. and Kuntzman, R.; *J. biol. Chem.*; **244**, (1969) 3671.
69. Murphy, P. J., Van Frank, R. M. and Williams, T. L.; *Biochem. biophys. Res. Commun.*; **37**, (1969) 697.
70. Rahman, H. and Parke, D. V.; *Biochem. J.*; **123**, (1971) 9.
71. Yamamoto, S., Lin, K. and Bloch, K.; *Proc. Nat. Acad. Sci. U.S.A.*; **63**, (1969) 110.
72. Gaylor, J. L. and Mason, H. S.; *J. biol. Chem.*; **243**, (1968) 4966.
73. Inano, H., Inano, A. and Tamaoki, B.-I.; *Biochim. biophys. Acta.*; **191**, (1969) 257.
74. Estabrook, R. W., Cooper, D. Y. and Rosenthal, O.; *Biochem. Z.*; **338**, (1963) 741.
75. Wilson, L. D., Harding, B. W. and Nelson, D. H.; *Biochim. biophys. Acta.*; **99**, (1965) 391.
76. Bryson, M. J. and Sweat, M. L.; *J. biol. Chem.*; **243**, (1968) 2799.
77. Matthijssen, C. and Mandel, J. E.; *Biochim. biophys. Acta.*; **146**, (1967) 613.
78. Matthijssen, C. and Mandel, J. E.; *Steroids*; **15**, (1970) 541.
79. Burnstein, S.; *Biochem. biophys. Res. Commun.*; **26**, (1967) 697.
80. Gustafsson, J. A., Lisboa, B. P. and Sjovall, J.; *Eur. J. Biochem.*; **5**, (1968) 437.
81. Gustafsson, J. A. and Lisboa, B. P.; *Steroids*; **14**, (1969) 659.
82. Voight, W., Thomas, P. J. and Hsia, S. L.; *J. biol. Chem.*; **243**, (1968) 3493.
83. Hutterer, F., Denk, H., Bacchin, P. G., Schenkman, J. B., Schaffner, F. and Popper, H.; *Life Sci.*; **9**, (1970) 877.
84. Ryan, K. J.; *J. biol. Chem.*; **234**, (1959) 268.
85. Axelrod, L. R., Matthijssen, C., Rao, P. N. and Goldzieher, J. W.; *Acta. endocr.*; **48**, (1965) 383.
86. Fishman, J. and Dixon, D.; *Biochemistry, N.Y.*; **6**, (1967) 1683.
87. Meigs, R. A. and Ryan, K. J.; *Biochim. biophys. Acta.*; **165**, (1968) 476.
88. Mirkin, B. L.; *Ann. Rev. Pharmac.*; **10**, (1970) 255.

89. Chakraborty, J., Hopkins, R. and Parke, D. V.; *Biochem. J.*; (1971) in press.
90. Kato, R., Vassanelli, P. and Chiesara, E.; *Biochem. Pharmac.*; **12**, (1963) 349.
91. Mitoma, C., Yasuda, D., Tagg, J. S., Neubauer, S. E., Calderoni, F. J. and Tanabe, M.; *Biochem. Pharmac.*; **17**, (1968) 1377.
92. Kato, R., Onoda, K. and Omori, Y.; *Jap. J. Pharmac.*; **18**, (1968) 514.
93. Wada, F., Hirata, K., Shibota, H., Higashi, K. and Sakamoto, Y.; *J. Biochem., Tokyo*; **62**, (1967) 134.
94. Salvador, R. A., Atkins, C., Haber, S. and Conney, A. H.; *Biochem. Pharmac.*; **19**, (1970) 1463.
95. Salvador, R. A., Atkins, C., Haber, S., Kozma, C. and Conney, A. H.; *Biochem. Pharmac.*; **19**, (1970) 1975.
96. Astrup, P., Kjeldsen, K. and Wanstrup, J.; *J. Atheroscler, Res.*; **7**, (1967) 343.
97. Shefer, S., Hauser, S. and Mosbach, E. H.; *J. Lipid Res.*; **9**, (1968) 328.
98. Einarsson, K. and Johansson, G.; *Eur. J. Biochem.*; **6**, (1968) 293.
99. Einarsson, K. and Johansson, G.; *FEBS Letters*; **4**, (1969) 177.
100. Johansson, G.; *Biochem. Pharmac.*; **19**, (1970) 2817.
101. Merola, A. J. and Arnold, A.; *Science*; **144**, (1964) 301.
102. Merola, A. J., Dill, R. R. and Arnold, A.; *Arch. Biochem. Biophys.*; **123**, (1968) 378.
103. Kritchevsky, D., Staple, E., Rabinowitz, J. L. and Whitehouse, M. W.; *J. Lipid Res.*; **4**, (1963) 188.
104. Saini, V. C. and Patrick, S. J.; *Biochim. biophys. Acta.*; **202**, (1970) 556.
105. Burnstein, S., Kimball, H. L., Klaiber, E. L. and Gut, M.; *J. clin. Endocr. Metab.*; **27**, (1967) 49.
106. Kupfer, D. and Peets, L.; *Experientia*; **24**, (1968) 893.
107. Conney, A. H., Jacobson, M., Schneidman, K. and Kuntzman, R.; *Life Sci.*; **4**, (1965) 1091.
108. Burnstein, S. and Bhavani, B. R.; *Endocrinology*; **80**, (1967) 351.
109. Southern, A. L., Tochimoto, S., Strom, L., Ratuschni, A., Ross, H. and Gordon, G.; *J. clin. Endocr. Metab.*; **26**, (1966) 268.
110. Kuntzman, R., Jacobson, M., Levin, W. and Conney, A. H.; *Biochem. Pharmac.*; **17**, (1968) 565.
111. Bledsoe, T., Island, D. P., Ney, R. L. and Liddle, G. W.; *J. clin. Endocr.*; **24**, (1964) 1303.
112. Kupfer, D. and Peets, L.; *Biochem. Pharmac.*; **15**, (1966) 573.
113. Conney, A. H. and Klutch, A.; *J. biol. Chem.*; **238**, (1963) 1611.
114. Kuntzman, R., Levin, W., Jacobson, M. and Conney, A.; *Life Sci.*; **7**, 215.
115. Welch, R. M., Levin, W. and Conney, A. H.; *J. Pharm. exp. Ther.*; **155**, (1967) 167.
116. Kuntzman, R., Levin, W., Jacobson, M. and Conney, A. H.; *Life Sci.*; **7**, (1968) 215.
117. Heinricks, W. L. and Colas, A.; *Biochemistry, N.Y.*; **7**, (1968) 2273.
118. von Bahr, C., Lisboa, B. P. and Orrenius, S.; *Naunyn-Schmiedebergs Arch. exp. Path. Pharmak.*; **264**, (1969) 420.
119. Levin, W., Welch, R. M. and Conney, A. H.; *J. Pharmac. exp. Ther.*; **159**, (1968) 362.
120. Watanabe, H.; *Steroids*; **13**, (1969) 189.
121. Furner, R. L. and Stitzel, R. E.; *Biochem. Pharmac.*; **17**, (1968) 121.
122. Driever, C. W. and Bousquet, W. F.; *Life Sci.*; **4**, (1965) 1449.

123. Castro, J. A., Greene, F. E., Gigon, P., Sasame, H. and Gillette, J. R.; *Biochem. Pharmac.*; **19**, (1970) 2461.
124. Radzialowski, F. M. and Bousquet, W. F.; *J. Pharmac. exp. Ther.*; **163**, (1968) 229.
125. Sarkar, N. S.; *FEBS Letters*; **4**, (1969) 37.
126. Sluyser, M.; *Biochim. biophys. Acta.*; **182**, (1969) 235.
127. James, D. W., Rabin, B. R. and Williams, D. J.; *Nature, Lond.*; **224**, (1969) 371.
128. Gessner, T., Acara, M., Baker, J. A. and Edelman, L. L.; *J. pharm. Sci.*; **56**, (1967) 405.
129. Novick, W. J. Jr., Stohler, C. M. and Swagzdis, J.; *J. Pharm. exp. Ther.*; **151**, (1966) 139.
130. Gerald, M. C. and Feller, D. R.; *Biochem. Pharmac.*; **19**, (1970) 2529.
131. Solymoss, B., Varga, S. and Classen, H. G.; *Eur. J. Pharmac.*; **10**, (1970) 127.
132. Solymoss, B., Krajny, M., Varga, S. and Werringloer, J.; *J. Pharmac. exp. Ther.*; **174**, (1970) 473.
133. Tephly, T. R. and Mannering, G. J.; *Molec. Pharmac.*; **4**, (1968) 10.
134. Wada, F., Shimakawa, H., Takasugi, M., Kotake, T. and Sakamoto, Y.; *J. Biochem., Tokyo*; **64**, (1968) 109.
135. Leibman, K. C.; *Molec. Pharmac.*; **5**, (1969) 1.
136. Hayakawa, T., Kanai, N., Yamada, R., Kuroda, R., Higashi, H., Mogami, H. and Jinnai, D.; *Biochem. Pharmac.*; **18**, (1969) 129.
137. Tochino, Y., Iwata, T. and Mineshita, T.; *Folia pharmac. Jap.*; **62**, (1966) 152.
138. Crawford, J. S. and Rudofsky, S.; *Brit. J. Anaesth.*; **38**, (1966) 446.
139. Short, R. V.; In: *'Hormones in Blood'*; Eds C. H. Gray and A. L. Bacherach. Academic Press, N.Y. (1961).
140. Hashimoto, I., Henricks, D. M., Anderson, L. L. and Melampy, R. M.; *Endocrinology*; **82**, (1968) 333.
141. Cessi, C.; *Boll. Soc. ital. Biol. sper.*; **28**, (1952) 1857.
142. Lathe, G. H. and Walker, M.; *Biochem. J.*; **68**, (1958) 6P.
143. Hsia, D. Y. Y., Dowben, R. M., Shaw, R and Grossman, A.; *Nature, Lond.*; **187**, (1960) 693.
144. Lauritzen, Ch. and Lehmann, W. D.; *J. Endocrin.*; **39**, (1967) 183.
145. Arias, I. M. and Gartner, L.; *Nature, Lond.*; **203**, (1964) 1292.
146. Creaven, P. J. and Parke, D. V.; *Fed. Eur. Biochem. Soc. Second Meeting Absts.*; **128**, (1965) 88.
147. Pulkkinen, M.; *Acta. physiol. scand.*; **66**, (1966) 120.
148. Neale, M. G. and Parke, D. V.; *Biochem. J.*; **113**, (1969) 12P.
149. Guarino, A. M., Gram, T. E., Schroeder, D. H., Call, J. and Gillette, J. R.; *J. Pharmac. exp. Ther.*; **168**, (1969) 224.
150. Juchau, M. R. and Fouts, J. R.; *Biochem. Pharmac.*; **15**, (1966) 89.
151. Blackham, A. and Spencer, P. S. J.; *Br. J. Pharmac.*; **37**, (1969) 129.
152. Rümke, Chr. L. and Noordhock, J.; *Eur J. Pharmac.*; **6**, (1969) 163.
153. Jori, A., Bianchetti, A. and Prestini, P. E.; *Eur. J. Pharmac.*; **7**, (1969) 196.
154. Neale, M. G.; *The Influence of pregnancy and oral contraceptive steroids on drug metabolism*; Thesis, University of Surrey, (1970).

CORTICOSTEROID BINDING PROTEINS OF LIVER CYTOSOL AND INTERACTIONS WITH CARCINOGENS*

Gerald Litwack, K. S. Morey† and B. Ketterer‡

Fels Research Institute and Department of Biochemistry, Temple University School of Medicine, Philadelphia, Pennsylvania 19140, U.S.A.

The subcellular fates of corticosteroids in liver were studied in a search for a specific biochemical function of the hormone that might be related to its action in stimulating protein synthesis; in particular, the stimulation of activity of enzymes with short half-lives, such as tyrosine aminotransferase (E.C. 2.6.1.5). Separation of subcellular fractions by differential centrifugation [1] and autoradiography [2] revealed that 45 min after intraperitoneal administration, a time when the hormone radioactivity was maximal in liver (Fig. 1) the distribution of cortisol radioactivity was, in the order of concentration: cytosol $\gg$ microsomal $>$ nuclear $>$ mitochondrial fractions. The peak of accumulation of radioactivity in all of these compartments occurred before there was a measurable increase in tyrosine aminotransferase activity in the cytosol as shown in Fig. 2. Radioactivity from cortisol was concentrated to a maximum by 45 min and declined thereafter, virtually disappearing by 240 min. Significantly, there was a decline in radioactivity in all of the compartments studied, including the nuclear fraction.

We have assumed that macromolecules responsible for concentration or binding within the cell do not derive from the cell surface

* Supported by Research Grants AM-08350 and AM-13531 from the National Institute of Arthritis and Metabolic Diseases, CA-10439 from the National Cancer Institute, and GB-8784 from the National Science Foundation.

† Present address: California State Polytechnic College, San Luis Obispo, California.

‡ Permanent address: Courtauld Institute of Biochemistry, Middlesex Hospital Medical School, London, W1.

or the cell membrane. Although there are no direct experiments to validate this assumption, Baxter and Tomkins [3] reported that p-chloromercuriphenyl sulphonic acid completely inhibits specific binding capacity for dexamethasone in cell-free extracts from HTC cells but does not readily enter most cells. Furthermore, this

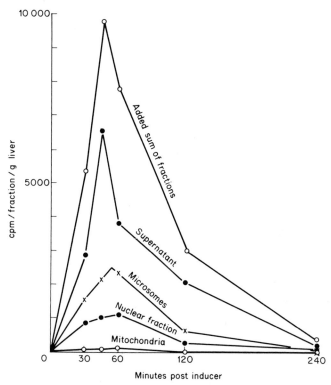

Fig. 1. Subcellular distribution of 4-^{14}C-cortisol administered with 60 mg unlabelled cortisol per kg as a function of time. Two μCi of the isotope were given. Each point plotted is the value of 1 to 4 observations. (From ref. 1 by permission of publisher.)

inhibitor does not affect the specific binding reaction when whole cells are incubated with ^{3}H-dexamethasone, so that it is unlikely that the binding reaction occurs on the cell surface. Previous experiments in this laboratory differentiated binding proteins of liver cytosol from corticosteroid binding proteins in serum [4]. In addition, Arias [5] communicates that in rat plasma, there is no antigen for the antibody to one of the binding proteins reported in this paper, a finding consistent with the localization of the protein primarily within the cell and not at its surface. Therefore, we concentrated our attention upon the compartment which contained most of the steroid, the cytosol fraction.

Changes induced in the endoplasmic reticulum by corticosteroids, although involving a much smaller amount of the hormone, are significant. Electron microscopy showed that very large changes occurred in the endoplasmic reticulum starting as early as 15 min after the administration of cortisol to the adrenalectomized male rat,

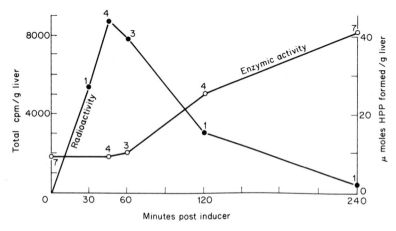

Fig. 2. The relationship between radioactivity and tyrosine aminotransferase activity in whole liver homogenate as a function of time after administration of inducer. 4-^{14}C-cortisol was administered together with unlabelled steroid inducer. (From ref. 1 by permission of publisher.)

signifying, perhaps, that sites at the translational level were responding to the hormone prior to effects on processes mediated by the nucleus [6]. In this connection, Rabin and his colleagues [7, 8] have demonstrated steroid hormone-dependent binding of polysomes to fractions of smooth endoplasmic reticulum. Investigations on the time course of incorporation *in vivo* of cortisol radioactivity into subfractions of the endoplasmic reticulum show that the smooth endoplasmic reticulum incorporates the major fraction of radio-activity, whereas the rough endoplasmic reticulum has little incorporating activity and the ribosomes do not bind cortisol radioactivity at all [9]. The hormone may bind to metabolizing enzymes in the smooth endoplasmic reticulum but there may be other sites for binding which could be occluded by the presence of ribosomes in the rough endoplasmic reticulum.

Aggregation of free liver ribosomes is a response to cortisol treatment of adrenalectomized animals but this change is not detected earlier than 3 hours after intraperitoneal administration of the hormone. Undoubtedly, this effect cannot explain the early effects of the hormone upon the cell [10].

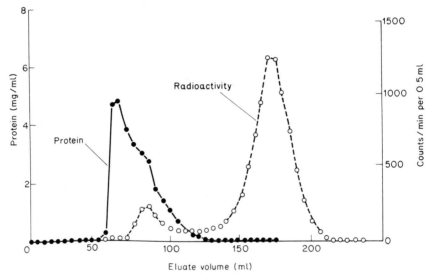

Fig. 3. Column chromatogram on Bio-Gel P-100 of 100,000 x g supernatant prepared from adrenalectomized rat liver 45 min after injection of inducing dose of cortisol with 4-^{14}C-cortisol. (From ref. 11 by permission of publisher.)

Although the interactions of corticosteroids with the endoplasmic reticulum are rapid and specific, reactions occurring in the cytosol may be among the earliest molecular fates of the hormone within the cell.

Macromolecular binding of cortisol radioactivity in liver cytosol

Separation of bound and unbound steroid radioactivity of the cytosol fraction is accomplished by gel filtration (Fig. 3). The bound radioactivity coinciding with the protein peak accounts for 6 to 13% of the total radioactivity. When this procedure was carried out at various times, and with either enzyme-inducing or physiological

Table 1
Time Dependence of (4-^{14}C) Hydrocortisone Binding to Cytoplasmic Proteins

Time after intraperitoneal injection (min)	Dose	Fraction of total intracellular labelled hormone bound (%)†	mμg hydrocortisone/mg protein
30	Inducing dose* + 8.4 μC	3.8	176
45	Inducing dose + 10 μC	7.0	225
45	Non-inducing dose + 8 μC	6.8	2
90	Inducing dose + 8 μC	4.2	112
180	Inducing dose + 8.62 μC	0.8	6

* Inducing dose = isotope *plus* 60 mg unlabelled hydrocortisone per kg; non-inducing dose = isotope only.

† $\dfrac{\text{Disintegrations/min bound to protein}}{\text{Total disintegrations/min in cell sap}} \times 100$.

(From ref. 11 by permission of publisher.)

Table 2
Enzymatic Treatment of Bound Radioactivity Eluted from Bio-Gel P-100 Columns

Enzymatic treatment*	% Binding by ultrafiltration	% Change
Experiment I		
Control (no enzyme)	66	
RNase†	61	(−8)
DNase‡	66	(0)
Trypsin§	46	(−30)
Experiment II		
Control	43	
+200 μg of trypsin	17	(−60)
+400 μg of trypsin	0	(−100)

* 60 mg of complex + 100 μg of enzyme; 4° for 18 hr with stirring.

† 20 μg of RNA, made acid-soluble per μg of enzyme per min; 38°.

‡ 21 μg of DNA, made acid-soluble per μg of enzyme per min; 38°.

§ 67 mμg of bovine serum albumin, made acid-soluble per μg of enzyme per min; 38°.

(From ref. 12 by permission of publisher. Copyright (1969) by the American Chemical Society.)

doses of the hormone, a large number of binding sites were shown to exist in the liver cytosol. There was a clear time dependence with a maximum of binding occurring in approximately 45 min, coinciding with the peak accumulation of hormone radioactivity. Independent of dosage, the same percentage of radioactivity appeared to be in the bound fraction (Table 1). Treatment of the bound fraction with

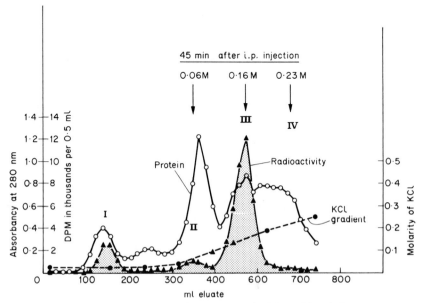

Fig. 4. Fractionation of protein bound radioactivity on DEAE-Sephadex A-50. A 2.8 × 70 cm column was used. A linear KCl gradient from 0 to 0.5 m was used for the elution. 2.9×10^7 DPM was applied 61% of which was recovered in the bound form. (From ref. 12 by permission of publisher. Copyright (1969) by the American Chemical Society.)

various enzymes for release of bound radioactivity suggested that the macromolecules were probably proteinaceous (Table 2).

The purification and properties of the major binding proteins of liver cytosol

When the bound fraction from liver cytosol, prepared 45 min after injection of isotopically labelled steroid, was chromatographed on a DEAE Sephadex A-50 column, three peaks of radioactivity (I, II, III) eluted as shown in Fig. 4. A fourth peak (IV, not shown here) eluted at 0.23 M KCl when a shallower gradient was used. This pattern suggested that the macromolecules represented by I and III contained most of the radioactivity at this time. I and III were isolated first and their properties examined. The protocol for the isolation of these proteins is shown in Fig. 5. This procedure allows for preparation of the two binding proteins in homogeneous condition. Binder I was shown to be homogeneous by analytical ultracentrifugation, disc-gel electrophoresis, isoelectric focusing, free

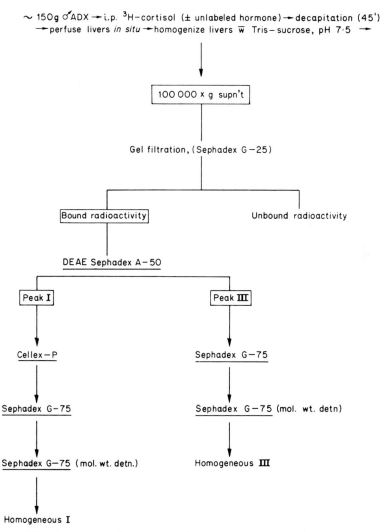

Fig. 5. Diagram for the procedures in purification of Binders I and III.

Table 3
Amino Acid Analyses of Binders I and III

Amino acid	Binder I		Binder III	
	Av. no. of residues*	Mol. wt × no. of residues	Av. no. of residues†	Mol. wt × no. residues
Aspartic acid	28	3724	4	532
Threonine	12	1428	4	476
Serine	12	1260	2	210
Proline	16	1840	3	345
Glutamic acid	36	5292	6	882
Glycine	20	1500	6	450
Alanine	24	2136	5	445
Valine	20	2340	6	702
Methionine	12	1788	1	149
Isoleucine	20	2620	5	655
Leucine	44	5764	8	1048
Tyrosine	12	2172	1	181
Phenylalanine	16	2640	2	330
Lysine	28	4088	7	1022
Histidine	4	620	2	310
Arginine	20	3480	2	348
Tryptophan	2	408		
	Total = 326	Total = 43100	Total = 64	Total = 8085
Corrected for peptide bonds (water of hydrolysis)		− 5850		− 1134
Corrected molecular weight		37250		6951

(From ref. 12 by permission of publisher. Copyright (1969) by the American Chemical Society.)

boundary electrophoresis and chromatographic criteria [10, 12, 13]. In the case of Binder III homogeneity was ascertained by chromatographic analysis and by isoelectric focusing [12]. The amino acid analyses of Binders I and III are presented in Table 3. Some characteristics of each of these proteins are listed in Table 4. Binder I and Binder III do not appear to be 'receptor' proteins on the basis of steroid specificity and kinetics of binding of steroid radioactivity. However, the case for Binder III is complex, since some

Table 4
Some Physical-Chemical Properties of Binders I and III

Property	I	III
$S_{20,w}$ (× 10^{-13} sec^{-1})	3.47	
$S^0_{20,w}$ (× 10^{-13} sec^{-1})	3.7	1.4
$D_{20,w}$	10.1 × 10^{-7} cm^2 sec^{-1}	24 × 10^{-7} cm^2 sec^{-1}
$D^0_{20,w}$	11.8 × 10^{-7} cm^2 sec^{-1}	
Partial specific volume ($\bar{v}$)	0.75	
Isoelectric point	8.9	5.4
$A_{280nm} : A_{260nm}$	1.54	0.68
Molecular weight		
Sedimentation–diffusion		
$S_{20,w}; D_{20,w}$	37,000	
$S^0_{20,w}; D_{20,w}$		4900
$S^0_{20,w}; D^0_{20,w}$	31,000	
Gel filtration	50,000 ± 6000	4000 – 5000
Gel filtration in 8 M urea	50,000	
Amino acid analysis	37,000	7000

evidence suggests a relationship between it and enzyme-inducing capacity of liver during development (see below).

Identity of Binder I with the dimethylaminoazobenzene binding protein and the bilirubin binding protein of liver cytosol

We have shown the corticosteroid Binder I to be identical with the dimethylaminoazo dye binding protein [14] isolated by Ketterer *et al.* [15]. ^{14}C-Dimethylaminoazobenzene was injected in oil 16 hours prior to an injection of ^{3}H-cortisol. Binder I was purified to homogeneity as described in Fig. 5, and the preparation, homogeneous by several criteria, showed perfect coincidence between the two isotopes of chromatography on Sephadex G-75. In addition,

Binder I had the same pI, $S_{20,w}$ and molecular weight values [14]. Comparison of the amino acid analyses of I [12] and of the dimethylaminoazobenzene binder [14] indicated identity [14]. Further proof of identity comes from mixing Binder I from our

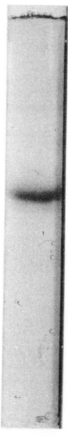

Fig. 6. SDS-urea disc gel electrophoresis of a mixture of the dimethylaminoazobenzene binding protein of Ketterer with the Binder I of Litwack.

laboratory and the azo dye binding protein from Ketterer's laboratory and subjecting the mixture to SDS-urea disc electrophoresis [16]. Only one protein band appears as shown in Fig. 6 equivalent to a molecular weight in the range of 23,000. This indicates that Binder I consists of 2 subunits of the same molecular weight. The same conclusion is reached after testing the antibody to the azo dye binding protein by immunodiffusion (Fig. 7). In this case a single line of identity is observed with both proteins. Preliminary experiments attempting to dilute out cortisol radioactivity by increasing 5-fold the dose of azo dye *in vivo* did not change the specific radioactivity from cortisol in combination with Binder I. This suggests, though does not prove, that there is more than one

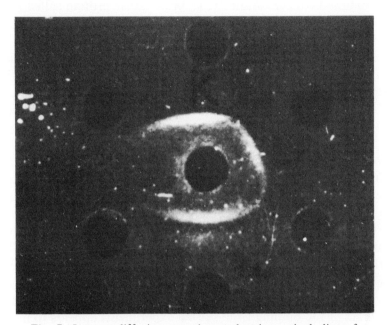

Fig. 7. Immunodiffusion experiment showing a single line of identity with Ketterer's dimethylaminoazobenzene binding protein and Litwack's Binder I against the antibody to the dimethylaminoazobenzene binding protein prepared from rabbit anti-sera.

binding site on the protein and the steroid binds to one site while the azo dye binds to a different one.

Binder I appears to be similar, if not identical to one of the azo dye binding h proteins of liver cytosol, probably the h_3 fraction described by Sorof and co-workers [17]. Heidelberger and collaborators [18] have partially purified a similar protein from mouse skin to which the carcinogenic hydrocarbons, 1,2,5,6-dibenzanthracene and 3-methylcholanthrene, were bound specifically, but the noncarcinogenic 1,2,3,4-dibenzanthracene was not bound. These investigators also demonstrated that this binder consists of 2 subunits of approximately 20,000 in molecular weight. Ketterer also has found a subunit weight in this range [19].

Arias and his collaborators have purified two proteins from liver cytosol which bind bilirubin and other anions [5, 20-22]. The larger molecular weight protein called the 'Y protein' by Arias has been shown to be identical with both the azo dye binder [15], and Binder I by immunodiffusion studies [5]. Arias' other protein called the 'Z protein' appears to be similar to Binder III [5]. The antibody to the Y protein does not react with the Z protein or with plasma.

Arias reports [5] that in a survey across the phylogenetic scale of bilirubin binding capacity, the Y protein, identical to Binder I, is present in all air breathing species examined, but not in aquatic gill breathers. The binding protein also appears to be lacking in azo dye-produced rat liver tumours [23].

Capacity of Binder I to bind 3-methylcholanthrene

Binder I has been shown to be a quantitatively important binding protein for 3-methylcholanthrene *in vivo* and *in vitro* [24]. This has been established by double labelling experiments and purification of I to homogeneity in an approach similar to that used to prove identity with the dimethylaminoazo dye binding protein [14]. Confirmation of the identity of I as a binder of 3-methylcholanthrene involved properties of the protein upon isoelectrofocusing, analytical ultracentrifugation and molecular sieve chromatography [24]. Part of the binding from *in vivo* experiments appears to involve covalent bonds since this portion of radioactive 3-methylcholanthrene or its metabolite is released by digestion with proteolytic enzymes but not by solvent extraction [24]. Thus Binder I may be one of the principal factors in determining the location of a large part of injected radioactive 3-methylcholanthrene in the cytosol fraction [25].

The relatively large concentration of this protein in liver cytosol and its ability to bind several small molecules: steroids, carcinogens and various anions, such as bilirubin suggests that it may be involved in the metabolism of these compounds and possibly in their removal from the liver cell. The question of whether this protein is a part of an enzyme is of interest since, in the case of corticosteroids, it binds unmetabolized corticosteroids as well as their anionic metabolites [26].

Both the azo dye and 3-methylcholanthrene (or their metabolites) also bind significantly to Binder II but not to III or IV. This observation is especially important because we believe Binder II has corticosteroid 'receptor' activity, as discussed below.

The carcinogen, acetylaminofluorene, or its metabolites, bind to proteins of liver cytosol *in vivo* and *in vitro* [27]. None of the proteins complexed with ^{14}C-acetylaminofluorene (or its metabolites), however, corresponds to any of the proteins in the corticosteroid binding series described here [28].

Some properties of Binder III

Binder III has a low molecular weight in the range of 5000 to 7000 as shown in Table 4 and, surprisingly, has a high ratio of 260 nm to 280 nm absorbance, suggesting the presence of a nucleotide(s). The purified Binder III, when isolated 45 min after injection of cortisol, appears to have bound to it a corticosteroid anionic metabolite in combination with some material which has the properties of a nucleotide [12]. The purified protein gives a positive orcinol reaction, a negative diphenylamine reaction and incorporates radioactivity from ^{14}C-labelled adenosine when it is injected together with the corticosteroid *in vivo* [29]. A molecular weight of Binder III, stripped of steroid and 260 nm absorbing material, is less than the bound form by approximately 1000 in molecular weight as determined in the analytical ultracentrifuge [23]. Further studies are in progress to determine the nature of this 260 nm absorbing component. The steroid may combine with the nucleotide-like material prior to binding to the protein since various treatments that dissociate the steroid from III dissociate the 260 nm absorbing component. Morris *et al.* [30] have confirmed the possible presence of a complex of steroid, polynucleotide and polypeptide in a partially purified fraction from liver cytosol having a molecular weight in the range of 5000. Our preliminary experiments suggest the presence of one to not more than a few nucleotide equivalents rather than a polynucleotide. Most of the estimated molecular weight of III can be accounted for by amino acid residues [12].

It is of interest that Arias and his collaborators have observed that his Z protein has a molecular weight in the range of Binder III and also binds bilirubin [5]. The function of Binder III is, as yet, unknown; however it may initially be associated loosely with a larger macromolecule since, in the original fractionation of free and bound steroid radioactivity by Bio Gel P-100, Binder III eluted close to the larger macromolecules. It was not included in Sephadex G-75 columns significantly until after it was purified.

Specificity of binding

The qualitative specificity of steroids and related compounds which bind to these proteins is shown in Table 5. These data have been obtained either from double-label studies with ³H-cortisol or ³H-corticosterone and ¹⁴C-labelled steroid under comparison, or by

Table 5

Specificity of Binding *in vivo* **as determined** *in vitro* **through Chromatography Step on DEAE Sephadex A-50**

Injected i.p. (45 min) (Physiol. doses of steroids to rats, ♂, ADX ¹⁴C or ³H)	Relative amount of radioactivity in chromatogram associated with binder			
	I	II	III	IV
Cortisol	+	++	+++	+
Corticosterone	++	+++	+++	+
Dexamethasone	+	++++	+	−
Cortisone	++	Low	+++	−
Deoxycorticosterone	+	Low to absent	+++	−
Oestradiol-17β*	+++	Low	−	
Testosterone	Low	+	++	++++
Progesterone	++	++	+++	+++
3-Methylcholanthrene†	+++	++	−	−
Dimethylaminoazobenzene†	++++	+	+	−
Acetylaminofluorene†	−	−	−	−

* Binding pattern is dose dependent (0.5-65 μg).
† After peak accumulation.

direct observation of the amounts of radioactivity from the radioactive steroid in question coinciding with Binders I, II, III and IV on the DEAE Sephadex chromatograms. The specificity for Binder I is such that it may not be considered a 'receptor' protein since its highest affinity is for oestradiol-17β, 3-methylcholanthrene and dimethylaminoazobenzene. Although I binds glucocorticoids, the order of binding preference is not the order of the biological potency established by other criteria [3, 30]. The steroid specificity for Binder III from DEAE Sephadex chromatograms also does not suggest physiologically related binding; however, it must be borne in mind that this small molecule may be associated with some other macromolecule, at present unknown, and the combination of the two, but not each alone, may have the appropriate specificity. Binder IV, which has not been emphasized thus far, is prominent in the DEAE Sephadex chromatogram labelled with corticosteroid, only when a shallow KCl gradient has been used and in this case it elutes at approximately 0.23 M KCl. Although IV binds corticosteroids, it binds radioactivity from progesterone and testosterone more avidly. Since testosterone is an anti-inducer for tyrosine aminotransferase in the HTC cell system [31], it seems possible that this protein may be involved in some glucocorticoid inhibitory capacity. However, we have not purified or characterized this fraction as yet. Binder II, on the other hand, appears to have an appropriate steroid specificity for what could be defined as a corticosteroid 'receptor' protein.

Fractionation and properties of binder II, a possible corticosteroid 'receptor'

Binder II, obtained from chromatography on DEAE Sephadex A-50 (Fig. 4), was fractionated further by isoelectrofocusing in a pH 3 to 10 gradient. The single peak so obtained ($pH_i \sim 6.7$) is still inhomogeneous. Fractionation procedures involving sucrose gradients tend to stabilize the binding between the protein and the radioactive corticosteroid. When the partially purified binder from isoelectro-focusing is subjected to molecular sieve chromatography on Sephadex G-75, the protein is separated into 3 partially resolved peaks; the middle one contains the radioactivity although much of the steroid dissociates in the process. The position of this protein on Sephadex G-75 corresponds to a molecular weight of about 67,000. Further fractionation has been hampered by the lability of the radioactive steroid-Binder II combination; however, since 3-methyl-cholanthrene binds to the same fraction more avidly, it is possible to follow the fractionation using the radioactive carcinogen as a marker. Further purification and characterization of II are in progress [32].

Time course of association of radioactivity with cytosol binders in vivo

The time course of association of radioactivity from tritiated cortisol with the various binders is shown in Fig. 8. The binding to Binder I increases very slightly at 5 min and does not show a significantly large increase until 45 min which is the peak of accumulation of radioactivity and also a point at which most of the radioactivity is in the form of anionic metabolites. This aligns with the previous statement that Binder I has a greater affinity for corticosteroid metabolites than it does for unchanged corticosteroids, although at 5-10 min the radioactivity associated with

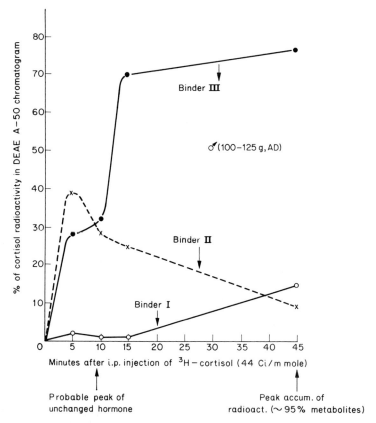

Fig. 8. Time course of radioactivity associated with Binders I, II and III in the DEAE-Sephadex A-50 chromatogram.

this binder is mainly unmetabolized corticosteroid. In fact, all 3 binders which have been studied in this respect, both *in vivo* and *in vitro,* have the capacity of binding unmetabolized steroids. The progress curve with Binder II shows a rapid approach to a steady state by 5 min after steroid injection. The radioactivity associated with this binder falls off rapidly until 45 min when the amount of binding is fairly low. This is in keeping with the fact that the radioactivity, associated with this binder throughout the experimental period, is largely in the form of unmetabolized steroid with a small amount of reduced hormone present. An anionic metabolite does not appear to be associated with this binder. If it is assumed that the binder is saturated at the steady state a dissociation constant can be calculated which would be uncorrected for the amount of steroid present in the cytosol bound to other macromolecules. This yields an apparent dissociation constant of about 2×10^{-8} M with respect to cortisol. This value should be considered cautiously since experiments involving relatively large amounts of unlabelled steroid have not been done in this format. However, this estimate fits very well within the framework of a 'receptor' since it is below the accepted physiological concentration of glucocorticoids in the cell.

The time course for Binder III shows a biphasic curve in which there is a shoulder at 5 min which may be close to the peak of accumulation of unmetabolized steroid and then a progressive increase of binding approaching saturation by 45 min although saturation does not appear to have been reached in this period. These data fit with the observations from *in vitro* experiments which show that this binder is capable of binding unmetabolized steroid, as well as with data from the purified binder from which an anionic metabolite of cortisol can be extracted [12]. Although the qualitative steroid specificity and the kinetics of binding suggest that III is not a 'receptor', judgment must be reserved on this point until after the development of enzyme induction capacity in the liver is compared with the development of ability of each binder to bind glucocorticoids.

Patterns of radioactivity associated with cytosol binders during development

In Fig. 9 are shown the results of *in vivo* experiments in which radioactive cortisol was injected into rats at various stages of development from 21 days after conception to 40 days after birth [33]. The radioactivity associated with Binder I is constant throughout this period, whereas there are complementary changes between Binders II and III. It might appear that Binder III and Binder II exist in a precursor-product relationship; however, this conclusion remains to be established. Binding of radioactivity to Binder II is fairly high by the time of birth, increases slightly at 15 days and then decreases sharply to 40 days after birth. On the other hand, binding of radioactivity to Binder III increases slightly after birth and then decreases again at 15 days and increases sharply up to 40 days. As shown in Fig. 10 [33] only the pattern of Binder III in any way aligns with the capacity of the liver to induce the enzyme, tyrosine aminotransferase. Therefore, it seems possible that Binder III could play a role in the development of the capacity for

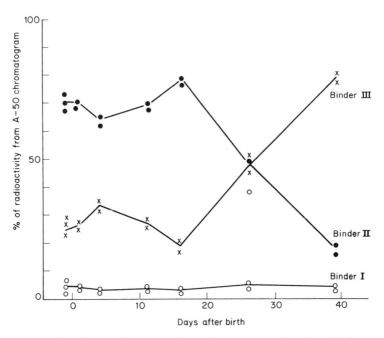

Fig. 9. Effect of age on the relative amounts of cortisol radioactivity associated with binding proteins from rat liver cytosol. (From ref. 33 by permission of publisher.)

enzymatic induction in the liver although this conclusion is certainly circumstantial at the present time. It should be emphasized that Binder III of itself does not show steroid binding specificity which would be expected of a 'receptor' macromolecule. However, our fractionation data suggest that Binder III may be bound to another macromolecule prior to fractionation by DEAE Sephadex A-50 chromatography. The macromolecule with which it may be associated at the early stages of fractionation has not been identified. The combination of the hypothetical macromolecule associated with Binder III could produce the appropriate steroid binding specificity for a 'receptor'. Binder II would be the ideal candidate in this context; however, there is no evidence to support this idea at the present time.

Binder II appears to be the probable corticosteroid 'receptor'. In such a role, it is significant that carcinogens bind to this

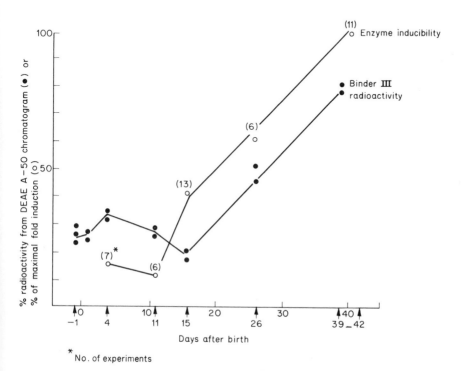

*No. of experiments

Fig. 10. The relationship between the radioactivity from cortisol associated with Binder III as a function of development and the development of the capacity of liver for tyrosine aminotransferase induction.

macromolecule, probably more strongly than do corticosteroids. The accepted hypothesis of 'receptor' function (demonstrated for oestrogens in the uterus [34], and corticosteroids in the thymus [35] states that it should carry the corticosteroid into the nucleus to perform some function involving gene expression. This possibility will be tested when II has been isolated. Meanwhile, if II functions in this manner, it may prove to be the essential vehicle in the early stages of chemical carcinogenesis in liver.

Acknowledgements

Research reported in this paper was supported by research grants AM-13531 and AM-08350 from the National Institute of Arthritis and Metabolic Diseases, CA-10439 from the National Cancer Institute and GB-8784 from the National Science Foundation.

Discussion

Tata (Mill Hill)
Could you qualify the criteria you use for distinguishing 'binders' from 'receptors'?

Litwack (Philadelphia)
I am using the term 'receptor' in the following sense: a macromolecule, in this case a protein, which binds corticosteroids with a specificity corresponding to their biological effectiveness; that binds them early (that is, long before the results of their actions are measurable); that is 'saturated' with steroid or reaches a homeostatic level of binding at a concentration within the cell, in this case within the cytoplasm, which is less than the accepted cellular concentration; and that binds primarily the unmetabolized hormone. The other proteins I have referred to also can bind the unmetabolized hormone at early times but they do not fulfil the rest of the criteria I have outlined. This is not to say that the functions of the other proteins are unimportant; they may be involved in transport, metabolism or in some other facet of hormonal function.

Tomkins (San Francisco)
Very often the question of the biological significance of steroid receptors is raised particularly with respect to their potential role in the action of the hormones themselves. Several types of evidence suggest that they are, in fact, involved. In our studies there is a very close correlation between the specificity of steroid action both quantitatively and qualitatively with the ability of various inducers and anti-inducers to associate with the glucocorticoid receptors in cultured hepatoma cells (HTC cells) (Tomkins, Martin, Stellwagen, Baxter, Mamont and Levinson; *Cold Spring Harbor Symp. quant. Biol.*; **35** (1970), 635).

Perhaps somewhat more convincing than these correlative studies are those derived from our work on cultured lymphoma cells. Physiological concentrations of the glucocorticoids are lethal to cloned lines of mouse lymphoma cells that we have been studying in conjunction with people from the Salk Institute. From sensitive lines, a number of steroid resistant clones can be isolated and preliminary studies (Baxter, Harris, Tomkins and Cohn; *Science;* **171**, (1971) 189) have shown that when cells become resistant to the steroids there is a decrease in their concentration of steroid receptor. More recent studies (Rosenau, Baxter, Rousseau and Tomkins, to be published) using more refined techniques, (Baxter and Tomkins; *Proc. Nat. Acad. Sci.;* (1971) in press) have shown that there is a drastic decrease in the concentration of steroid receptors in steroid-resistant variants derived from sensitive lines. These arguments strongly suggest that the receptors are truly involved in the biological action of the steroid hormones.

Tata (Mill Hill)

I noticed that Binders I and III had opposite affinities for oestradiol and testosterone and would like to ask if you noticed any sex specificity in this respect?

Litwack (Philadelphia)

As I mentioned in my talk, using high specifically-labelled sex hormones, we are now able to show that there is binding to all four Binders and this occurs with both sex hormones (oestradiol-17β-6,7-^{3}H and testosterone-1,2-^{3}H), so that I and III really do not have opposite affinities in this regard. The data in Table 5 were obtained with injection of 65 mg of the oestradiol so that there was apparent dilution of III by non-radioactive hormone. Labelling is seen when a small mass of high specific radioactivity (40 Ci per mmol) oestradiol is injected. Dr S. Singer in my laboratory has found slight differences between the sexes in the amounts of hormone taken up by the liver. That is, more oestradiol is taken up by adrenalectomized male liver than by adrenalectomized female liver, and more testosterone appears to be taken up by adrenalectomized female liver than by adrenalectomized male liver. There seems to be more oestradiol bound in adrenalectomized female liver cytosol *in vivo* than in adrenalectomized male liver cytosol; there seems to be more testosterone bound in adrenalectomized male liver cytosol *in vivo* than in adrenalectomized female liver cytosol. There are also sex-related differences in binding of sex hormones to various Binders in the DEAE-Sephadex A-50 chromatogram and these will be reported at a later time. These data apply to adrenalectomized animals and we have no data as yet on untreated or castrated animals. Unfortunately, we do not observe a striking sex dependency similar to that reported by Professor Rabin and his colleagues for polysome binding to smooth endoplasmic reticulum.

King (London)

If Binder II is the true receptor, how do you explain its equal binding of cortisol and progesterone in view of their different biological effects?

Litwack (Philadelphia)

That is a good question. Of course, we do not yet know the binding constants which we hope to have after the protein is isolated. This information would give us a better idea of the true specificity of steroid binding. It may be worth mentioning that J. D. Baxter and G. M. Tomkins [3] showed that 11-β-hydroxyprogesterone and 17-α-hydroxyprogesterone, both of which are suboptimal inducers of tyrosine aminotransferase in the HTC system completely interfered with 'specific' binding of ^{3}H-dexamethasone. Perhaps more to the point, H. H. Samuels and G. M. Tomkins [31] reported that progesterone could interfere substantially with the cortisol induction of tyrosine aminotransferase in the HTC system. In addition, B. P. Schaumburg and E. Bojeson [36] indicated that progesterone possessed about the same activity as cortisol in inhibiting the uptake of corticosterone by thymus cells, a method they used to determine corticosteroid receptor activity of these cells. Therefore, while I cannot answer your question satisfactorily, the observation is not without precedent where specific corticosteroid functions are involved.

King (London)

Where does corticosteroid-binding globulin run in your systems? Sekeris [37] has reported the presence of large amounts of it in liver cytosol.

Litwack (Philadelphia)

Some time ago, using double-label experiments, we reported that the serum cortisol binding proteins did not co-chromatograph with cortisol binding proteins of liver cytosol [4]. Other experiments leading to the conclusion that serum binding proteins (e.g. trans-cortin) were distinct from the Binders reported in this paper were mentioned also. Sekeris' group has isolated a glycoprotein from liver cytosol with a pH of 4.2 [38] which may be the one to which you refer. We have determined the pH values of Binders I, II and III by isoelectrofocusing to be 8.9, about 6.7 and 5.4 respectively. The pH of Binder IV is undetermined, and its elution position in chromato-grams obtained with DEAE-Sephadex A-50 might indicate that its pH value is smaller than that of Binder III. Thus Sekeris' protein is possibly similar, on the basis of pH, to Binder IV which we believe, for reasons of specificity, is probably not a corticosteroid receptor. However, since we have not yet isolated and characterized Binder IV, we cannot comment further on its resemblance to the fraction reported from Sekeris' laboratory. Beyond the points made above I might refer to the work of R. S. Gardner and G. M. Tomkins [39] who, on the basis of their experiments with the HTC cell system, were unable to detect the presence of transcortin. Finally, the most telling piece of evidence to distinguish transcortin from the proteins reported in this paper is the fact that transcortin seems to bind cortisol more avidly than the intracellular proteins from liver cytosol.

Lasnitzki (Cambridge)

Dr Litwack, we found in a different system, that testosterone and hydrocortisone inhibited the action of 3-methylcholanthrene. Do you think that this could have been due to a competition between the hormones and the carcinogen for Binder II?

Litwack (Philadelphia)

That is a most interesting observation. It is clear from the specificity data I presented, that Binder II binds both of these hormones and 3-methylcholanthrene to an even greater extent. Unfortunately, we have not yet done competition studies with this carcinogen so that I cannot answer your question. We have, for what it is worth, done a preliminary competition study with Binder I *in vivo*, trying to swamp out specific cortisol radioactivity with high doses of the carcinogen, dimethylaminoazobenzene; the carcinogen was bound to Binder I without having much effect on diluting out the binding of radioactive cortisol, from which we can entertain tentatively the idea of two separate binding sites on I. But, this does not help us very much with your question regarding Binder II. If it proves to be the liver corticosteroid 'receptor', I would expect to find competition between glucocorticoids and carcinogens, especially if the receptor functions in some mechanism of transport to the nucleus.

Cohen (Open University)

Why is there so much Binder I, and dexamethasone-binder in HTC cells (Tomkins)? This argues against a nuclear effect.

Litwack (Philadelphia)

There is a substantial amount of Binder I in liver cells; we have estimated its concentration to be in the range of 0.05% of the cytosol proteins from our data on purification and correction, probably with a large error, for losses during isolation. Arias, from data on dye-binding estimates his Y protein, demonstrated to be identical to Binder I, to be as much as 3% of the total cytoplasmic protein in liver [22] which seems high. Assuming your comment on HTC cells refers to the P2 fraction [39] my guess is that one of the functions of Binder I and possibly P2 is, at least in part, in concentrating the hormone in the cell. There may be additional functions of this protein but we have no hard facts about what they might be. With regard to your comment concerning a nuclear effect, we have no evidence concerning the site of action of the postulated 'receptor' protein and I am not yet convinced that in the liver it is essential to refer to genetic information in order to produce an hormonal effect. However, that remains to be worked out. More recent data on Binder I is about to be published [40].

Slater (Brunel)

You showed a graph in which the changes in Binder II and Binder III during the early weeks of life were recorded. Binder II decreased and Binder III increased at about the same time that rats are normally weaned. Do you think there is some steroid factor in milk that is responsible for this change. Lathe in Leeds has isolated certain milk steroids that affect the level of liver glucuronyl transferase for example?

Litwack (Philadelphia)

That is a very interesting question and one which we have not considered at all. Actually, the major change with which we were concerned was the relationship, if any, of steroid binding with the development of the capacity of liver for enzyme induction. The best parallel is with Binder III during development, although total binding (determined by gel filtration of the cytosol fraction on Sephadex

G-25 columns) roughly aligns with the development of enzyme induction capacity. Steroid binding is very low 24 hours before birth and increases about 8 to 10 fold within 24 hours after birth.

References

1. Litwack, G., Sears, M. L. and Diamondstone, T. I.; *J. Biol. Chem.*; **238**, (1963) 302.
2. Litwack, G. and Baserga, R.; *Endocrinology*; **80**, (1967) 774.
3. Baxter, J. D. and Tomkins, G. M.; *Schering Symposium* (Germany), (1970).
4. Fiala, E. S. and Litwack, G.; *Biochim. biophys. Acta*; **124**, (1966) 260.
5. Arias, I. M.; personal communication.
6. Rancourt, M. W. and Litwack, G.; *Expt. Cell Res.*; **51**, (1968) 413.
7. Williams, D. J. and Rabin, B. R.; *FEBS Letters*; **4**, (1969) 103.
8. James, D. W., Rabin, B. R. and Williams, D. J.; *Nature, Lond.*; **224**, (1969) 371.
9. Mayewski, R. J. and Litwack, G.; *Biochem. biophys. Res. Commun.*; **37**, (1969) 729.
10. Litwack, G. and Singer, S; In 'Biochemical Actions of Hormones'; Ed. G. Litwack. Vol. **2**, Academic Press, (1971) in press.
11. Litwack, G., Fiala, E. S. and Filosa, R. J.; *Biochim. biophys. Acta*; **111**, (1965) 569.
12. Morey, K. S. and Litwack, G.; *Biochemistry*; **8**, (1969) 4813.
13. Litwack, G; In: 'Topics in Medicinal Chemistry'; Eds J. L. Rabinowitz and R. M. Myerson. Interscience Publishers, John Wiley & Sons, Inc. (New York), **1** (1967) 3.
14. Litwack, G. and Morey, K. S.; *Biochem. biophys. Res. Commun.*; **38**, (1970) 1141.
15. Ketterer, B., Ross-Mansell, P. and Whitehead, J. K.; *Biochem. J.*; **103**, (1967) 316.
16. Shapiro, A. L., Vinuella, E. and Maizel, J. V.; *Biochem. biophys. Res. Commun.*; **28**, (1967) 815.
17. Sorof, S., Young, E. M., McBride, R. A. and Coffey, C. B.; *Cancer Res.*; **30**, (1970) 2029.
18. Tasseron, J. G., Diringer, H., Frohwith, N., Mirvish, S. S. and Heidelberger, C.; *Biochemistry*; **9**, (1970) 1636.
19. Ketterer, B.; personal communication.
20. Reyes, H., Levi, A. J., Gatmaitan, Z. and Arias, I. M.; *Proc. Nat. Acad. Sci.*; **64**, (1969) 168.
21. Levi, A. J., Gatmaitan, Z. and Arias, I. M.; *J. Clin. Invest.*; **48**, (1969) 2156.
22. Fleischner, G. and Arias, I. M.; *Am. J. Med.*; **49**, (1970) 576.
23. Louis, C. J. and Blunck, J. M.; *Cancer Res.*; **30**, (1970) 2043.
24. Singer, S. and Litwack, G.; *Cancer Res.*; **31**, (1971), in press.
25. Bresnick, E., Liebelt, R. A., Stevenson, J. G. and Madix, J. C.; *Cancer Res.*; **27**, (1967) 462.
26. Singer, S., Morey, K. S. and Litwack, G.; *Physiol. Chem. Physics*; **2**, (1970) 117.
27. Barry, E. J., Malejka-Giganti, D. and Gutmann, H. R.; *Chem.-Biol. Interactions*; **1**, (1969/70) 139.
28. Keats, C. J., Singer, S. and Litwack, G.; unpublished experiments.
29. Morey, K. S. and Litwack, G.; unpublished experiments.

30. Morris, D. J., Sarma, M. H. and Barnes, F. W.; *Endocrinology*; **87**, (1970) 486.
31. Samuels, H. H. and Tomkins, G. M.; *J. Mol. Biol.*; **52**, (1970) 57.
32. Filler, R. S. and Litwack, G.; unpublished experiments.
33. Singer, S. and Litwack, G.; *Endocrinology*; **88**, (1971) 126.
34. Jensen, E. W., Suzuki, T., Kawashima, T., Stumpf, W. E., Jungblut, P. W. and DeSombre, E. R.; *Proc. Nat. Acad. Sci. U.S.A.*; **59**, (1968) 632.
35. Wira, C. and Munck, A.; *J. Biol. Chem.*; **245**, (1970) 3436.
36. Schaumburg, B. P. & Bojeson, E.; *Biochim. Biophys. Acta*; **170**, (1968) 172.
37. Sekeris, C. E.; *Advances in the Biosciences*; **7**, (1971) in the press.
38. Beato, M., Schmid, W., Braendle, W., and Sekeris, C. E.; *Steroids*; **16**, (1970) 207.
39. Gardner, R. S. & Tomkins, G. M.; *J. Biol. Chem.;* **244**, (1969) 4761.
40. Litwack, G., Ketterer, B. and Arias, I. M.; *Nature, Lond.*; in press.

STEROIDS AND THE DEVELOPMENT
OF MAMMARY EPITHELIAL CELLS

Yale J. Topper and Takami Oka

National Institute of Arthritis and Metabolic Diseases,
National Institute of Health, Bethesda, Maryland, 20014

Enzyme: DPNH-Cytochrome C reductase (EC 1.6.99.3).
Non-standard abbreviations: AIB = α-Amino-isobuytil acid. RER = Rough endoplasmic reticulum.

Mammary gland tissue from immature mice [1], adult virgin mice [2] and pregnant mice [3] can be stimulated to differentiate *in vitro*. Additions of insulin, glucocorticoid and prolactin to the synthetic culture medium are required for the complex sequence of cellular events which culminates in the synthesis of secretory proteins such as casein [3]. The interplay of these hormones during development of mouse mammary epithelial cells, *in vitro*, is the subject of this discussion, with particular emphasis on the roles of the steroids.

Epithelial cells within the mammary gland of the mature, virgin mouse undergo little proliferation. During pregnancy, extensive proliferation *does* occur, representing one of the major developmental processes taking place during this period. It has been shown that insulin stimulates epithelial proliferation within pregnant mouse mammary explants, and that the extent of this stimulation is independent of glucocorticoid and prolactin [2]. Insulin also stimulates proliferation of epithelial cells within explants derived from mature, virgin mice [2]. This was surprising, since these cells, as stated above, do not divide in the intact, mature virgin animal even in the presence of a functioning pancreas. The apparent discrepancy between these observations prompted a more detailed comparative study of the responses to insulin of pregnant and mature virgin mouse mammary tissue.

131

Materials and Methods

The previously described [3] organ-culture technique employing mammary gland explants was used. Such explants contain predominantly epithelial and fat cells. In order to find out whether or not the observed effects related to epithelial cells, the tissue was treated with collagenase, and the epithelial cells were separated from the lysed fat cells by centrifugation [4]. From this we think that these results probably reflect responses of the epithelial cells.

Insulin (crystalline beef insulin, a gift from the Eli Lilly Co.) was used at a calculated final concentration of 10^{-7} M. In the presence of bovine serum albumin (final concentration, 2.5%), which minimizes loss of insulin by adsorption on glassware, the same effects were manifested at a calculated insulin concentration of 10^{-9} M. Medium 199 (obtained from Microbiological Associates), containing fructose instead of glucose, was used in all experiments.

The incorporation of ^{3}H-thymidine into DNA was determined by a modification of a method previously described; no carriers were added [2]. Accumulation of ^{14}C-AIB by mammary explants was measured according to Friedberg *et al.* [5]. DNA was determined according to Dische [6]. DPNH-cytochrome C reductase was assayed by the method of Ernster *et al.* [7]. Rough endoplasmic reticulum (RER) and free ribosomes were isolated according to Ganoza and Williams [8]. RNA was measured by the method of Mejbaum [9]. ^{3}H-Uridine incorporation into RNA was determined according to Green and Topper [10].

The pregnant mice used in these studies were midway through their first pregnancy. The virgin animals ranged from 3.5 to 5 months of age. All animals were of the 3CH/HeN strain.

Results

The rate of incorporation of tritiated thymidine into trichloroacetic acid-insoluble materials within the explants has been used to measure DNA synthesis by the epithelial cells. This is based on the observed correspondence between the time course of ^{3}H-thymidine incorporation and mitotic indices in the epithelium [2], on autoradiographic studies [11] which demonstrated silver grains in greater numbers over epithelial nuclei (compared to other nuclei), and on the observation that fat cells do not make DNA under the influence of insulin [12].

Figure 1 shows that DNA synthesis by pregnant explants is relatively active during the first 6 hours in the presence (I) and absence (NH) of insulin, and that it declines more slowly in the next 6 hours with insulin than without it. While without insulin, DNA synthesis continues to decline, with insulin it plateaus between 12-18

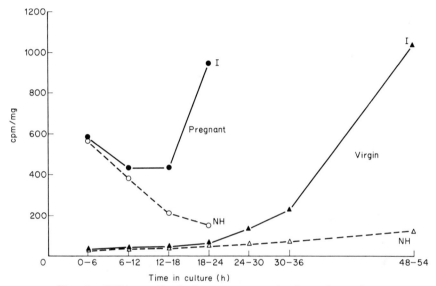

Fig. 1. DNA synthesis in mammary gland explants from pregnant and virgin mice. Incubations were carried out in the absence (NH) or presence (I) of insulin, and methyl-^{3}H-thymidine (20 Ci/mM) was added (final concentration, 1 μCi/ml) for 6-hour periods during the culture, as indicated. For details of isotope determinations, see Materials and Methods. Each point represents the average of 3 determinations.

hours, thereafter rapidly increasing to a maximum ([2], not shown here) between 18-24 hours. The very low initial extent of DNA synthesis by virgin explants is maintained during the first 24 hours, both with and without insulin. The synthesis without insulin increases slightly during the second day, but the level of DNA synthesis with insulin increases markedly after 36 hours. Pregnant tissue, then, responds to insulin, in terms of DNA synthesis, at least 18 hours before mature virgin tissue does, and the corresponding maxima occur about 24 hours apart [2].

To determine whether exogenous insulin is necessary during the first 24 hours in order that mature virgin tissue respond to the hormone during the second day, the experiments illustrated in Fig. 2 were performed. Tissue was incubated in the absence of insulin for different lengths of time before the insulin was added. The rates of DNA synthesis are approximately the same in all systems for the first

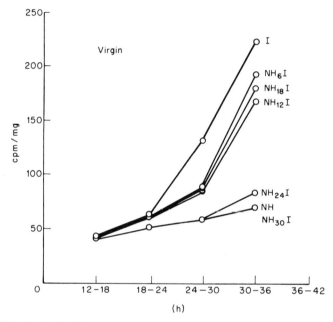

Fig. 2. Delay between the onset of insulin treatment and the DNA-synthesis response. Virgin mammary gland tissues was cultured for varying lengths of time in hormone-free (NH) medium before exposure to insulin (I). Cultures were pulsed with methyl-^{3}H-thymidine as described in the legend to Fig. 1.

24 hours. The rates in the NH_6I, $NH_{12}I$, and $NH_{18}I$ systems are the same, between 24-30 hours, and only somewhat slower than in the system with insulin present throughout. However, between 24-36 hours, the slopes in all four cases are essentially identical. It appears that, while mature virgin tissue may be slightly sensitive to insulin during the first 18 hours, as reflected by DNA synthesis, an important process which is independent of exogenous insulin is implicated in the eventual acquisition of greatly enhanced insulin-sensitivity.

In order to determine whether the difference between the epithelial cells of pregnant and mature, virgin animals described above related uniquely to DNA synthesis, a comparison of insulin-responsiveness in terms of the rate of accumulation of the non-metabolizable amino acid, α-amino isobutyric acid (AIB), was

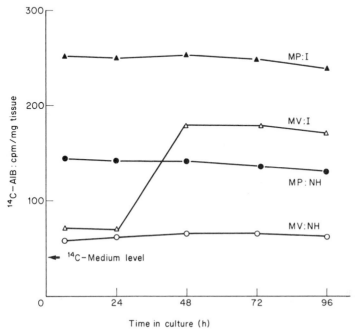

Fig. 3. The accumulation of ^{14}C-AIB during 96 hours of culture. Mammary gland explants prepared from mid-pregnant (MP) and virgin (MV) mice were cultured in the absence (NH) or in the presence (I) of insulin. ^{14}C-AIB (0.1 μCi/ml) was present for 3 hours ending at the times indicated, and accumulation was measured (cf. Materials and Methods). Each point represents the average of 3 determinations.

made. In Fig. 3, the rate of accumulation of AIB at various times during 96 hours of culture is depicted. The rate of accumulation of the amino acid by pregnant explants is constant over the entire 4-day culture period in the presence, and absence, of insulin. The difference in accumulation with, and without, insulin is manifested immediately and remains constant during this time. The rate of accumulation by mature virgin explants in the absence of insulin is also constant during 4 days. During the first day, the rate of accumulation by mature virgin tissue in the presence of the hormone is constant, and is only slightly larger than in the absence of insulin. By the end of the second day, however, insulin exerts a marked effect on the rate in the virgin explants. More detailed time studies showed that the insulin effect is first detected between 24-28 hours. This enhanced rate of accumulation is maintained during the next 2

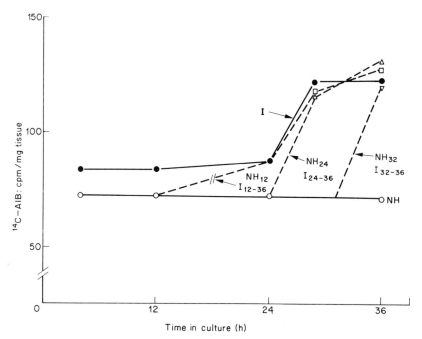

Fig. 4. Effect of culture in the absence of insulin on the subsequent insulin-stimulated accumulation of AIB by virgin explants. After culture in the absence (NH) of insulin, virgin explants were transferred to insulin (I) medium at the times indicated. AIB accumulation was measured as described in the legend to Fig. 3.

days. Similar results are obtained when corresponding epithelial cell-connective tissue complexes are used instead of explants. This indicates that the effects reflect responses of the epithelial cells, and that the development of insulin-responsiveness in terms of this parameter does not require the presence of the fat cells.

The experiments presented in Fig. 4 are designed to determine whether incubation of mature virgin tissue in the absence of insulin for different lengths of time has an effect on the rate of response to the hormone added at later points in time. It can be seen that prior incubation for 12 or 24 hours in the absence of insulin essentially has no effect on these kinetics. The duration of the lag-period, and the events which lead from hormone-insensitivity to sensitivity are, therefore, again seen to be independent of exogenous insulin. Even amounts of insulin much larger than the standard $5\mu g/ml$ dose do not affect the kinetics. Moreover, once the virgin tissue becomes insulin-sensitive *in vitro*, it, like pregnant tissue, responds to insulin at a level of 10^{-9} M in the presence of bovine serum albumin. This is not to say that the delay in response of virgin mouse mammary gland to insulin necessarily means that such tissue is totally incapable of being affected by the hormone initially. Possibly one or more early effects, not detectable by the methods employed, may well be occurring during the so-called insensitive period.

It has been shown [5] that mammary epithelial cells from the pregnant mouse are initially sensitive to insulin *in vitro* but that freshly explanted virgin tissue is virtually insensitive. After about 1 day in culture the mature virgin tissue acquires sensitivity to the hormone comparable to that of pregnant tissue. Acquisition of the ability to respond to insulin is largely independent of exogenous insulin. The events which lead to insulin-sensitivity *in vitro*, in virgin tissue, are probably not identical to those which produce sensitivity *in vivo* during pregnancy. Thus, altered levels of some hormones may play a role in the intact animal during pregnancy. The following observations provide further information in this context.

Pregnancy rapidly elicits critical changes in mouse mammary epithelium. By the second day the cells exhibit insulin-sensitivity *in vitro* in terms of AIB accumulation, and active proliferation has been initiated *in vivo* [13]. Since the blood levels of corticosteroids [14], progesterone and prolactin increase markedly soon after inception, the possibility that these hormones participate in the acquisition of insulin-sensitivity by mammary epithelial cells *in vivo* was entertained. Table 1 shows the results of experiments in which these hormones were administered to groups of mature, virgin mice, followed by assay, *in vitro*, of the effect of insulin on ^{3}H-thymidine incorporation into DNA. It can be seen that only the tissue which has been pre-treated with hydrocortisone *in vivo* is responsive to insulin during the first 24 hours of culture. Furthermore, in this system, the rate of incorporation of ^{3}H-thymidine into DNA had almost reached its peak by the end of the first day, a situation reminiscent of pregnant tissue [2]. The results of a similar experiment, employing the AIB-accumulation assay *in vitro*, are shown in Table 2. Again, it is apparent that only pre-treatment with

Table 1

Incorporation of ^{3}H-thymidine into DNA, *in vitro*, after Treatment with Hormones, *in vivo*

Mature, virgin animals were injected intramuscularly once on each of 3 successive days with (*a*) 0.15 M saline, or (*b*) 10 μg hydrocortisone dissolved in 1% ethanol in 0.15 M saline, or (*c*) 10 μg progesterone in ethanol-saline, or (*d*) 300 μg prolactin dissolved in 0.15 M saline. Twenty-four hours after the third injection, the mammary glands were excised, and placed in organ culture with (I) and without (NH) insulin. Labelling periods with ^{3}H-thymidine (0.1 μCi/ml; S.A. 6.7 Ci/mM) lasted 24 hours. Incorporation into DNA was measured as described in Materials and Methods. Each value represents the mean of 3 separate determinations.

| Treatment, *in vivo* | Conditions, *in vitro* | Labelling period (hours) | |
| | | 0-24 | 0-48 |
		cpm/mg tissue	
Saline	NH	61	117
	I	97	550
Prolactin	NH	43	179
	I	55	633
Progesterone	NH	70	155
	I	89	660
Hydrocortisone	NH	160	172
	I	354	836

hydrocortisone leads to insulin-sensitivity, as manifested during the first day of culture.

Assuming that insulin is a primary mitogenic agent *in vivo* during pregnancy, the evocation of insulin-sensitivity, as described above, would be expected to lead to proliferation of mammary epithelial cells in intact virgin animals treated with hydrocortisone. It is recognized that such an effect would only indirectly implicate insulin as a proliferative hormone. Nevertheless, the results shown in Table 3 agree with the aforementioned expectation. After removal of the fat cells by collagenase treatment, the cell-pellet derived from the hydrocortisone-treated animals contained 50% more DNA than the

Table 2

Accumulation of [14]**C-AIB** *in vitro,* **after Treatment with Hormones,** *in vivo*

The animals used in these experiments were the same as those described in the legend to Table 1. ^{14}C-AIB accumulation was measured as described in Materials and Methods.

Treatment, *in vivo*	Conditions, *in vitro*	Accumulation period (hours)		
		1-4	21-24	25-28
		cpm/mg tissue		
Saline	NH	78	75	86
	I	80	81	172
Prolactin	NH	59	66	62
	I	56	72	128
Progesterone	NH	63	74	65
	I	77	80	122
Hydrocortisone	NH	94	92	93
	I	136	150	163

corresponding fraction derived from saline-treated animals. Prolactin has very little effect. A combination of hydrocortisone and prolactin has an effect no greater than that of hydrocortisone alone. Also, Table 3 demonstrates that the glucocorticoid augments the extent of ^{3}H-thymidine incorporation into the epithelium by a factor of 10. Again, prolactin has virtually no effect.

The *in vivo-in vitro,* and the *in vivo-in vivo* experiments strongly suggest that glucocorticoids are involved in endowing mammary epithelial cells with insulin-sensitivity at the onset of pregnancy. One cannot infer from these results, however, that the steroids exert this effect by direct impingement on mammary tissue. Yet, the results of experiments in which hydrocortisone was added *in vitro* do give credence to this possibility. Figure 5 shows the time courses of the incorporation of ^{3}H-thymidine into DNA by virgin tissue, in the

Table 3
DNA Synthesis, *in vivo*, **after Treatment with Hormones,** *in vivo*

Mature virgin animals were injected subcutaneously once on each of 3 successive days with (*a*) saline, or (*b*) 50 μg hydrocortisone in 1% ethanol-saline, or (*c*) 300 μg prolactin in saline. ^{3}H-Thymidine (5 μCi/25 gm body weight) in 0.1 ml saline was injected subcutaneously 6 hours after the last hormone injection. The animals were sacrificed 24 hours later. The mammary glands were excised, collagenased [4], and the epithelial pellets analysed for DNA content and isotope incorporation into DNA as described in Materials and Methods. In each category duplicate determinations were done on each of 3 animals.

Treatment	DNA content O.D.$_{610}$ x 10^3/mg tissue	Incorporation of ^{3}H-thymidine cpm/mg tissue
Saline	0.93	0.66
	1.01	0.87
	0.90	0.60
Prolactin	1.15	0.60
	1.18	1.07
	1.15	0.99
Hydrocortisone	1.55	11.1
	1.45	8.0
	1.52	8.3
Hydrocortisone and prolactin	1.54	9.2
	1.32	6.1
	1.60	10.0

presence of insulin alone (I-system), or insulin and hydrocortisone (IF-system). In the I-system, the lag-period is seen to be about 24 hours, and the peak rate of incorporation is reached after about 48 hours. This, it will be recalled, is characteristic of virgin tissue cultured in the presence of insulin alone. Tissue in the IF-system responds more quickly. The lag-period is shorter, and the peak-rate of incorporation occurs 12 hours earlier. Tissue in the presence of hydrocortisone, but in the absence of insulin, reacted no differently from tissue in the absence of both hormones (not shown). When pregnant tissue is used, the time courses in the two systems are nearly superimposable. The peaks are attained after about 24 hours of culture. These results indicate that hydrocortisone, *in vitro*,

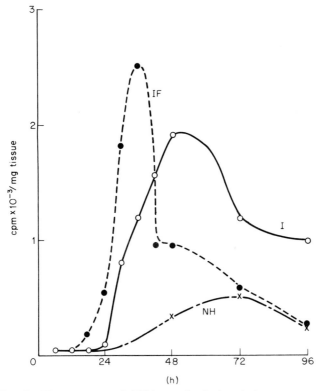

Fig. 5. Time course of DNA synthesis in virgin mammary explants. Virgin mouse mammary explants were cultured in the absence of hormones (NH), in the presence of insulin (I) or in the presence of insulin and hydrocortisone (5 μg/ml) (IF). The tissue was labelled with methyl-³H-thymidine (1 μCi/ml, S.A. 6.15 Ci/mM) during 6-hour periods ending at the times indicated. Incorporation of radioactivity into DNA was determined as described in Materials and Methods.

accelerates the acquisition of insulin-sensitivity by virgin mammary cells.

The developmental pinnacle of the mammary gland is reached during lactation. During this period the tissue produces enormous quantities of proteins and other products, destined for export into the milk. The synthesis of these secretory proteins requires the presence of rough endoplasmic reticulum (RER). Electron-microscopic examination of cultured mouse mammary epithelial cells reveals that glucocorticoids play a key role in the fabrication of these organelles [15]. The observations to be described represent an extension of these ultrastructural studies.

Rough endoplasmic reticulum was isolated from the epithelial fraction of cultured pregnant mammary explants, by centrifugation

Table 4
Effect of Various Hormones on DPNH-cytochrome C reductase

Pooled explants from several pregnant mice were cultured for 60 hours in the presence of the hormones shown. The final concentration of each hormone was 5 $\mu g/ml$. At the end of the culture period the explants were weighed and collagenased. The epithelial fractions were homogenized in cold 0.25 M sucrose, and the homogenates were centrifuged at 5500 x g for 20 min at 4°. The supernatant fluids were assayed for the reductase. Similar relative values were obtained in several experiments.

Hormones	DPNH-cytochrome C reductase % increase over zero-time control
Insulin	44
Hydrocortisone	130
Insulin + hydrocortisone	360
Insulin + corticosterone	300
Insulin + aldosterone	380
Insulin + hydrocortisone + prolactin	320
Insulin + corticosterone + prolactin	450
Insulin + aldosterone + prolactin	380

in a discontinuous sucrose gradient. Two types of analysis were performed on the RER.

(1) DPNH-cytochrome C reductase activity was determined; contribution from possible mitochondrial contamination was precluded by addition of CN to the assay mixture [7]. This determination reflects the membrane component of the RER.

(2) The RNA content was appraised. This is largely a reflection of the ribosomal component of the RER.

Table 4 shows the effect of various hormones on the DPNH-cytochrome C reductase activity after 60 hours of culture. Note that insulin itself has very little effect, but that the hydrocortisone effect is largely dependent on insulin. Corticosterone, the mouse glucocorticoid, is almost as potent as hydrocortisone. Aldosterone, which can substitute for glucocorticoid in the augmentation of casein synthesis [16], also exerts a large stimulatory effect on this membrane enzyme. Prolactin does not enhance the insulin-steroid systems.

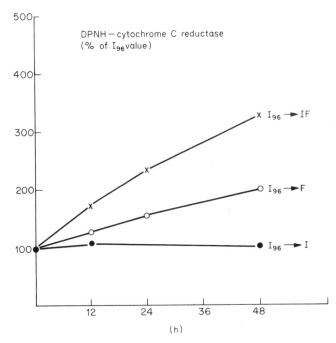

Fig. 6. Hormone effects on DPNH-cytochrome C reductase. Mammary explants from pregnant mice were cultured for 96 hours in the presence of insulin. The explants were then transferred to media containing only insulin (I), only hydrocortisone (F) (5 μg/ml) or both insulin and hydrocortisone (IF). Enzyme activities were determined, at the times indicated, by the method described in the legend to Table 4. Each point represents the average of 2 separate experiments.

In the next series of experiments, a double-incubation technique was used. This method has been very useful in achieving functional [17] and morphological [18] synchronization of the alveoli. After 4 days in an insulin medium, the alveolar cell number has doubled, but these cells (I-cells) no longer proliferate, no detectable casein is made, and very little RER is observed in electron micrographs. After 4 days in an insulin-hydrocortisone medium the same situation prevails, except that all the cells (IF-cells) have a rich supply of RER uniformly distributed in the cytoplasm. I-cells have been shown [18] to respond to the addition of hydrocortisone and prolactin by first forming visible RER, followed by the synthesis of casein. Figure 6 demonstrates that the addition of hydrocortisone to I-cells produces an increase in membrane-bound DPNH-cytochrome C reductase, and that, again, this effect is at least partially dependent on insulin.

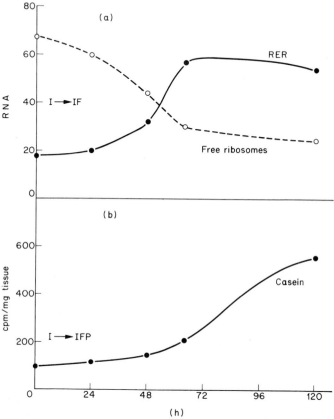

Fig. 7. Time course of RER formation and casein synthesis. Mammary explants from pregnant mice were cultured in the presence of insulin for 96 hours. The explants were then transferred to medium containing insulin and hydrocortisone (IF), or to medium containing these 2 hormones and prolactin (IFP). At the indicated times the explants were weighed and treated with collagenase. RER and free ribosomes were isolated and analysed for RNA as described in Materials and Methods. Casein synthesis was estimated by labelling with $^{32}P_i$ (15 μCi/ml) for 4-hour periods ending at the times indicated [3]. Each point represents the average of duplicate determinations.

The time course for RNA-content of RER, after the addition of hydrocortisone to I-cells, is shown in Fig. 7a. No increase is detectable during the first 24 hours. Recall that an increase in membrane-associated DPNH-cytochrome C reductase was detectable

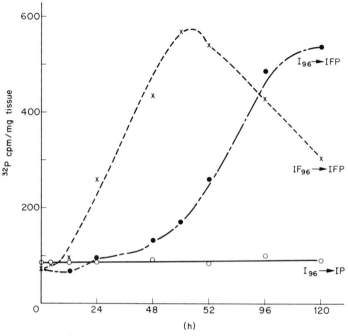

Fig. 8. Time course of casein synthesis. Mammary explants from pregnant mice were cultured for 96 hours in the presence of insulin (I), or in the presence of insulin and hydrocortisone (IF). The I system was then changed to an insulin-prolactin system (IP) or to an insulin-hydrocortisone-prolactin system (I → IFP). The IF system was changed to an IFP system (IF → IFP). Casein synthesis was estimated by labelling with $^{32}P_i$ during 4-hour periods ending at the times indicated [3]. Each point represents the average of duplicate determinations.

in the first 12 hours. Thus, various components of the RER appear to be assembled into the organelles in an asynchronous way. It can also be seen that as the RNA content of membrane-bound ribosomes increases, there is a corresponding decrease in the RNA content of free ribosomes. Apparently hydrocortisone does not increase the total number of ribosomes, but leads to a redistribution of them. This is consistent with an earlier observation [10] which indicated that hydrocortisone has no effect on the extent of ^{3}H-uridine incorporation into total epithelial RNA.

Figure 7b depicts the time course of casein synthesis after hydrocortisone and prolactin are added to I-cells. As expected, casein synthesis emerges after the RNA content of RER begins to increase

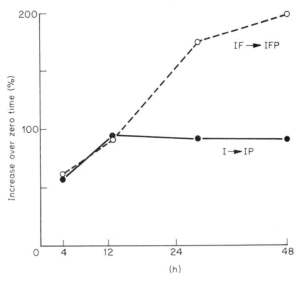

Fig. 9. Hormone effects on the rate of ^{3}H-uridine incorporation into RNA. Mammary explants from pregnant mice were
cultured with insulin (I) or insulin and hydrocortisone (IF).
During the 92-96 hour period, aliquots of the tissues were
labelled with ^{3}H-uridine (0.5 μCi/ml, S.A. 8 Ci/mM); the
radioactivity values obtained correspond to the zero-time
values referred to in the ordinate. At the end of 96 hours
prolactin (5 μg/ml) was added to each system. The tissues were
then labelled with ^{3}H-uridine for 4-hour periods ending at the
times indicated. Isotope incorporation into RNA of the
epithelial-cell fraction was determined as described in Materials
and Methods.

in response to hydrocortisone. This is consistent with a previous observation [18] that prolactin produces its effects on ultrastructure after hydrocortisone has promoted RER formation, visible in the electron microscope.

It is interesting to compare the time courses of casein synthesis after adding prolactin to IF-cells, and after adding hydrocortisone and prolactin to I-cells. Figure 8 demonstrates that casein synthesis is accelerated by more than a day in the IF-cells treated with prolactin. This is presumably because IF-cells have an extensive RER, whereas I-cells are virtually devoid of these membranes [18]. The temporal increment for casein formation corresponds to the time required for RER formation in the I-cells. The decline of casein synthesis in the IF-IFP system is probably not due to the length of the culture period (cf. I → IFP system), but to an observed stasis, corresponding to an accumulation of proteinaceous material within the alveolar lumina [11]. Note also that when prolactin alone is added to I-cells no casein is formed.

Figure 9 compares the effects of prolactin (P) on the incorporation of ^{3}H-uridine into total RNA of IF-cells and I-cells. During the first 12 hours, prolactin stimulates incorporation by I-cells to the same extent as by IF-cells. Subsequently the rate of incorporation by IP-cells does not increase, while the rate by the IFP cells continues to increase. It has been shown [18] that prolactin does not cause polarization of cell organelles until RER has been formed under the influence of insulin and hydrocortisone. It will also be remembered that casein is not formed in the absence of hydrocortisone, i.e., by IP-cells. Thus the effects of prolactin on the epithelial cells are largely dependent on prior exposure to hydrocortisone. Nevertheless, the hydrocortisone-independent action of prolactin [10] is an intriguing phenomenon which warrants further study.

Conclusions

The full development of mouse mammary epithelial cells *in vitro* requires the presence of insulin, a glucocorticoid such as hydrocortisone (aldosterone will also serve), and prolactin. The steroid(s) plays a pivotal, poly-functional role in the conversion of the non-proliferating non-secretory cells, present in the mature, virgin mouse, into the proliferating pregnant cells which evolve into secretory cells.

Insulin is believed to act as a direct mitogenic agent on the epithelial cells during pregnancy. The cells in the mature, virgin mouse have, however, been shown to be insensitive to insulin. This is, presumably, why virtually no proliferation occurs in the mature, virgin animal. The isolated tissue can acquire insulin-sensitivity in the absence of any added hormones. In the intact animal, however, the acquisition of insulin sensitivity depends upon initiation of pregnancy, and is probably not hormone-independent. It has been observed, that by the second day of pregnancy the cells are insulin-sensitive when assayed *in vitro*, and have undergone considerable proliferation *in vivo*. It has also been reported [14] that the levels of corticosteroids in the blood have increased several-fold by this time. Accordingly, a possible role of these steroids in conferring insulin-sensitivity *in vivo* has been studied. The results of experiments performed *in vivo* and *in vitro* strongly suggest that glucocorticoids do, indeed, confer such sensitivity by direct impingement on mammary tissue.

Glucocorticoids also promote RER formation in the incipiently secretory mammary epithelial cells. These steroids increase the level of the membrane-associated DPNH-cytochrome C reductase, and participate in the formation of visible RER. When explants are transferred from an insulin-medium to an insulin-hydrocortisone medium, there is no increase in the number of ribosomes, but they are redistributed so that the majority become membrane-bound. It is not known whether hydrocortisone plays an active role in the attachment of ribosomes to the newly-formed membranes in these cells. Corticosterone has been reported [19] to promote such attachment in liver preparations.

The interplay of glucocorticoids and insulin is brought into relief by the observation that insulin, and therefore insulin sensitivity, is required for hydrocortisone to realize its full potential as a promoter of RER formation. Glucocorticoid somehow makes it possible for the cells to respond to insulin, which, in turn synergizes with the glucocorticoid in the fabrication of the membranes. This relationship at least partially explains the paucity of RER in the mammary epithelium of the mature, virgin mouse. Still another part, played by glucocorticoids in the development of mammary epithelium, relates to the actions of prolactin. Unless the cells have been previously exposed to hydrocortisone and insulin, prolactin treatment leads to an aborted effect on RNA synthesis, and no detectable casein synthesis ensues.

It is evident that the steroids in question play multiple roles in the maturation of mammary epithelial cells, and that the interplay among the various hormones is intricate.

Discussion

Allison (Northwick Park)

I believe that you have some evidence that DNA synthesis is required for the expression of the differentiated function in your cells, namely casein synthesis. Do you know whether a full cycle of DNA synthesis, followed by cell division, regularly occurs?

Topper (Bethesda)

The alveolar cell-number doubles *in vitro* in the presence of insulin when pregnant mammary explants are used.

Tata (Mill Hill)

Did you observe an enhanced rate of turnover of ribosomes during the period of re-distribution between bound and free ribosomes following steroid treatment?

Topper (Bethesda)

The steroid treatment does not appear to cause an enhanced rate of turnover of ribosomes.

Falconer (Nottingham)

We use a pseudopregnant rabbit as a model system to investigate the effects of hormones on lactogenesis. In these animals in mid pseudopregnancy a single intraductal injection of prolactin will initiate both increased DNA synthesis and cell division, possibly two periods of DNA synthesis, but only one cell division.

Have you ever seen DNA synthesis or cell division in your cultured mammary tissue after addition of prolactin to the medium?

Topper (Bethesda)

We have never observed a proliferative effect of prolactin on mouse mammary explants.

Forsyth (Shinfield)

Why is it that it seems impossible to initiate a second wave of DNA synthesis in mammary gland explants *in vitro*?

Topper (Bethesda)

I do not know.

Slater (Brunel)

Your findings that the number of cells per alveolus almost doubles in the mouse *in vitro* system are remarkably similar to the findings *in vivo* in the rat when there is a wave of mitosis in the mammary gland shortly after parturition. Does a similar localized burst of mitosis occur in mouse mammary gland *in vivo*?

Topper (Bethesda)

Yes, it has been reported that a wave of mitosis occurs in the mouse mammary gland shortly after parturition.

References

1. Voytovich, A. E. and Topper, Y. J.; *Science*; **158**, (1967) 1326.
2. Stockdale, F. E. and Topper, Y. J.; *Proc. Nat. Acad. Sci. U.S.A.*; **56**, (1966) 1283.
3. Juergens, W. G., Stockdale, F. E., Topper, Y. J. and Elias, J. J.; *Proc. Nat. Acad. Sci. U.S.A.*; **54**, (1965) 629.
4. Lasfargues, E. Y.; *Anat. Rec.*; **127**, (1957) 117.
5. Friedberg, S. H., Oka, T. and Topper, Y. J.; *Proc. Nat. Acad. Sci. U.S.A.*; **67**, (1970) 1493.
6. Dische, Z.; *Microchemie*; **8**, (1930) 4.
7. Ernster, L., Siekevitz, P. and Palade, G. E.; *J. Cell Biol.*; **15**, (1962) 541.
8. Ganoza, M. C. and Williams, C. A.; *Proc. Nat. Acad. Sci. U.S.A.*; **63**, (1969) 1370.
9. Mejbaum, W.; *Z. Physiol. Chem.*; **258**, (1939) 117.
10. Green, M. R. and Topper, Y. J.; *Biochim. biophys. Acta*; **204**, (1970) 441.
11. Stockdale, F. E., Juergens, W. G. and Topper, Y. J.; *Develop. Biol.*; **13**, (1966) 266.
12. Lockwood, D. H., Voytovich, A. E., Stockdale, F. E. and Topper, Y. J.; *Proc. Nat. Acad. Sci. U.S.A.*; **58**, (1967) 658.
13. Oka, T. and Topper, Y. J.; unpublished results.
14. Venning, E. H.; *Endocrinology*; **9**, (1946) 557.
15. Mills, E. S. and Topper, Y. J.; *Science*; **165**, (1969) 1127.
16. Turkington, R. W., Juergens, W. G. and Topper, Y. J.; *Endocrinology*; **80**, (1967) 1139.
17. Turkington, R. W., Lockwood, D. H. and Topper, Y. J.; *Biochim. biophys. Acta*; **148**, (1967) 475.
18. Mills, E. S. and Topper, Y. J.; *J. Cell Biol.*; **44**, (1970) 310.
19. James, D. W., Rabin, B. R. and Williams, D. J.; *Nature, Lond.*; **224**, (1969) 371.

BASIC BIOCHEMISTRY AND CONTROL OF PRODUCTION OF CYCLIC AMP*

K. J. Hittelman and R. W. Butcher

*Department of Biochemistry, School of Medicine,
University of Massachusetts, Worcester, Massachusetts*

In 1957, Rall, Sutherland, and Berthet, [1] reporting the effects of epinephrine and glucagon on phosphorylase activation in liver homogenates, stated that:

'. . . the response of the homogenates to the hormones occurred in two stages. In the first stage, a particulate fraction of homogenates produced a heat-stable factor in the presence of hormones; in the second stage, this factor stimulated the formation of liver phosphorylase in supernatant fractions of homogenates in which the hormones themselves were inactive.'

When subsequently isolated and characterized, this unknown 'factor' proved to be cyclic adenosine-3',5'-monophosphate, or cyclic AMP [2, 3, 4]. Its discovery in biological systems and its implication as a courier of biochemical information in hormonal control mechanisms provided the first step into a field of research which has now seen immense amounts of activity. As we shall see, the fruits of this work have been a better, though by no means complete, understanding of a large number of hormone/effector systems in which intracellular levels of cyclic AMP have been shown to play a key role in the physiological response of the effector to the hormone [5-10].

Intracellular concentrations of cyclic AMP
Intracellular concentrations of cyclic AMP reflect the relative activities of at least two enzymes which function in opposition to

* Supported by Grant AM-13904 from the National Institutes of Health.

153

each other (Fig. 1). Production of cyclic AMP is catalysed by adenyl cyclase [11-14]. This enzyme has been detected in almost every mammalian tissue in which it has been sought and is also present in the tissues of many lower organisms [15, 16]. Magnesium and ATP are required for its activity [2] and so the substrate is probably

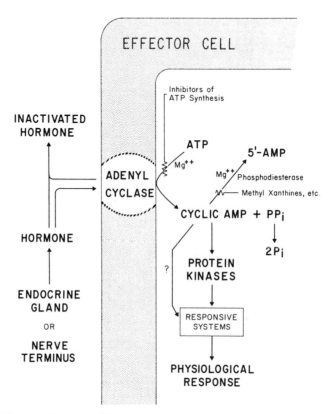

Fig. 1. Hormone-effector cell interactions and the metabolism
of cyclic AMP.

Mg-ATP. In addition to cyclic AMP, one mole of pyrophosphate is formed per mole of ATP utilized [12].

Adenyl cyclase was first described in detail by Sutherland and Rall and their co-workers in 1962 [11-14]. At that time, it was realized that the cyclase was not a simple soluble enzyme, but might be a component of a non-mitochondrial membrane. This suspicion has been borne out, of course, and with the single exception of the soluble enzyme from *Brevibacterium liquefaciens* [17], all adenyl cyclases which have been studied have been found to be associated with membranes. In the case of certain types of muscle, the cyclase system appears to be bound to the membranes of the sarcoplasmic reticulum [18]. The transverse tubular segments of this reticulum can, of course, be argued to be extensions of the plasma membrane. In all other cases, adenyl cyclase activity has been found to be associated at least in part with the plasma membranes [16].

To date, in spite of intense efforts, adenyl cyclase has defied all attempts to isolate it in a highly purified form. For one thing, its catalytic activity seems to be extremely labile. But another important factor in the failure to obtain a pure preparation of this enzyme may be a semantic problem rather than a biochemical one. For we do not yet know how to define 'adenyl cyclase'. Is it only a complex protein catalyst—possibly a lipoprotein component of the plasma membrane—which is difficult to isolate because of its chemical nature? Or must we include as part of the cyclase itself—possibly in the role of regulatory subunits—the hormone receptor moieties which a large body of experimental evidence suggests are an integral part of the cyclase insofar as they wield such control over the catalytic activity? Unfortunately, the answers to these questions would not seem to be immediately forthcoming.

Regulation of the intracellular concentration of cyclic AMP is a function shared with adenyl cyclase by one or more specific cyclic adenosine-3',5'-monophosphate phosphodiesterases. This enzyme, first described by Sutherland and Rall [3], hydrolyses the 3'-phosphate ester bond of cyclic AMP to yield 5'-AMP. Like adenyl cyclase, phosphodiesterase seems to be ubiquitous. It requires a divalent cation for catalytic activity (usually Mg^{++}), as demonstrated by its inhibition by ethylenediaminetetraacetic acid (EDTA) [19].

In contrast to adenyl cyclase, phosphodiesterase appears to exist in the cell in either (or both) a soluble or a particulate form [20, 21]. The enzyme has been purified by a number of investigators [21-24], and its characteristics have been reported in detail. It generally shows greater affinity for cyclic AMP than for other cyclic nucleotides, and the K_m's, previously found for phosphodiesterases from a variety of sources, lie in the range of about 10^{-4} M cyclic AMP [25].

Recently, it has been reported that several different cell types contain two different phosphodiesterases [25-28]. These differ in both molecular weight and the K_m for cyclic AMP. In addition to the enzymes of K_m, about 10^{-4} M enzymes with K_m's of about 10^{-6} M were found. The higher molecular weight enzyme appeared to have a lower affinity for cyclic AMP [29], and in addition, was the only one to show catalytic activity with cyclic guanosine monophosphate (GMP) as substrate [30]. The physiological significance of these observations is still to be explained.

Phosphodiesterase appears to be present in cells at far greater activity than is adenyl cyclase [25]. This observation, if it reflects accurately the state of the intact cell, has profound implications with respect to the regulation of intracellular concentrations of cyclic AMP. How might we explain the ability of cyclic AMP to carry out its missions in the face of seemingly insurmountable odds? At present, three possible explanations present themselves:

(1) Adenyl cyclase and phosphodiesterase are somehow separated from each other by compartmentalization within the cell. Rall and his co-workers have presented some evidence for such a possibility in brain tissue [31]. Segregation of the enzymes producing and destroying cyclic AMP might permit accumulation of the nucleotide to the extent that its functions could be carried out. However, invoking compartmentalization raises another problem, and that is, how to account for the rapid destruction of cyclic AMP once its role as second messenger has been fulfilled.

(2) Cyclic AMP-mediated events are triggered by relatively small changes in the intracellular concentration of cyclic AMP. In many instances, this is very likely the case. It has been demonstrated in the case of hormone-stimulated lipolysis, a process known to be under the control of cyclic AMP, that as the cyclic AMP concentration increased from 180 to 300 pmoles/gm in rat epididymal fat pads, the rate of glycerol release (i.e., lipolysis) increased from about 0.25 to 3.25 μmoles/gm/hr [7, 32]. Any further increase in cyclic AMP was without further effect on glycerol release. It is thus entirely within reason to suspect that even in the face of a very high phosphodiesterase activity, a hormone-stimulated adenyl cyclase might be able to increase the intracellular cyclic AMP concentration sufficiently to trigger the desired physiological effects.

(3) It is possible that phosphodiesterase is under some sort of control which directs its activity in a reciprocal manner to that of adenyl cyclase. Both citrate and ATP can inhibit phosphodiesterase [19, 33]. Although this may simply be a metal chelation effect, it

could conceivably be of regulatory significance. Additionally, Cheung has presented some evidence to show that phosphodiesterase activity may be affected by a protein activator [25], but much work remains to be done to establish this as a regulatory function.

Figure 1 summarizes the relationship between adenyl cyclase and phosphodiesterase and illustrates the three primary possibilities for control of intracellular cyclic AMP levels: (1) modulation of the activity of adenyl cyclase; (2) modulation of the activity of phosphodiesterase; or (3) a concerted modulation of the activities of both of these enzymes simultaneously. Additionally, there is the factor of leakage of cyclic AMP out of cells, a process which may play a role in limiting the extent to which the nucleotide can accumulate intracellularly. Although our present state of knowledge does not allow us to select which of these is at work in the cell—and, indeed, it may vary depending upon the cell—there is an over-whelming body of evidence which suggests that one of the primary controls occurs at the level of adenyl cyclase, and this control is generally a result of hormonal activation of the cyclase system.

The second messenger hypothesis

In retrospect, the description quoted above by Rall *et al.* [1] of a two-stage response to hormones seems almost prophetic. In 1961, Rall and Sutherland [34] expanded their concept of the role of cyclic AMP to include those instances in which hormone-induced changes might be due to *decreased* intracellular concentrations of cyclic AMP. And by 1965, a sufficient number of hormone-target systems had been tested so that Sutherland *et al.* [35] could formally propose the 'Second Messenger Hypothesis.'

According to this hypothesis (Fig. 2), a neurohormone or circulating hormone (first messenger) impinges upon a target cell, specifically, at the adenyl cyclase system. This complex is called the first target system. As a result of the interaction between the hormone and its receptor, adenyl cyclase activity is affected in such a way as to bring about a change in the intracellular level of cyclic AMP. In effect, the information originally contained in the hormone is translated intracellularly through changes in cyclic AMP levels, and it is in fact the altered level of intracellular cyclic AMP that changes the metabolic behavior of the cell so that it can be said to have 'responded to the hormone'. Furthermore, some tissues, such as thyroid, adrenal cortex, anterior pituitary, and gonads, may respond to an increase in intracellular cyclic AMP by increasing the rate at which they secrete their own hormones; and thus these hormones qualify for the title of 'third messenger'.

One of the most striking implications of the second messenger hypothesis, as has been frequently discussed by others, is that a

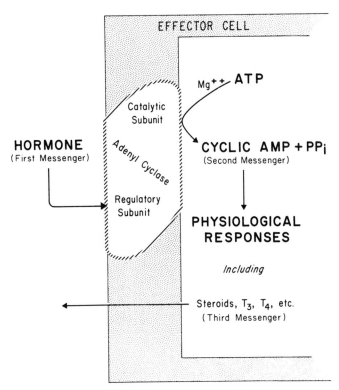

Fig. 2. The second messenger system.

single, small, ubiquitous molecule—cyclic AMP—can induce as wide a variety of physiological responses as there are different types of cells to respond. This apparent versatility, of course, is merely a reflection of the different enzyme profiles of different cells, and any given cell will respond to a hormone by using that metabolic machinery which it has available. Specificity of response to a hormone must thus reside with the regulatory subunits of adenyl cyclase at the cell surface, a topic of much current research interest. Anything further we could say at this time would only echo the sentiment of Rall and

Sutherland who stated in 1961 that they were '. . . impressed with the degree of biochemical differentiation among the tissues of a given animal, which allows a single substance to call forth glucose from one tissue and corticosteroids from another' [34].

Scope of the second messenger

It is now known that in many tissues, one of the earliest detectable responses to hormones is an increased intracellular cyclic AMP concentration. Table I presents a partial list of these tissues, along with some of the hormones affecting them and the direction of change of cyclic AMP. The overt physiological responses resulting from these hormones acting on their target tissues, though not listed, are implied, for the table is meant primarily to illustrate the second messenger function of cyclic AMP in a variety of hormone/effector systems.

In addition to the systems shown in Table I, where changes in intracellular cyclic AMP have been measured directly in intact tissues, there are a number of other instances wherein cyclic AMP has been implicated as a second messenger, although direct evidence is lacking. Usually, the indirect evidence that cyclic AMP may be involved in physiological control in a tissue comes from three types of experiments.

First, one can demonstrate that in the presence of phospho-diesterase inhibitors, physiological changes occur which mimic the response to a hormone [16]. It is then inferred that the changes observed are a consequence of increased intracellular cyclic AMP concentrations resulting from inhibition of the phosphodiesterase. Presumably, the cyclic AMP which accumulates in the presence of such inhibitors is a magnification of a low endogenous rate of cyclization of ATP by adenyl cyclase. As there is little direct evidence that the phosphodiesterase inhibitors increase cyclic AMP through other mechanisms, such experiments constitute a fair indication of the involvement of cyclic AMP in the normal response of the tissue to hormone.

The well-known synergistic effect, which exists between phospho-diesterase inhibitors and certain hormones, speaks further to this point. For in those cases where phosphodiesterase inhibitors can be shown to act synergistically with a hormone on a physiological response (e.g., lipolysis [36]), the synergism is found to be the result of the effect on intracellular cyclic AMP levels [37, 38].

A second method which has been used to implicate cyclic AMP as a mediator of effector response patterns is the demonstration of hormone-sensitive adenyl cyclase activity in broken-cell preparations [16]. Such experiments have provided strong evidence for the involvement of cyclic AMP in hormone-induced physiological responses. While in general the activities of broken-cell preparations of adenyl cyclase have accurately reflected those of intact cells, this

Table 1

Some Target Tissues in which Hormones are known to Affect Intracellular Cyclic AMP Levels

Tissue	Hormone	Change in cyclic AMP	References
Adipose, brown	Catecholamines	increase	75,76
Adipose, white	Catecholamines	increase	37,38
	Glucagon	increase	38
	ACTH	increase	38
	TSH	increase	38
	Secretin	increase	77
	Insulin	decrease	32
	Prostaglandin	decrease	48
Adrenal cortex	ACTH	increase	78
Anterior pituitary	Vasopressin	increase	79
	Prostaglandin	increase	80
Bone	Parathyroid hormone	increase	81
	Prostaglandin	increase	81
Cardiac muscle	Catecholamines	increase	82,93,94
	Glucagon	increase	92
Kidney, cortex	Parathyroid hormone	increase	81
	Prostaglandin	increase	48
Kidney, medulla	Vasopressin	increase	81,83
Liver	Catecholamines	increase	35
	Glucagon	increase	35
	Insulin	decrease	84
Ovary (corpus luteum)	LH	increase	85
Pancreas (islets)	Glucagon	increase	86
	Epinephrine	decrease	86
Parotid	Catecholamines	increase	16
Platelets	Prostaglandins	increase	87
	Catecholamines	decrease	87
Skeletal muscle	Catecholamines	increase	88
Skin (frog)	α-MSH	increase	89
	Norepinephrine	decrease	89
	Melatonin	decrease	89
Smooth muscle	Catecholamines	increase	37,90,95
Testes	LH (ICSH)	increase	91

is not always the case. One notable exception was adrenocortical carcinoma described by Ney *et al.* [39], in which it was found that cyclic AMP levels were insensitive to ACTH in the intact tissue, but adenyl cyclase in homogenates did respond to the hormone.

The third, and perhaps most direct approach, involves the use of cyclic AMP or its derivatives to mimic effects of hormones. As cyclic AMP itself does not easily penetrate cells, derivatives designed to be more lipid soluble are used instead [40]. The derivative most frequently used in such studies is $N^6, O^{2'}$-dibutyryl cyclic AMP. It has been shown in several studies that this agent evoked the same qualitative response patterns in intact cells which were evoked by relevant hormones. Consequently, it appears that the action of the hormone itself is mediated by cyclic AMP, and direct administration of the nucleotide or its derivatives merely short-circuits a step in the normal route of the hormone action. It is well to remember, however, that in most such experiments nucleotide concentrations used were several orders of magnitude greater than those commonly found in tissues. Thus, caution must be exercised in describing a physiological role of cyclic AMP when the possibility exists that toxic as well as physiological effects may have been observed.

In general, however, conclusions from experiments indirectly implicating cyclic AMP as a mediator in hormone response patterns have subsequently been verified by direct observation of altered cyclic AMP levels in the tissue in response to hormonal stimulation. And, of course, the converse is true as well, *viz.*, in systems known to use cyclic AMP as a mediator in the response pattern to hormone, phosphodiesterase inhibitors or cyclic AMP derivatives have the same qualitative effect as the hormone itself, and hormonal sensitivity of adenyl cyclase in broken-cell preparations can usually be demonstrated.

It is well to note at this point that results of several types of experiments used to link hormonal effects to cyclic AMP levels—e.g., direct measurement of cyclic AMP, inhibitor studies, temporal studies, the use of various cellular and subcellular preparations, and so forth—are subject to an alternative explanation. None of these experiments eliminates the possibility that cyclic AMP, instead of eliciting the response to the hormone, is in some way produced simultaneously with the physiological effect, but however, does not elicit it. In this light, experiments in which cyclic AMP or its derivatives are used to evoke a response attain a special significance, for this approach constitutes the only direct demonstration that cyclic AMP itself lies directly on line between the hormone receptor and expression of the physiological response.

An exemplary system: white adipose tissue

Of the many tissues which show changes in intracellular cyclic AMP concentrations as a part of their response to hormones, one of the most exploited is white adipose tissue. It is in many ways an ideal tissue for such studies. Available in quantity, it can be used intact, or relatively homogeneous isolated-cell preparations can be made easily and rapidly, or ghosts or broken cells can be used. In all of these preparations, some degree of hormone sensitivity of the adenyl cyclase can be retained. Thus, either changes in intracellular cyclic AMP concentrations or the activities of adenyl cyclase and phosphodiesterase can be studied under a variety of conditions. In addition, lipolysis, lipogenesis, and glucose utilization, three of the primary indicators of the physiological state of this tissue, can be easily monitored in intact-cell preparations under a wide variety of conditions.

There are many substances which can be used to induce alterations of cyclic AMP concentrations in adipose tissue. For purposes of discussion, these can be divided into two groups, lipolytic hormones and pharmacological agents, and these can be further categorized on the basis of whether they increase or decrease intracellular cyclic AMP concentrations. The lipolytic hormones include the catechol-amines, ACTH, TSH, LH, and glucagon and the antilipolytic hormones include insulin and prostaglandins. In the case of the lipolytic hormones, the polypeptides may not have physiological functions. Pharmacological agents include lipolytic compounds such as the methyl xanthines, and antilipolytics such as nicotinic acid, phenylisopropyl adenosine, and β-adrenergic antagonists.

For several years after the demonstration of the involvement of cyclic AMP in phosphorylase activation, this remained its only well-defined role. However, there were several indications that cyclic AMP might be involved in hormone-activated lipolysis. Vaughan [41] found that phosphorylase activation occurred in parallel with increased lipolytic activity in adipose tissue treated with lipolytic hormones, and her data thus suggested a cyclic AMP-mediated effect of these hormones. Indeed, not too long thereafter Klainer *et al.* [14] demonstrated an epinephrine-sensitive adenyl cyclase system in homogenates of rat epididymal fat pads. It was later found [36] that caffeine, now well known and widely used as an inhibitor of the phosphodiesterase, not only stimulated lipolysis by itself, but acted synergistically with epinephrine to accelerate both free fatty acid and glycerol release from rat epididymal fat pads. And finally, it was reported [42] that cyclic AMP activated triglyceride lipase in subcellular preparations of epididymal fat.

Cyclic AMP was more directly demonstrated to be involved in the mechanism of hormone-stimulated lipolysis in 1965 when, a very close correlation was found between tissue cyclic AMP levels and the rate of release of free fatty acids into the medium in response to epinephrine administration [37]. In subsequent experiments, ACTH, LH, TSH, and glucagon were all found to act through cyclic AMP in exerting their lipolytic effects [38]. β-Adrenergic antagonists, which blocked the actions of catecholamines on free fatty acid release were also found to inhibit the effects of epinephrine on cyclic AMP levels [38]. The general picture which evolves from such studies is one of a very strong qualitative and quantitative correlation between the rate of lipolysis and the intracellular cyclic AMP concentration.

It is important to note two further points. First, not all adipose tissues are sensitive to the wide array of hormones which affect rat epididymal fat. For instance, lipolysis in human adipose tissue seems responsive only to catecholamines [43], whereas rabbit fat responds only to ACTH [44]. In such cases, where lipolysis is stimulated by one hormone but not another, the hormone which induces lipolysis also caused increases in cyclic AMP levels; conversely, inactive hormones did not affect cyclic AMP levels.

Secondly, none of the evidence thus far discussed, relating cyclic AMP to the lipolytic mechanism, necessarily establishes a cause and effect relationship. Hence the temporal sequence of the events occurring between hormone administration and release of free fatty acids from the tissue becomes of great significance. Indeed, it has been shown that tissue cyclic AMP levels change before there is any evidence of lipolysis [37, 38], and thus increasing cyclic AMP levels trigger lipolysis and not *vice versa.*

Although adipose tissues from various sources differ with respect to the lipolytic hormones to which they are sensitive—and also in the *degree* of sensitivity to these hormones—there is a note of consistency which can be sounded: lipolytic hormones which increase cyclic AMP in fat cells do so by increasing the activity of adenyl cyclase. The alternative control point—inhibition of phospho-diesterase activity—does not seem to be affected by these hormones.

Both insulin and prostaglandins exhibit antilipolytic activity. Although the first report of the antilipolytic action of insulin attributed the effect to its influence on glucose metabolism [45], subsequent studies showed the effect to be independent of the presence of glucose [46]. It was then demonstrated that insulin caused a rapid and marked decrease in cyclic AMP levels in epinephrine-stimulated rat epididymal fat pads incubated either in the presence or absence of glucose [32].

The precise mechanism by which insulin effects a decrease in intracellular cyclic AMP levels is not yet known. Initially, studies were directed at elucidating a possible inhibitory effect of the hormone on adenyl cyclase, but such efforts were hampered when it did not prove possible to elicit an effect of insulin on cyclic AMP production in broken-cell preparations. More recently, Loten and Sneyd [28] have presented evidence that insulin may act by affecting the phosphodiesterase, rather than adenyl cyclase. They showed the rat epididymal adipocytes have two phosphodiesterases which differ in K_m by a factor of about 50, and in V_{max} by a factor of about 4. When adipocytes were incubated with insulin, homogenized, and the phosphodiesterase activity subsequently estimated, it was found that the V_{max} of the low-K_m enzyme was increased, while the K_m of the high-K_m enzyme was decreased. Overall, this would be expected to have the effect of increasing the phosphodiesterase activity of the cell. Loten and Sneyd propose this as the mechanism whereby insulin decreases intracellular levels of cyclic AMP [28].

It was reported a number of years ago [47] that prostaglandin E_1 (PGE_1) inhibited the lipolytic effects of several hormones in adipose tissue. This antilipolytic action was subsequently shown to be caused by decreased intracellular cyclic AMP levels, and adipocytes were found to respond quite rapidly to very low concentrations of PGE_1 [48, 49, 50].

Prostaglandins pose one of the more intriguing puzzles with respect to regulation of intracellular cyclic AMP levels, for although it is clear that their antilipolytic effect results from their ability to lower cyclic AMP levels in adipocytes, they have the effect of *increasing* cyclic AMP in other tissues. This duality in the effects of prostaglandins is reminiscent of the α- and β-adrenergic activities of catecholamines [51, 52]. As is the case with insulin, then, it must be admitted that the precise mechanism whereby prostaglandins decrease cyclic AMP in adipose tissue is unknown. Here, again, experiments with broken-cell preparations have not provided conclusive results, and neither a direct inhibition of adenyl cyclase nor a stimulation of phosphodiesterase have been observed in adipocytes. There are, however, suggestions that in adipose tissue prostaglandins may act by inhibiting adenyl cyclase. Perhaps the most persuasive of these is the finding that PGE_1 inhibited lipolysis induced by the methyl xanthines [53]. Since the latter agents inhibit phosphodiesterase, the resultant accumulation of cyclic AMP produced by a low endogenous cyclization rate ultimately triggers lipolysis. One way to inhibit the lipolytic mechanism under such circumstances would be to inhibit adenyl cyclase, and the antilipolytic action of PGE_1 can be explained in this way.

Among the pharmacological agents which can affect intracellular cyclic AMP levels, perhaps the best known are the methyl xanthines. One of these—caffeine—was shown by Vaughan and Steinberg [36] both to stimulate lipolysis by itself, and to act synergistically with epinephrine in doing so. It had already been shown that phosphodiesterase was inhibited by methyl xanthines [20], and the picture was completed with the demonstration that xanthines stimulated lipolysis by causing elevated intracellular cyclic AMP levels [54]. The kinetics of methyl xanthine inhibition of the phosphodiesterase have been evaluated, and in most cases are competitive [20]. This is perhaps not surprising in light of the very close structural similarity between the xanthines and the adenine moiety of cyclic AMP.

Another substance which may be classified as a pharmacological lipolytic agent is $N^6,O^{2'}$-dibutyryl cyclic AMP. Its use was described earlier with respect to methods of illuminating the possible role of cyclic AMP in effector response patterns. Presumably, its mechanism of action is identical to that of cyclic AMP, and it is possible that, through metabolic changes within the cell, the dibutyryl derivative is indeed transformed into cyclic AMP itself. The dibutyryl derivative, however, is resistant to attack by phosphodiesterase.

Papaverine is an alkaloid found in crude opium powder, and it has been used therapeutically as an antispasmodic and vasodilator because of its activity as a smooth muscle relaxant. It has recently been shown that it is also a muscle phosphodiesterase inhibitor [55], thus permitting an increase in the intracellular cyclic AMP concentration which was presumed to cause the accompanying decrease in tonus [56]. Curiously, however, papaverine has not been demonstrated to be lipolytic in intact adipose tissue, even though as a phosphodiesterase inhibitor it would be expected to show such activity.

It might appear that this drug exhibits tissue-selective behaviour in its modification of the second messenger mechanism, and such a quality would be of great therapeutic interest. However, Beavo *et al.* [57] have recently shown that such an interpretation must be viewed cautiously. In studies using isolated fat cells, they found that not only was papaverine bound to albumin in the reaction mixture—and thus its effective concentration decreased—but by virtue of its high lipid solubility it may be 'concentrated' in the lipid phase of the cells. This latter phenomenon could have further contributed to the lowering of the effective papaverine concentration at the site of the phosphodiesterase. Only in fat-cell homogenates was papaverine effective as a phosphodiesterase inhibitor, and this effect could be markedly reduced by addition of albumin [57].

At least in part, then, the failure of papaverine to elicit lipolysis in experiments with isolated fat cells is due to the presence of albumin. However, its lipophilic nature and probable concentration in cellular lipids must also be considered, a phenomenon which raises the interesting question of tissue-selective therapy in the second messenger system (see below).

Nicotinic acid and phenylisopropyladenosine (PIA) are two pharmacological agents which exhibit antilipolytic activity. Nicotinic acid was observed to inhibit free fatty-acid release *in vivo* and *in vitro* [58], and this effect has been shown in isolated fat cells to be associated with decreased intracellular cyclic AMP concentrations [38, 59]. The exact mechanism of action of nicotinic acid is not known, but it has been suggested that its effect may be due to stimulation of phosphodiesterase activity [60].

Like nicotinic acid, PIA has also been shown to inhibit lipolysis [61]. This action is due to its decreasing intracellular cyclic AMP levels [62] by an as yet unknown mechanism.

The β-adrenergic antagonists are the only antilipolytic agents whose site of action is fairly well understood. These compounds act by antagonizing the effects of catecholamines on adenyl cyclase [16]. Presumably, they do so by preventing the hormone from binding to the regulatory subunit of the enzyme.

The β-adrenergic antagonists are different from other antilipolytic agents in three major respects. First, they are specific in antagonizing only the catecholamines. Other antilipolytic agents, such as insulin, prostaglandins, PIA and nicotinic acid, lower cyclic AMP levels in response to a wide variety of hormones. Secondly, β-adrenergic antagonists are effective in broken-cell preparations in which phosphodiesterase activity can be greatly minimized, while the non-specific agents seem to work only on intact cells. And thirdly, the β-adrenergic antagonists must be used at higher concentrations than the non-specific agents.

Other factors involved in lipolysis

The factors influencing lipolysis which have been discussed thus far are what can be termed fast-acting agents; that is, their effects are detectable within seconds or minutes after administration. In contrast, it has been demonstrated that there are other agents which affect lipolysis but these only act after a longer lag period. Growth hormone or growth hormone plus a glucocorticoid, for instance, have marked effects on lipolysis, and it has been suggested [63, 64] that these hormones are acting to increase the amount of adenyl cyclase in the fat-cell membrane. Such a contention is supported by the observation that inhibitors of protein synthesis abolish the effects of these hormones [63]. Additionally Krishna *et al.* [65] and Goodman [63] have presented evidence that thyroid hormone increases the lipolytic potential of adipose tissue, but apparently in a manner independent of the protein synthetic mechanism of the cell.

Another topic of great current interest is the site of action of cyclic AMP. The preceding discussion has dwelt primarily on the synthesis and degradation of cyclic AMP and the end result of changes in its intracellular concentration, with little attention paid to the intervening events. In 1968, Walsh *et al.* [66] reported that the site of action of cyclic AMP in phosphorylase activation was not at phosphorylase *b* kinase, but, rather, that cyclic AMP activated another protein kinase which phosphorylated phosphorylase *b* kinase at the expense of the terminal phosphate of ATP. It has subsequently been shown that many tissues have cyclic AMP-dependent protein kinases [67, 68]. Indeed activation of adipose tissue lipase can be accomplished by purified protein kinases from skeletal muscle [69, 70].

The relationship of the protein kinases to the overall scheme of cyclic AMP metabolism and to the physiological response is illustrated in Fig. 1. There is currently some speculation that the *only* action cyclic AMP has in effector response patterns is to activate protein kinases. Nevertheless, this has not yet been shown to be the case experimentally, and so Fig. 1 also shows a bypass of protein kinases to illustrate those instances in which cyclic AMP may affect responsive systems other than by activation of protein kinase.

Thus there appears to be a great deal of similarity amongst different tissues as to the site of action of cyclic AMP, as illustrated by the wide distribution of cyclic AMP-dependent protein kinases. If it does develop that all effects of cyclic AMP are mediated through protein kinases, our view of the nucleotide will have to change from thinking of it as an agent which has a multitude of actions to viewing it as having the role of activating specific protein kinases.

The second messenger system and drug therapy

We have now seen that the rate of lipolysis in adipose tissue is controlled by intracellular cyclic AMP levels, and that in turn the cyclic AMP levels are controlled by a number of factors both within and without the cell. It must be emphasized here that adipose tissue was used as an example merely because so much information is available. It seems probable that all tissues which respond to hormones *via* the second messenger system have equally complex characteristics.

What, then, are the possibilities for the pharmacological exploitation of the second messenger system on the basis of the generalized understanding we have of it? It has been pointed out earlier [71] that there are three major avenues of approach which can be considered for thereapeutic intervention in the second messenger system: (*a*) at the level of adenyl cyclase; (*b*) at the level of phosphodiesterase; and (*c*) by circumventing both adenyl cyclase and phosphodiesterase and instead mimicking or inhibiting the action of cyclic AMP.

The nature of adenyl cyclase—particularly the selectivity of its activation process as determined by specific hormone receptor moieties—makes it an outstanding candidate as a point of therapeutic intervention, and there are potentially several circumstances under which one would like to alter the activity of the enzyme. These would include what one might call direct lesions of the second messenger system, in which part of this system *per se* is faulty, and indirect lesions, in which factors normally impinging on the second messenger system become deranged. The ACTH-insensitive adreno-cortical tumor of Ney *et al.* [39] discussed above illustrates what we may call a direct lesion, while a disease such as hyperparathyroidism [72] illustrates an indirect lesion.

Obviously, methods for controlling direct and indirect derange-ments of the second messenger system might be quite different. In a direct disorder where, for example, an adenyl cyclase appears to be insensitive to a hormone which normally activates it, one would like to have an agent available which could replace the hormone, perhaps by acting at the catalytic subunit rather than at a faulty regulatory subunit. Such an effect, of course, would have to be elicited in a highly tissue-specific manner, for administration of an agent which generally increased adenyl cyclase activity would precipitate an endocrine crisis. On the other hand, in a disorder such as hyperparathyroidism, where adenyl cyclase activity in responsive tissues is always high because of constant hormonal stimulation, one might seek an analogue of parathyroid hormone which, though inactive in stimulating the cyclase, nevertheless competes with the hormone for binding sites on the regulatory subunit. The converse of this latter type of treatment for lesions of the second messenger system is extensively used today in the form of the hormone replacement therapy.

There are some drugs currently available which affect the activity of adenyl cyclase, at least insofar as its activity is coupled to α- and β-adrenergic receptors. Additionally, there are catecholamine deriva-tives, such as isoproterenol, which appear to be relatively specific for β receptors, rather than affecting both α and β receptors, as frequently seems to be the case with the naturally occurring catecholamines. With these drugs, we have the ability to either increase or decrease intracellular levels of cyclic AMP by affecting adenyl cyclase activity in tissues with adrenergic innervation. However, both the adrenergic receptor antagonists and the catechol-amine derivatives have the distinct disadvantage of lacking any specificity for a particular target organ. The β-adrenergic antagonists provide a good illustration of this. Certainly they are quite effective in inhibiting lipolysis, for example, but their action is not limited to adipose tissue, and all β-adrenergic receptors in the organism are presumably affected to some degree by administration of a dose of such an agent.

A second site at which it is possible to affect the second messenger system is the phosphodiesterase. In a way, successful therapeutic intervention at this level would seem to be even more difficult to achieve than at the level of adenyl cyclase, if only because the activities of phosphodiesterases of different tissues are not yet known to be affected by specific inhibitory or stimulatory agents as is the case with adenyl cyclase. Insulin may be an exception to this [28], but because of its other hormonal activities it is an unlikely candidate as a therapeutic activator of phosphodiesterase. The methyl xanthines apparently have little or no tissue specificity, and so are of doubtful promise as selective phosphodiesterase inhibitors. Imidazole will stimulate phosphodiesterase activity [20] in cell-free preparations, but it would probably do so indiscriminately if it acted in intact cells.

A third point at which drug therapy can be aimed is the actual site of action of cyclic AMP. In a sense, this type of intervention has been successfully executed experimentally *in vitro* innumerable times by use of derivatives of cyclic AMP which mimic its effects. As discussed above, this site of action is in many cases a cyclic AMP-dependent protein kinase, and thus presumably any agent which could activate the kinase would serve the function of cyclic AMP. Conversely, any agent which would affect a protein kinase in such a way as to make it insensitive to cyclic AMP would block the action of the second messenger, and there is a suggestion that such an agent may be formed biologically [73]. It should also be noted that a protein inhibitor of cyclic AMP-dependent protein kinase has also been reported [74]. However, as was the case with agents which affect adenyl cyclase or phosphodiesterase, specificity of the desired effect is again the major problem with drugs intended to affect the protein kinases. This would presumably also be the case with drugs designed to affect the action of cyclic AMP-dependent protein kinases on the particular proteins whose activity they in turn govern.

It would seem that if we are to be able, some day, to control in a specific manner disease processes which may involve cyclic AMP, a necessary approach for the pharmacologist must be to attempt to achieve some degree of tissue specificity in the drugs he devises. In this light perhaps we should not dismiss papaverine out of hand, if only for the lesson it may teach us. And that is that even though the second messenger system itself may be ubiquitous in nature, and thus appear to be largely refractory to successful therapeutic intervention, there are so many other striking differences between cells of various types that the exploitation of these differences by the pharmacologist may eventually lead us to a rational therapeutic approach to metabolic lesions involving the second messenger system.

References

1. Rall, T. W., Sutherland, E. W. and Berthet, J.; *J. biol. Chem.*; **224**, (1957) 463.
2. Rall, T. W. and Sutherland, E. W.; *J. biol. Chem.*; **232**, (1958) 1065.
3. Sutherland, E. W. and Rall, T. W.; *J. biol. Chem.*; **232**, (1958) 1077.
4. Cook, W. H., Lipkin, D. and Markham, R.; *J. Am. Chem. Soc.*; **79**, (1957) 3607.
5. Haynes, R. D., Jr., Sutherland, E. W. and Rall, T. W.; *Recent Progress in Hormone Research*; **16**, (1960) 121.
6. Sutherland, E. W. and Rall, T. W.; *Pharmacol. Rev.*; **12**, (1960) 265.
7. Butcher, R. W., Robison, G. A., Hardman, J. G. and Sutherland, E. W.; *Advances Enz. Reg.*; **6**, (1968) 357.
8. Sutherland, E. W.; *J. Am. med. Ass.*; **214**, (1970) 1281.
9. 'Role of Cyclic AMP in Cell Function'; Eds Greengard, P. and Costa, E. *Advances in Biochem. Psychopharmacol.*; **3**, (1970).
10. Robison, G. A., Sutherland, E. W. and Butcher, R. W.; *Cyclic AMP*; Academic Press, New York, (1971).
11. Sutherland, E. W., Rall, T. W. and Menon, T.; *J. biol. Chem.*; **247**, (1962) 1220.
12. Rall, T. W. and Sutherland, E. W.; *J. biol. Chem.*; **237**, (1962) 1228.
13. Murad, F., Chi, Y.-M., Rall, T. W. and Sutherland, E. W.; *J. biol. Chem.*; **237**, (1962) 1233.
14. Klainer, L. M., Chi, Y.-M., Friedberg, S. L., Rall, T. W. and Sutherland, E. W.; *J. biol. Chem.*; **237**, (1962) 1239.
15. Sutherland, E. W., Jr. and Davoren, P.; In: *Biochemical Aspects of Hormone Action*; Ed. A. B. Eisenstein. Little, Brown and Co., Inc., Boston, (1964) p. 149.
16. Robison, G. A., Butcher, R. W. and Sutherland, E. W.; In: *Fundamental Concepts in Drug-Receptor Interactions*; Ed. D. J. Triggle. Academic Press, New York, (1970) p. 59.
17. Hirata, M. and Hayaishi, O.; *Biochim. biophys. Acta*; **149**, (1967) 1.
18. Rabinowitz, M., De Salles, L., Meisler, J. and Lorand, L.; *Biochim. biophys. Acta*; **97**, (1965) 29.
19. Cheung, W. Y.; *Biochemistry*; **6**, (1967) 1079.
20. Butcher, R. W. and Sutherland, E. W.; *J. biol. Chem.*; **237**, (1962) 1244.
21. De Robertis, E., Arnaiz, G. R. D. L., Alberici, M., Butcher, R. W. and Sutherland, E. W.; *J. biol. Chem.*; **242**, (1967) 3487.
22. Chang, Y. Y.; *Science*; **160**, (1968) 1.
23. Menahan, L. A., Hepp, K. D. and Wieland, O.; *Eur. J. Biochem.*; **8**, (1969) 435.
24. Cheung, W. Y.; *Anal. Biochem.*; **28**, (1969) 182.

25. Cheung, W. Y.; In: 'Role of Cyclic AMP in Cell Function'; Eds P. Greengard and E. Costa. *Advances in Biochem. Psychopharmacol.*; **3**, (1970) p. 51.
26. Brooker, G., Thomas, L. J., Jr. and Appleman, M. M.; *Biochemistry*; **7**, (1968) 4177.
27. Loten, E. G.; *Proc. Univ. Otago Med. Sch.*; **48**, (1970) 44.
28. Loten, E. G. and Sneyd, J. G. T.; *Biochem. J.*; **120**, (1970) 187.
29. Jard, S. and Bernard, M.; *Biochem. biophys. Res. Commun.*; **41**, (1970) 781.
30. Thompson, W. J. and Appleman, M. M.; *Biochemistry*; **10**, (1971) 311.
31. Rall, T. W. and Sattin, A.; In: 'Role of Cyclic AMP in Cell Function'; Eds P. Greengard and E. Costa. *Advances in Biochem. Psychopharmacol.*; **3**, (1970) p. 113.
32. Butcher, R. W., Sneyd, J. G. T., Park, C. R. and Sutherland, E. W., Jr.; *J. biol. Chem.*; **241**, (1966) 1652.
33. Cheung, W. Y.; *Biochem. biophys. Res. Commun.*; **23**, (1966) 214.
34. Rall, T. W. and Sutherland, E. W.; *Cold Spring Harb. Symp. quant. Biol.*; **26**, (1961) 347.
35. Sutherland, E. W., Oye, I. and Butcher, R. W.; *Recent Prog. Horm. Res.*; **21**, (1965) 623.
36. Vaughan, M. and Steinberg, D.; *J. Lipid Res.*; **4**, (1963) 193.
37. Butcher, R. W., Ho, R. J., Meng, H. C. and Sutherland, E. W.; *J. biol. Chem.*; **240**, (1965) 4515.
38. Butcher, R. W., Baird, C. E. and Sutherland, E. W.; *J. biol. Chem.*; **243**, (1968) 1705.
39. Ney, R. L., Hochella, N. J., Grahame-Smith, D. G., Dexter, R. N. and Butcher, R. W.; *J. clin. Invest.*; **48**, (1969) 1773.
40. Posternak, T., Sutherland, E. W. and Henion, W. F.; *Biochim. biophys. Acta*; **65**, (1962) 558.
41. Vaughan, M.; *J. biol. Chem.*; **235**, (1960) 3049.
42. Rizack, M. A.; *J. biol. Chem.*; **239**, (1964) 392.
43. Carlson, L. A., Butcher, R. W. and Micheli, H.; *Acta Med. Scand.*; **187**, (1970) 525.
44. Braun, T. and Hechter, O.; In: 'Adipose Tissue: Regulation and Metabolic Functions'; Eds B. Jeanrenaud and D. Hepp. Acadamic Press, New York, (1970) p. 11.
45. Gordon, R. S. and Cherkes, A.; *Proc. Soc. Exptl. Biol. Med.*; **97**, (1958) 150.
46. Jungas, R. L. and Ball, E. G.; *Biochemistry*; **2**, (1963) 383.
47. Steinberg, D., Vaughan, M., Nestel, P. J., Strand, O. and Bergstrom, S.; *J. Clin. Invest.*; **43**, (1964) 1553.
48. Butcher, R. W. and Baird, C. E.; *J. biol. Chem.*; **243**, (1968) 1713.
49. Butcher, R. W. and Baird, C. E.; *Proc. IVth Internatl. Cong. Pharmacol.*; **4**. Schwabe and Co., Basel, (1970) p. 42.
50. Butcher, R. W.; In: 'Role of Cyclic AMP in Cell Function'; Eds P. Greengard and E. Costa. *Advances in Biochem. Psychopharmacol.*; **3**, (1970) p. 173.
51. Robison, G. A., Butcher, R. W. and Sutherland, E. W.; *Ann. N.Y. Acad. Sci.*; **139**, (1967) 703.
52. Robison, G. A. and Sutherland, E. W.; *Circulation Res.* (Supplement I); **26** and **27**, (1970) I-147.
53. Steinberg, D. and Vaughan, M.; In: 'Proceedings of the Second Nobel Symposium'; Eds S. Bergstrom and B. Samuelsson. Interscience, New York, (1966) p. 109.

54. Beavo, J. A., Rogers, N. L., Crofford, O. B., Hardman, J. G., Sutherland, E. W. and Newman, E. V.; *Molec. Pharmacol.*; **6**, (1970) 597.
55. Triner, L., Vulliemoz, Y., Schwartz, I. and Nahas, G. G.; *Biochem. biophys. Res. Commun.*; **40**, (1970) 64.
56. Triner, L., Overweg, N. I. A. and Nahas, G. G.; *Nature Lond.*; **225**, (1970) 282.
57. Beavo, J. A., Rogers, N. L., Crofford, P. B., Baird, C. E., Hardman, J. G., Sutherland, E. W. and Newman, E. V.; *Ann. New York Acad. Sci.*; In press.
58. Carlson, L. A. and Bally, P. R.; In: 'Handbook of Physiology'. Section 5, Adipose Tissue; Eds A. E. Renold and G. F. Cahill, Jr. Am. Physiol. Soc.; Washington, (1965) p. 557.
59. Butcher, R. W.; In: 'Proceedings of Nicotinic Acid Workshop'; Flims, Switzerland. Ed. K. F. Gey. Huber Publ., Berne, 1970.
60. Schwabe, U. and Ebert, R.; *Arch. Pharmakol. Exp. Pathol.*; **263**, (1969) 251.
61. Westermann, E. and Stock, K.; In: 'Adipose Tissue: Regulation and Metabolic Functions'; Eds B. Jeanrenaud and D. Hepp. Academic Press, New York, (1970) p. 47.
62. Butcher, R. W. and Jasnos, J.; Unpublished observations.
63. Goodman, H. M.; *Endocrinol.*; **86**, (1970) 1064.
64. Moskowitz, J. and Fain, J. N.; *J. biol. Chem.*; **245**, (1970) 1101.
65. Krishna, G., Hynie, S. and Brodie. B. B.; *Proc. Nat. Acad. Sci. U.S.A.*; **59**, (1968) 884.
66. Walsh, D. A., Perkins, J. P. and Krebs, E. G.; *J. biol. Chem.*; **243**, (1968) 3763.
67. Walsh, D. A., Krebs, E. G., Reimann, E. M., Brostrom, M. A., Corbin, J. D., Hickenbottom, J. P., Soderling, T. R. and Perkins, J. P.; In: 'Role of Cyclic AMP in Cell Function'; Eds P. Greengard and E. Costa. *Advances in Biochem. Psychopharmacol.*; **3**, (1970) p. 265.
68. Kuo, J. F. and Greengard, P.; *Proc. Nat. Acad. Sci. U.S.A.*; **64**, (1969) 1349.
69. Corbin, J. D., Reimann, E. M., Walsh, D. A. and Krebs, E. G.; *J. biol. Chem.*; **245**, (1970) 4849.
70. Huttunen, J. K., Steinberg, D. and Mayer, S. E.; *Proc. Nat. Acad. Sci. U.S.A.*; **67**, (1970) 290.
71. Sutherland, E. W., Robison, G. A. and Butcher, R. W.; *Circulation*; **37**, (1968) 279.
72. Chase, L. R. and Aurbach, G. D.; *Proc. Nat. Acad. Sci. U.S.A.*; **58**, (1967) 518.
73. Murad, F., Rall, T. W. and Vaughan, M.; *Biochim. biophys. Acta*; **192**, (1969) 430.
74. Posner, J. B., Hammermeister, K. E., Bratvold, G. E. and Krebs, E. G.; *Biochemistry*; **3**, (1964) 1040.
75. Butcher, R. W. and Baird, C. E.; In: 'Drugs Affecting Lipid Metabolism'; Eds W. L. Holmes, L. A. Carlson and R. Paoletti. Plenum Publ. Corp., New York, (1969) p. 5.
76. Hittelman, K. J. and Butcher, R. W.; Unpublished observations.
77. Butcher, R. W. and Carlson, L. A.; *Acta physiol. scand.*; **79**, (1970) 559.
78. Grahame-Smith, D. G., Butcher, R. W., Ney, R. L. and Sutherland, E. W.; *J. biol. Chem.*; **242**, (1967) 5535.
79. Fleischer, N., Donald, R. A. and Butcher, R. W.; *Am. J. Physiol.*; **217**, (1969) 1287.

80. Zor, U., Keneko, T., Schneidner, H. P. G., McCann, S. M., Lowe, I. P., Bloom, G., Borland, B. and Field, J. B.; *Proc. Nat. Acad. Sci. U.S.A.*; **63**, (1969) 918.

81. Chase, L. R., Fedak, S. A. and Aurbach, G. D.; *Endocrinol.*; **84**, (1969) 761.

82. Namm, D. H. and Mayer, S. E.; *Molec. Pharmacol.*; **4**, (1968) 61.

83. Brown, E., Clarke, D. L., Roux, U. and Sherman, G. H.; *J. biol. Chem.*; **238**, (1963) 852.

84. Jefferson, L. S., Exton, J. H., Butcher, R. W., Sutherland, E. W. and Park, C. R.; *J. biol. Chem.*; **243**, (1968) 1031.

85. Marsh, J. M., Butcher, R. W., Savard, K. and Sutherland, E. W.; *J. biol. Chem.*; **241**, (1966) 5436.

86. Turtle, J. R. and Kipnis, D. M.; *Biochem. biophys. Res. Commun.*; **28**, (1967) 797.

87. Robison, G. A., Arnold, A. and Hartmann, R. C.; *Pharmacol. Res. Commun.*; **1**, (1969) 325.

88. Posner, J. B., Stern, R. and Krebs, E. G.; *J. biol. Chem.*; **240**, (1965) 982.

89. Abe, K., Robison, G. A., Liddle, G. W., Butcher, R. W., Nicholson, W. E. and Baird, C. E.; *Endocrinol.*; **85**, (1969) 674.

90. Bueding, E., Bülbring, E., Gercken, G., Hawkins, J. T. and Kuriyama, H.; *J. Physiol. (London)*; **193**, (1967) 187.

91. Butcher, R. W., Baird, C. E. and Sutherland, E. W.; Unpublished observations.

92. Mayer, S. E., Namm, D. H. and Rice, L.; *Circulation Res.*; **26**, (1970) 225.

93. Robison, G. A., Butcher, R. W., Oye, I., Morgan, H. E. and Sutherland, E. W.; *Molec. Pharmacol.*; **1**, (1965) 168.

94. Hammermeister, K. E., Yunis, A. A. and Krebs, E. G.; *J. biol. Chem.*; **240**, (1965) 986.

95. Bueding, E., Butcher, R. W., Hawkins, J., Timms, A. R. and Sutherland, E. W.; *Biochim. biophys. Acta*; **115**, (1966) 173.

THE EFFECT OF CYCLIC AMP ON MEMBRANE-BOUND PROTEIN-KINASES AND PHOSPHATASES IN MAMMALIAN TISSUES

R. Rodnight and M. Weller

Department of Biochemistry, Institute of Psychiatry,
British Postgraduate Medical Federation,
University of London

Abbreviations: Cyclic AMP = Adenosine, $3'5'$ (cyclic) mono-phosphate. ATPase = Adenosine triphosphatase.

Protein kinases, activated by cyclic AMP, occur in several locations in the mammalian cell. They mediate the transfer of the γ-phosphoryl group of ATP to serine hydroxyl groups in cellular proteins which may or may not be enzymes. The most widely investigated kinase of this nature is that involved in the control of glycogen metabolism [1] and in this case, the acceptors are enzymes. In the nucleus non-enzymic proteins, including histones, have been identified as acceptors for the nuclear protein kinase [2]. Protein kinase-like activity also occurs in cell membrane fragments [3] and in neurotubular sub-units [4] but in these latter two cases the nature of the acceptor proteins are unknown. In the cytoplasm, nucleus and probably in the membrane, protein phosphatases occur in close association with the kinases and their acceptors [1, 5, 6]. These and other macromolecular complexes involved in protein phosphorylation and dephosphorylation may prove to be of fundamental importance in regulating a variety of cellular processes.

The coupled action of protein kinases and phosphatases on intracellular proteins is probably mainly responsible for the slow, but steady, turnover of protein-bound phosphorylserine which can be demonstrated in a variety of tissues by isotopic methods both *in vivo* and *in vitro* [7, 8]. In respiring slices of cerebral cortex, this turnover has the distinctive feature that under suitable conditions its rate can be increased by depolarization of the tissue by brief application of electrical pulses, an observation first made by Heald [9] using techniques developed by McIlwain [10] and since confirmed in a number of subsequent studies in this (Table 1) and other laboratories [14]. It is of particular interest that the increase in turnover appears to be confined to subcellular fractions of the tissue derived from the cell membrane [11], suggesting a special role for a membrane-bound phosphoprotein in the events accompanying depolarization and the restoration of neuronal excitability.

These observations in a cell-containing system prompted a study of protein phosphorylation in membrane fragments of neuronal origin using $[\gamma^{32}P]ATP$ as precursor, as a result of which we were able to demonstrate the presence in the membrane of intrinsic protein kinase activity, later shown to be stimulated by cyclic AMP [3, 15]. A possible link between these observations in membrane fragments and those in the intact tissue is provided by the discovery of Kakiuchi, Rall and McIlwain [16] that depolarization of brain slices, by similar methods to those found to increase phosphoprotein turnover, results in a striking increase in the intracellular concentration of cyclic AMP in the tissue. The increased turnover could therefore be secondary to the release of cyclic AMP. Thus it is reasonable to postulate that cyclic AMP, as well as acting as an intracellular messenger, may also be concerned in regulating the phosphorylation of a membrane protein (or proteins) involved in neuronal function.

At present there is very little, if any, evidence to suggest what functions of the membrane are likely to be mediated or controlled by cyclic AMP-regulated protein phosphorylation. We need to know more of the complexity of the phosphorylating system, the nature of its activation by cyclic AMP and of the physiological and pharmacological factors which may modify it. The present paper reports a little progress along this road, but leaves the major questions still unanswered. In passing it may be noted that the membrane-located phosphorylating system is tightly bound to the membrane structure and has yet to be successfully dissociated into its components or indeed from the bulk of the insoluble membrane proteins [6]. By contrast, the cytoplasmic and nuclear protein

Table 1

The Effect of Electrical Pulses on Phosphoprotein Labelling in Brain Slices

Ref.		N	Labelling of phosphoprotein ±S.E.M.			P
			Without pulses	With pulses	Percent change	
[9]	c.p.m./µg alkali labile P / c.p.m./µg Pi in medium	8	41	56	+37	<0.01
[11]	d.p.m. × 10^{-2}/µmol phosphorylserine P	7	57 ± 6.1	74 ± 6.4	+30	<0.01
[12]	d.p.m. × 10^{-2}/µmol phosphorylserine P	6	256 ± 21	304 ± 25	+19	<0.01
[13]	c.p.m. in alkali labile P / c.p.m. in acid soluble P	16	10.8 ± 0.6	13.0 ± 0.8	+23	<0.0025
	As above, without ouabain	9	10.8 ± 0.3	12.6 ± 0.4	+17	<0.05
	As above, with 10 µM ouabain	9	11.3 ± 0.3	13.0 ± 0.4	+16	<0.05
[13]	d.p.m./µmol phosphorylserine P / d.p.m./µmol and soluble P	16	0.172 ± 0.01	0.202 ± 0.01	+18	<0.05

All results refer to slices of guinea pig cerebral cortex respiring in oxygenated salines and stimulated according to ref. [9].

kinase-phosphatase systems may be readily extracted from the tissue in a soluble form, thus facilitating purification and study of their components.

The methods we have used in this work are described in detail elsewhere. Briefly, preparations rich in fragments of the neuronal membrane were made from crude ox-brain microsomes [17] or synaptosomes [18] and enzyme activities measured as given in [3] and [6]. The latter involves the isolation by electrophoresis of [^{32}P] phosphorylserine from acid hydrolysates of labelled membrane protein and determination of its radioactivity by standard procedures. From the specific radioactivity of the [^{32}P] ATP used the rate of phosphorylation can be calculated. This method is reasonably specific and accurate, but only recovers about 50% of the total protein-bound phosphorylserine in the membrane; the values quoted for kinase activity have not been corrected for these losses.

Demonstration of an intrinsic turnover of protein-bound phosphorylserine in membrane fragments

It was important to investigate this aspect of the problem first, since, in contrast to the clear evidence in cell-containing systems, there was no evidence from the initial study of membrane fragments [15] that the ^{32}P incorporated into membrane protein was actually turning over. In theory, therefore, the observed transfer could have been due entirely to a rephosphorylation of serine hydroxyl groups, which had become dephosphorylated by protein phosphatases from other parts of the cell during subcellular fractionation, or possibly to an exchange reaction. Later research [6] has indicated that both rephosphorylation of vacant sites and genuine turnover are involved, and that turnover arises, as suspected, from intrinsic phosphatase activity, which is also tightly bound to the membrane and associated with the same acceptor protein as the kinase. This has been shown in two ways:

First, using the alkali-labile phosphate content of the membrane protein as a measure of protein-bound phosphorylserine (see ref. [8] for a justification of this assumption), a small net transfer of phosphate from ATP to membrane protein could be demonstrated. Quantitatively, however, this net transfer was only about 50% of the amount of ^{32}P transferred to the alkali-labile phosphate fraction with [^{32}P] ATP as the phosphorylating agent. On incubation of the membrane fragments without ATP but otherwise under identical conditions, a net loss of alkali-labile phosphate was observed which was apparently enzymically mediated and just accounted for the discrepancy in the two values for kinase activity. Second, labelled membrane preparations washed free of excess [^{32}P] ATP, on reincubation at physiological pH were found to release ^{32}P from [^{32}P] phosphorylserine in a time- and Mg^{2+}-dependent reaction which was abolished by denaturing the membrane protein.

In the subcellular system we are studying, intrinsic phosphatase activity is clearly the rate-limiting step in the turnover of protein-bound phosphorylserine, otherwise little incorporation of ^{32}P would be expected. This accounts, in part at least, for the curvilinear shape of the time course of phosphorylation noted in the previous work [8, 15, 19] (Fig. 1a). It seems that during the first few minutes of the reaction, phosphorylation of vacant serine hydroxyl groups is occurring, but as the membrane protein approaches the fully phosphorylated state, transfer becomes increasingly dependent on the rate at which protein phosphatase activity is dephosphorylating sites which are already phosphorylated. This interpretation is particularly well supported by the observation [6] that after preincubation of the membrane fragments with non-radioactive ATP for short periods of time so as to phosphorylate the vacant sites, the labelling of protein from [^{32}P] ATP follows a linear time course at about half the initial rate observed in the untreated preparation (Fig. 1b).

Protein phosphatase activity in the membrane fragments is inhibited by univalent cations [6]. It is interesting that in the case of Na^+ and K^+ there is a marked difference in the dependence of the inhibition on cation concentration in the range 10-100 mM: the slope is much steeper with Na^+ than with K^+, although at 10 mM-concentration, K^+ is the more potent inhibitor. Phosphatase activity is also inhibited by theophylline (K_i about 10 mM) and by a relatively high concentration of cyclic AMP (0.6 mM), but not by 5'-AMP. Mn^{2+}, but not Ca^{2+}, stimulates the activity.

Since the phosphatase activity is rate-limiting, the inhibition of ^{32}P incorporation by the chlorides of univalent cations (see ref. [15, 19] and Fig 1a) needs re-appraising. Assuming that ^{32}P-incorporation, over the first minute of incubation, approximates to the potential rate of the kinase reaction, the major action of Na^+ appears to be on the phosphatase enzyme since it gives hardly any inhibition of labelling until after incubation for 3 min; K^+, on the other hand, inhibits kinase activity to some extent, even at 10 mM. This effect is increased threefold in the presence of cyclic AMP. LiCl (at 100 mM) inhibits both enzyme activities to a greater extent than either Na^+ or K^+.

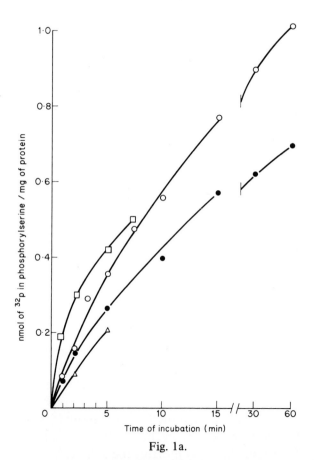

Fig. 1a.

Fig. 1. Time course of phosphorylation of membrane protein by the intrinsic kinase system in tris buffer at pH 7.4 and 20°C with 1 mM [^{32}P] MgATP. *a*. Untreated preparations with various additions (for details see [3, 6, 19]). ○, control with no addition; ●, with 100 mM NaCl; △, with 100 mM KCl; □, with 100 μM cyclic AMP. *b*. Before and after treatment with unlabelled MgATP (1 mM) for 10 min [6]. ○, before treatment; ● after treatment.

Action of cyclic AMP on the labelling of protein in membrane fragments

Is the stimulation of the phosphorylation of membrane protein by cyclic AMP in broken-cell preparations likely to be of physiological significance in the intact cell, or is it a pharmacological curiosity?

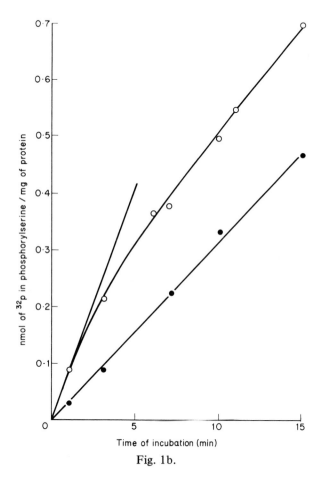

Time of incubation (min)

Fig. 1b.

The doubt arises because of the relatively small magnitude of the effect and its rapid decline as phosphorylation proceeds. For example, in the original report [3] stimulation was approximately twofold after incubation for 1 min, but hardly evident after 7 min (Fig. 1a). This pattern has now been confirmed in a number of different preparations. For instance, in comparison to the effect of the cyclic nucleotide on the soluble protein kinase in brain studied by Miyamoto, Kuo and Greengard [20], (which is virtually cyclic AMP dependent) the effect on the membrane-bound system is much less impressive. On the other hand, the concentration of cyclic AMP required for maximal stimulation in the membrane system is only 10 μM and some effect is observed at 0.02 μM (Fig. 2), indicating a similar sensitivity to that reported for other more extensively studied protein kinases. In discussing this question it will be convenient to

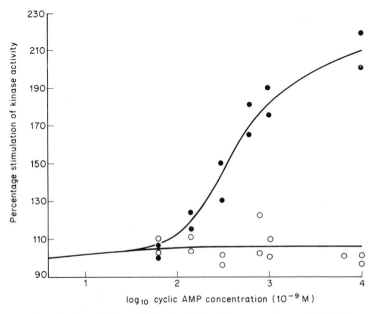

Fig. 2. Sensitivity of the intrinsic kinase system at 20°C to cyclic AMP (●) and N^6-2^1-O-dibutyryl cyclic AMP (○).

consider the two features of the stimulated time course separately: first, the magnitude of the stimulation over the first minute or so of incubation, and second, the rapid decline of the effect with time.

Relevant to the first point is the question as to whether the observed transfer of ^{32}P to membrane protein is the result of phosphorylation of intrinsic protein by one or more protein kinases in the membrane fragments. If the latter is the case, the extra activity observed in the presence of cyclic AMP may be due to activation of another distinct kinase rather than a stimulation of the basal activity. It is admittedly difficult at this stage to exclude entirely heterogeneity in the activity we measure, since the membrane fragments contain a variety of enzymes utilizing ATP as a substrate and are to some extent derived from more than one cell type. Moreover, the preparations do contain a protein kinase which is capable of phosphorylating added phosvitin and which is not stimulated by cyclic [21], although unlike the intrinsic system this enzyme is readily easily dissociated from the membrane [22]. There are, however, some cogent reasons for accepting, as a working hypothesis, that the major part of the phosphorylating activity observed both with and without cyclic AMP is the result of a single system. Cellular heterogeneity can be reasonably discounted since the preparations of synaptosome membranes [18], which have been used for the majority of the experiments, are relatively low in fragments of glial membranes and the endoplasmic reticulum. The pH optima of the stimulated and unstimulated activities, as well as their dependence on Mg^{2+}-concentration, are very similar [21]. Further, by assuming a single system and taking into account the rate-limiting action of the phosphatase enzyme Weller derived a theoretical expression for the time course of phosphorylation which agrees well with the observed time course.

Granted, therefore, that we are probably mainly observing the activity of one kinase system, can we account for the appreciable labelling which occurs in the absence of cyclic AMP? A possible explanation may be that the membrane fragments, which are known to contain adenyl cyclase [23], synthesize enough cyclic AMP to activate the kinase under the incubation conditions used to study protein phosphorylation. Preliminary work has indeed shown that cyclic AMP is formed from the ATP in the reaction mixture concomitantly with the phosphorylation of membrane protein. At 20°C (the temperature at which we normally study protein phosphorylation), the rate is of the order of 1-2 nmol of cyclic AMP/mg of protein/hour in the presence of theophylline and about one-third of that in its absence [21]. It is true that these quantities are only just sufficient to give a medium concentration in the range stimulating the reaction, but it is perhaps reasonable to suggest that the synthesis occurs in the vicinity of the kinase enzyme and that the latter is able to bind and utilize the nucleotide without major release to the medium. Also relevant to this hypothesis is the observation that the membrane preparations may contain very small amounts of bound cyclic AMP. However, treatment of a membrane preparation with phosphodiesterase, while effective in decreasing the initial rate of phosphorylation, also markedly decreased the stimulation given by added cyclic AMP.

The rapid decline in cyclic AMP stimulation with time can be more readily explained than the lack of any obvious dependence on the nucleotide. It is not due to phosphodiesterase activity in the membrane since the fall-off in the effect was not modified by greatly increasing the concentration of cyclic AMP in the medium [3]. Rather it appears to be related to the same factor which determines fall-off in the unstimulated time course, namely the rate-limiting effect of the phosphatase enzyme. This conclusion is well illustrated by the following three observations [21]: (*a*) preincubation of membrane fragments with non-radioactive ATP greatly decreased the stimulation of ^{32}P-incorporation given by cyclic AMP on the subsequent addition of labelled ATP; (*b*) addition of cyclic AMP to the reaction mixture after incubation with ATP for 10 min resulted in no stimulation of phosphorylation over the following minute; and (*c*) preincubation in the absence of ATP for 10 min, with the aim of partially dephosphorylating the membrane protein, greatly increased the stimulation of kinase activity given by cyclic AMP when measured 10 min after the addition of labelled ATP. Presumably in the latter case the rate-limiting action of the phosphatase enzyme was delayed because of the additional time needed to fully re-phosphorylate the acceptor protein.

Other evidence supporting this interpretation of the stimulated time course has come from observations [21] on membrane preparations treated with sodium iodide by a procedure originally introduced by Japanese workers [24] to enhance the activity of the membrane-bound Na^+- and K^+- activated adenosine triphosphatase; this was incidentally found by us [25] to abolish about 90% of the intrinsic protein kinase activity. We now find that the magnitude of the stimulation by cyclic AMP of the residual 10% of the kinase activity in the treated preparations increases instead of decreases with time of incubation. In fact, the stimulated time course is virtually linear over the first 10 min of incubation suggesting that the residual activity over this period involved rephosphorylation of serine hydroxyl without the intervention of phosphatase activity. Consistent with this conclusion, is a preliminary observation that treatment with sodium iodide has an even greater effect in decreasing intrinsic phosphatase activity than kinase activity. The action of sodium iodide is probably to dissociate the complex, but so far it has not proved possible to re-constitute activity by recombination of the various fractions produced by the treatment [6].

The effect of putative transmitters and drugs on protein phosphorylation in membrane fragments

A number of neurohormones and other agents known to stimulate the formation of cyclic AMP in cell-containing preparations from brain [26] have been examined for their possible effects on protein

Table 2
Inhibitory Effect of Some Compounds on Intrinsic Protein Kinase Activity in Membrane Preparations from Brain

Compound	Concentration (mM)	Protein kinase activity at 1 min as percentage of control	
		Cyclic AMP:	
		Absent	Present
Strychnine HCl (N = 6)	1	68 ± 10	59 ± 14
Theophylline	5	53 50 (Duplicates)	55 58 (Duplicates)
Caffeine	20	56 61 (Duplicates)	—
Adenosine	1	33 34 (Duplicates)	—
Adenosine	0.1	87 88 (Duplicates)	—

Kinase activity was determined with and without 100 μM-cyclic AMP by procedures given in [3] and [6].

phosphorylation in the subcellular system [3, 21]. Incorporation of ^{32}P over the first minute of the reaction was taken as a measure of the kinase activity sensitive to cyclic AMP. The substances tested included catecholamines, serotonin, acetylcholine, histamine, insulin, thyroxine, prostaglandins and the tris salts of γ-aminobutyric, glutamic, aspartic and cysteic acids. None of these compounds showed any significant effect in stimulating phosphorylation, either in the presence or absence of theophylline. This was not altogether surprising since other workers [27] have noted the relative insensitivity to activation by such agents, of adenyl cyclase activity in broken-cell preparations from brain.

The intrinsic kinase system in membrane fragments has also been found to be relatively unaffected by the inclusion of a variety of centrally acting drugs in the reaction mixture [6], both with and without the addition of cyclic AMP. Compounds giving no significant stimulation or inhibition within the range ±20% (usually at 1 mM-concentration) included several barbiturates, chlorpromazine, amphetamine, morphine, cocaine, procaine, atropine, ouabain, reserpine, desimipramine and ethanol. Kinase activity was, however, consistently inhibited by strychnine hydrochloride (1 mM), theophylline (5 mM), caffeine (20 mM) and adenosine (1 mM) (Table 2). The magnitude of the inhibition given by theophylline (K_i about 5 mM) was very similar to that exhibited by this compound towards the membrane-bound phosphodiesterase which hydrolyzes cyclic AMP. (The soluble diesterase in brain [28] is considerably more sensitive to inhibition by methylxanthines.)

Discussion

Bound protein kinase activity stimulated by cyclic AMP has been found in membrane fragments prepared from non-nervous tissues (Table 3). However, brain yielded the preparations which exhibited the highest rate of transfer. It is noteworthy that, of the two cerebral preparations studied, the microsomes were more active than fragments of synaptosome membranes, an observation which makes it difficult to sustain a unique role for the system in synaptic function. This difference in kinase activity between the two preparations may have a further significance since the synaptosome membranes were richer in Na^+ and K^+ activated ATPase activity than the microsomes. It is therefore difficult to believe that the two activities are necessarily associated in membrane fragments of the same origin. Surprisingly, however, no stimulation by cyclic AMP of kinase activity was observed in a microsomal fraction from skeletal muscle. The fraction was prepared by a procedure [32] which yields a membrane preparation rich in Ca^{2+}-activated ATPase characteristic of the sarcoplasmic reticulum, but lacking the typical Na^+-, K^+-activated ATPase of the sarcolemma. On the other hand, a preparation of sarcoplasmic vesicles from heart muscle [31] exhibited the usual sensitivity to cyclic AMP. In general, all that can be concluded from these comparative observations is that they suggest that membrane-bound, protein kinase activity reflects some

Table 3

Intrinsic Protein Kinase Activity in Membrane Preparations From Different Tissues [21]

Ref.	Source	Kinase activity without cyclic AMP (pmol of ^{32}P in phosphorylserine/ mg of protein) Incubation time		Percent stimulation by 10 μM cyclic AMP Incubation time	
		1 min	10 min	1 min	10 min
	Guinea-pig				
[15]	Brain	185 (Duplicates) 200	598 598	43	0
[29]	Liver	14 (Duplicates) 15	52 45	60	24
[30]	Kidney	25 (Duplicates) 24	108 96	70	20
[31]	Heart	36 (Duplicates) 40	100 93	70	24
[32]	Skeletal muscle	28 (Duplicates) 24	66 80	0	0
	Ox				
[17]	Brain microsomes (N = 7)	76 ± 27	350 ± 90	126 ± 16	16 ± 5
[18]	Synaptosome membranes (N = 9)	62 ± 20	300 ± 95	90 ± 7	9 ± 3

fundamental process of the cell membrane which has special significance in neural tissues.

At one stage, an obvious candidate for this process was indeed the active transport of univalent cations, the rate of which is known to increase concomitantly with the increased turnover of phospho-protein on depolarization of neural tissues with electrical pulses [33]. Moreover in two studies, ouabain, an inhibitor of cation transport was reported [11, 14] to reverse the increased phospho-protein turnover on stimulation. However, using more refined techniques we have recently been unable to substantiate these earlier observations (Table 1). Also there is now a wealth of evidence to discount the hypothesis that a serine hydroxyl group accepts phosphate from ATP as a stage in the hydrolysis of the latter by the Na^+ and K^+-activated ATPase. Further, while it does appear that inhibition of this enzyme system by di-isopropylphosphofluoridate [34] is associated with the phosphorylation of a serine hydroxyl at the active centre there is no evidence that phosphorylation of a serine residue by ATP in some other part of the system plays any part in controlling its activity. For instance, cyclic AMP was not found to have an influence on the Na^+- and K^+-activated hydrolysis of ATP by membrane preparations, nor was any significant labelling of serine found in an acyl-labelled subunit of the enzyme system, isolated from a membrane preparation by gel filtration after incubation with $[^{32}P]$ATP [35, 36].

In the absence of any clear correlation with active transport of cations, it is tempting to postulate that the protein acceptor for kinase activity is not an enzyme but a structural component of the membrane involved in control of the passive permeability of the membrane to cations and water. Relevant to this hypothesis is the work of Orloff and Handler [37] who found that in toad bladder and rabbit renal tubule, increases in permeability to Na^+ and water (induced by vasopressin applied to the mucosal side) appear to be mediated through the release of cyclic AMP. It would be of interest to investigate whether vasopressin in this situation causes an increased turnover of protein-bound phosphorylserine in the mucosal membrane, analogous to the changes occurring on the application of depolarizing pulses to cortical slices from brain. However, there are obvious difficulties in accepting, even as a working hypothesis, the idea that permeability changes are the direct result of changes in the phosphorylated state of a membrane protein. The turnover of protein-bound phosphate in the membrane is very slow (of the order of 5 nmol/mg of protein/hour), whereas the increase in Na^+-permeability associated with depolarization is extremely rapid and in any case does not involve an immediate consumption of energy.

Is it possible that the phosphorylated state of a membrane protein conditions, in some less direct way, the permeability response? Suppose, for example, that the structural integrity and ability of the membrane to alter its permeability on receipt of the appropriate stimulus depends upon the maintenance of a membrane protein in a phosphorylated state. There is in fact circumstantial evidence, from the work of the Cambridge school on the perfused squid axon, suggesting that the permeability response to electrical excitation, while not requiring an immediate consumption of energy, does in the long run depend on a slow metabolic process in the membrane. Baker, Hodgkin and Shaw [38] noted that although axons perfused with salt solutions containing no energy source could conduct impulses for several hours, they eventually became exhausted as the interior of the axon lost K^+ and gained Na^+; however, replacement of the perfusing fluid with fresh solution of the correct K^+ content only led to a partial recovery, suggesting in Caldwell's words 'the exhaustion of a membrane process normally maintained by metabolism in the axoplasm' [39]. It is an intriguing possibility that a failure to maintain protein phosphorylation in the axolemma may be a factor in this loss of responsiveness of the permeability mechanism.

In applying such a hypothesis to the change in phosphoprotein-P turnover induced by electrical stimulation of brain slices we have to consider first, why the response is so relatively rapid (being complete after stimulation for only 5-10 sec) and, secondly, why the turnover rate actually increases. The rapidity may be related to the fact that electrical stimulation under the conditions used, leads within a few seconds to a fairly major disturbance of the balance between energy production and utilization in the slice, due to the greatly increased demands of the sodium pump mechanism; this is seen mainly in a decline in the steady-state concentration of creatine phosphate in the tissue, and although the total ATP-concentration hardly changes it is reasonable to assume that local changes do occur, particularly in the region of the plasma membrane. This departure from steady-state conditions may have secondary consequences for the protein kinase system in the membrane, depleting it of its phosphoryl-donor and leading to a transient dephosphorylation of membrane protein through continuing phosphatase action. The increase in turnover actually observed may then reflect a recovery process aimed at restoring the permeability mechanism by rephosphorylating the membrane protein under the influence of the cyclic AMP released during stimulation.

Implicit in this interpretation are two postulates. First, that during normal cerebral functioning *in vivo* the incessant cycle of increase and decrease in permeability to Na^+ does not involve parallel cyclic changes in the phosphorylated state of the putative membrane protein concerned in the permeability response; under equilibrium conditions the protein remains optimally phosphorylated. Secondly, if equilibrium breaks down and the supply of energy to the membrane is restricted, the needs of the Na^+- and K^+-activated ATPase and adenyl cyclase take priority over those of the protein kinase system. Accurate data for the K_m with respect to ATP concentration for the cyclic AMP-stimulated component of the kinase system are not available, but preliminary observations suggest a value around 0.5 mM. The upper limit of the K_m for the Na^+- and K^+-activated ATPase was recently given as 0.18 mM ATP, but at very low ATP concentrations, a value of 3.3 μM has been quoted [40]. We have observed that at ATP/protein ratios of 25 pmol/μg or less, no detectable transfer of ^{32}P to protein-bound phosphorylserine occurs in membrane fragments, all of the ATP being used by the transport enzyme [17]. Thus, depending upon the extent of the local changes in ATP concentration occurring at the membrane during stimulation it appears possible that the ATP available for the kinase system might become a limiting factor.

In conclusion, the extremely tentative and exploratory nature of these speculations must be stressed. As indicated earlier, we need to know much more about phosphorylated proteins in the membrane generally, and also the nature of such factors as Ca^{2+} and the cyclic nucleotides, which may control the influence the turnover of protein-bound phosphorylserine.

Acknowledgements

We are grateful to the U.S. Public Health Service for financial support (Grant No. NS 05502).

References

1. Holzer, H.; *Adv. Enzymol.*; **32**, (1969) 297.
2. Langan, T. A.; *J. biol. Chem.*; **244**, (1969) 5763.
3. Weller, M. and Rodnight, R.; *Nature, Lond.*; **225**, (1970) 187.
4. Goodman, D. B. P., Rasmussen, H., Di Bella, F. and Guthrow, C. E. Jr.; *Proc. Nat. Acad. Sci. U.S.A.*; **67**, (1970) 652.
5. Meisler, M. H. and Langan, T. A.; *J. biol. Chem.*; **244**, (1969) 4961.
6. Weller, M. and Rodnight, R.; *Biochem. J.*; **124**, (1971) 393.
7. Agren, G.; *Uppsala Universitets Arsskrift.*; **5**, (1958) 5.
8. Rodnight, R.; In: 'Handbook of Neurochemistry'; **5**. Ed. A. Lajtha. Plenum Press, New York, (1971). In Press.
9. Heald, D. J.; *Biochem. J.*; **66**, (1957) 659.
10. McIlwain, H. and Rodnight, R.; 'Practical Neurochemistry'; J. & A. Churchill, London, (1962) 155.
11. Trevor, A. J. and Rodnight, R; *Biochem. J.*; **95**, (1965) 889.
12. Jones, D. A. and Rodnight, R.; *Biochem. J.*; **121**, (1971) 597.
13. Reddington, M. and Rodnight, R.; Unpublished observations.
14. Ahmed, K., Judah, J. D. and Wallgren, H.; *Biochim, biophys. Acta.*; **69**, (1963) 428.
15. Rodnight, R. and Lavin, B. E.; *Biochem. J.*; **101**, (1966) 495.
16. Kakiuchi, S., Rall, T. W. and McIlwain, H.; *J. Neurochem.*; **16**, (1969) 485.
17. Rodnight, R.; *Biochem. J.*; **120**, (1970) 1.
18. Rodnight, R., Weller, M. and Goldfarb, P. S. G.; *J. Neurochem.*; **16**, (1969) 1591.
19. Weller, M.; *M. Phil Thesis*; (1969) London University.
20. Miyamoto, E., Kuo, J. F. and Greengard, P.; *J. biol. Chem.*; **244**, (1969) 6395.
21. Weller, M. and Rodnight, R.; (1971b) Unpublished.
22. Decsi, L. and Rodnight, R.; *J. Neurochem.*; **12**, (1965) 791.
23. DeRobertis, E., Rodriguez de Lovez Arnaiz, G., Alberici, M., Butcher, R. W. and Sutherland, E. W.; *J. biol. Chem.*; **242**, (1967) 3487.
24. Nakao, T., Tashima, K., Nagano, K. and Nakao, M.; *Biochem. biophys. Res. Commun.*; **19**, (1965) 755.
25. Weller, M. and Rodnight, R.; *Biochem. J.*; **111**, (1968) 16P.
26. McIlwain, H.; (1971) This symposium, p. 237.
27. Rall, T. W. and Gilman, A. G.; *Neurosciences Res. Prog. Bull.*; **8**, (1970) 225.
28. Butcher, R. W. and Sutherland, E. W.; *J. biol. Chem.*; **237**, (1962) 1244.
29. Sedgwick, B. and Hubscher, G.; *Biochim. biophys. Acta*; **106**, (1965) 63.
30. Stanbury, J. B., Morris, M. C., Corrigan, H. J. and Larithe, W. E.; *Endocrinology*; **67**, (1960) 353.
31. Fanburgh, B. and Gergly, J.; *J. biol. Chem.*; **240**, (1965) 2721.
32. Rubin, B. and Katz, A.; *Science*; **158**, (1967) 1189.
33. McIlwain, H. and Bachelard, H. S.; In: 'Biochemistry and the Central Nervous System'; 4th Ed. J. & A. Churchill, London, 1971.
34. Bonting, S. L.; In: 'Membranes and Transport' Ed. E. E. Bittar. Wiley-Interscience, London, 1970, p. 343.
35. Alexander, D. R. and Rodnight, R.; *Biochem. J.*; **119**, (1970) 44P.
36. Alexander, D. R.; *Ph.D. Thesis*; London University, (1971).

37. Orloff, J. and Handler, J.; *Am. J. Med.*; **42**, (1967) 757.
38. Baker, P. F., Hodgkin, A. L. and Shaw, T. I.; *J. Physiol.*; **164**, (1962) 330.
39. Caldwell, P. C.; *Physiol. Rev.*; **48**, (1968) 1.
40. Kanazawa, T., Saito, M. and Tomomura, Y.; *J. Biochem. (Tokyo)*; **67**, (1970) 693.

EFFECT OF 3', 5'- CYCLIC AMP ON GENE EXPRESSION IN *ESCHERICHIA COLI*

D. Schlessinger, Y. Ohnishi, M. Kuwano and L. Silengo

Department of Microbiology, Washington University
School of Medicine, St. Louis

Non-standard abbreviation: mRNA = messenger RNA; cAMP = 3',5'-cyclic AMP.
Code number of enzymes: EC 3.2.1.23, β-galactosidase.

The disparity between the known roles of cyclic AMP (cAMP) in bacteria and higher cells has been puzzling. In mammalian cells, as participants of this Symposium have been reminding us, a number of effects are exerted independent of the transcription process, presumably by activating latent enzymatic machinery—or possibly latent messenger RNA. In contrast, for the best characterized systems in bacteria, cyclic AMP helps to determine the repertoire of gene transcription open to the cell [1-5].

The possibility exists that *E. coli* may not always be an adequate model for higher cells, but granted the evidence for some effects of cyclic AMP, independent of transcription in higher cells, there might also be such effects in bacteria.

We have been attempting to estimate, by a genetic approach, the extent of involvement of cyclic AMP in cellular metabolism, and whether any of its function extends beyond the positive initiation of transcription at certain gene loci. Here we report the existence and some properties of bacterial mutants completely dependent on cAMP for growth.

To briefly reiterate the views of the role of cyclic AMP in *E. coli.*: 'catabolite repression', the inhibition of formation of certain messenger RNA species by products of catabolism, is antagonized by cAMP. It is itself required for the induction of a number of dispensible proteins, including flagellin and β-galactosidase.

According to the pre-eminent studies of Pastan and co-workers [1-5] and of Beckwith, Schwartz and Zubay [6, 7], this action is exerted through a complex of a specific receptor protein and the cyclic nucleotide at a site on DNA; the complex potentiates transcription by RNA polymerase from that region. In mutants with a defective receptor protein, little if any β-galactosidase can be induced, and in mutants with low adenyl cyclase levels, fermentation of lactose requires cyclic AMP in the growth medium.

Because mutants that have lost most cyclase activity can grow [8, 9], it has seemed likely that cyclic AMP is only involved in promoting synthesis of 'non-vital' enzymes—i.e., those not critical for general growth processes. However, the 'cyclase-less' mutants were obtained as non-fermenting colonies on indicator agar plates, or as non-motile cells. In other words, these mutants had to grow in absence of cyclic AMP in order to be isolable. Thus, if cyclic AMP were indispensible for growth, these adenyl cyclase mutants would necessarily be leaky or incomplete. Some support for this notion is given by studies of the inducibility of β-galactosidase in a wild-type strain and two standard adenyl cyclase-less strains. In absence of cyclic AMP, neither the mutant GPI [8] nor mutant 5336 [9] can make enough β-galactosidase to grow on lactose. However, both strains show measureable induction of the enzyme in presence of a gratuitous inducer, IPTG (isopropyl-β,D-galactopyranoside). In a series of trials in media containing salts, glycerol and casein hydrolysate, the differential rate of synthesis of enzyme in response to inducer was compared with and without cAMP. In absence of cyclic AMP, the relative level was 2-12% for mutant GPI and 1-2% for 5336 (cf. comparable data for 5336 in ref. [9]). This suggests that these 'cyclase-less' strains may be leaky or otherwise able to maintain a limited level of cytoplasmic cyclic AMP that could support a hypothetical system critically dependent on cAMP.

We have therefore tried to isolate, by screening colonies after mutagenesis, mutants that require cyclic AMP for growth. To increase the likelihood that a mutation would be effective, we started from the two strains with low cyclase level, GPI and 5336.

Cells dependent on 3',5'-cyclic AMP for growth did indeed arise. Their frequency was about 1 in 2000 among survivors of mutagenic treatment, which is typical for mutation of one or a few gene loci in *E. coli.* These mutants cannot grow on any medium tested (agar containing minimal salts, salts fortified with casein hydrolysate, yeast extract, or rich nutrient broth), unless supplemented with 10^{-3} M 3′,5′-cyclic AMP.

Some of the cAMP-requiring (*car*) mutants barely grow in liquid medium, even in presence of cyclic AMP. All are very temperature-sensitive. Here we describe some details, primarily about one of the hardiest, called S107.

The levels of cAMP required by *car* mutants for maximal growth are very high (10^{-3} M). This can be because uptake of cyclic AMP is poor; similar levels are required for maximal induction of β-galacto-sidase in the cyclase-less strain [9]. Alternatively, cAMP might be used as a nutrient by these mutants. It could conceivably provide either 5′-AMP, by phosphodiesterase action, or ribose-5-phosphate, by adenine ribosidase action. Neither AMP nor ribose-5-phosphate can ordinarily enter cells, and a mutant unable to make one of them might accept cAMP instead. However, such a mutant should accept adenine or adenosine instead of 5′-AMP [10], and ribose or ribitol instead of ribose-phosphate [11], using kinases to produce the required compounds. Instead, neither AMP, adenine, adenosine, ribose nor ribitol can replace cAMP for S107.

Furthermore, if dependence and temperature sensitivity are caused by a single mutation (see below), the possibility is remote that nutritional deficiencies are alleviated by cAMP in the dependent mutants, for the mutants are temperature sensitive at 42°C even in presence of the nucleotide. By a similar argument, the mutation is unlikely to be a second, more complete lesion in adenyl cyclase activity.

Genetic analysis of car *strains*

Genetic analysis by P1 phage-mediated transduction shows that the temperature sensitivity and cAMP requirement of S107 are closely linked. The transductions were carried out as follows.

The donor strain was a prototroph; the recipients in various trials were two *car* strains, S106 and S107, which are also adenyl cyclase-less and require methionine, isoleucine-valine, and thiamine. Thus, the crosses are of *ilv*⁺ *adc*⁺ *car*⁺ *thi*⁺ x *ilv adc car thi*. In each case, P1 phage from the donor was mixed with recipient cells [23] and plated on minimal medium containing cAMP, methionine, and thiamine. The transductants therefore are *ilv*⁺. When a total of 400 were analysed, most had also regained adenyl cyclase, since *ilv* and *adc* are closely linked [8]. However, 20% of the transductants could also grow without cAMP and were no longer temperature-sensitive. Thus, the *car* and *adc* alleles are in very near genes.

The genetic analysis by phage-mediated transduction is consistent with the simple notion that *car* strains contain two mutations involved in the phenotype: the adenyl cyclase-less allele and an allele that simultaneously renders the cell temperature-sensitive and cAMP-requiring. However, it is still possible that temperature-sensitivity and cAMP-dependence are caused by two closely-linked mutations. It would be strange for all the three cAMP-dependent strains we have studied, to have picked up an additional, ts-allele; but further experimentation is required to establish definitively whether one or two alleles are involved.

In many transductants, the capacity to ferment lactose and to grow without cAMP (adc^+) had been regained, but the cells were still temperature-sensitive. In support of this, one temperature-sensitive transductant of S107 was analysed in more detail, and was found to be fully inducible for β-galactosidase without an external source of cAMP (i.e., adc^+). But at 42°C, as expected, the strain behaved like S107 grown in presence of cAMP at 42°C; growth and RNA synthesis slowed down, and β-galactosidase remained inducible.

In other words, mutation in *car* strains renders the cells temperature-sensitive and introduces cAMP-dependence in an *adc* strain. Probably *car* strains always require cAMP, but are indifferent to whether their source of cAMP is endogenous (in an adc^+ strain) or exogenous (in a cyclase-less strain).

Growth and RNA metabolism in S107

One might anticipate that a mutant affected in its cyclic AMP requirements would show a lesion in a critical process associated with RNA metabolism. In primary experiments to test this possibility, *car* mutants were examined at 30°C. In presence of cyclic AMP, S107 grew exponentially, as expected (Fig. 1); but when a culture of S107 cells was washed free of cyclic AMP and maintained at 30°C, cells continued to form protein for many hours. The synthesis of RNA also continued. However, after 1 to 4 hours, growth and the accumulation of RNA were linear (for growth, see Fig. 1; for RNA, see below). In other words, the capacity to form new RNA and protein tend to become fixed at the level the cells had achieved in presence of cyclic AMP.

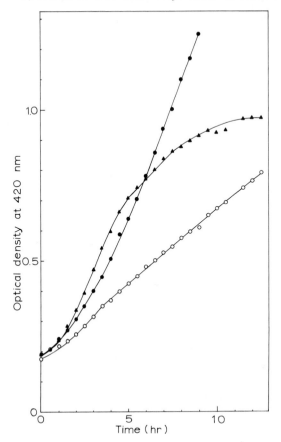

Fig. 1. Growth curve of S107 at 30°C in presence of cAMP, and at 30°C in absence of cAMP. A culture of S107 was grown in glucose minimal salts medium fortified with 0.2% casamino acids and 10^{-3} M cAMP. At about 10^8 cells/ml, 5 ml portions were centrifuged and washed once with medium to remove cAMP. Cells were then suspended in presence (—●—) or absence (—○—) of cAMP at 30°C, or in presence of cAMP at 42°C (—▲—), and growth monitored by increase in optical density.

S107 at high temperature showed a related phenotype, as expected. When the temperature of a culture growing in presence of cyclic AMP was raised to 42°C, the synthesis of RNA continued, but gradually reached a slower, constant rate. At 30°C, pulse-labelling in absence of cAMP similarly became linear. In Fig. 2, this is expressed as a constant level of incorporation in pulse-labelling experiments, compared to the exponentially increasing rate in the cells kept at 30°C with cAMP.

For several reasons it seems that whatever the temperature-sensitive substance in S107 proves to be, it is probably not the cyclic AMP binding protein (CRP [5] or CAP [7] protein) required for the synthesis of β-galactosidase and other catabolite-repressible enzymes.

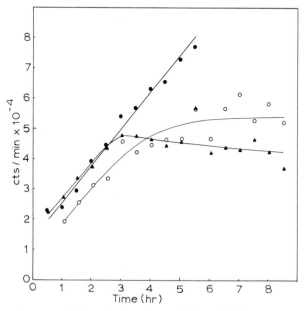

Fig. 2. Rate of RNA synthesis in S107 at 30°C in presence or absence of cyclic AMP, and at 42°C in presence of cAMP. A culture of S107 was washed free of cAMP as in Fig. 1 and grown further at 30°C (—●—) or 42°C (—▲—) in presence of cAMP, or at 30°C in absence of cAMP (—○—). At each indicated time, a 0.2 ml portion of culture was incubated with 0.5 μC (0.01 μg) ^{3}H uracil for 2 min. Each sample was then precipitated with 10% trichloroacetic acid, plated and counted.

First of all, the gene for CRP maps very near the locus for streptomycin resistance in *E. coli* (Pastan, personal communication). However, introduction of streptomycin resistance into S107 by transduction with P1 phage from a streptomycin-resistant donor strain cured none of 20 transductants of S107 of their temperature sensitivity or cAMP dependence. Instead (see above), the *car* allele maps near the *ilv* locus, at a great distance from the streptomycin locus on the *E. coli* chromosome. Secondly, even long after the temperature-sensitive phenotype is expressed at 42°C, in S107, β-galactosidase can be induced. Thus, the CRP protein is apparently intact in S107 by both genetic and biochemical evidence.

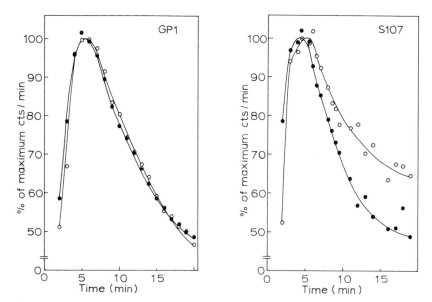

Fig. 3. Formation and breakdown of RNA after rifampicin addition to GPI or S107. For each of four cultures (GPI or S107 incubated 4 hours at 30°C with (—●—) or without (—○—) 10^{-3} M cAMP), RNA was pulse-labelled by addition of ^{3}H uracil as in Fig. 2. At 2 min, 200 μg/ml rifampicin was added to each culture, and acid-insoluble RNA estimated on portions of each culture at the times indicated. At intervals, DNA formation was estimated as alkali-stable cts/min, and amounted to about 5% of the incorporation at 5 min [24]. The values for incorporation into DNA were about the same in the two cultures of GPI and in the two cultures of S107, and have been subtracted from the plotted data. The maximum incorporation in each culture was greater than 3000 cts/min. The maximum values have been set to 100% and the other values normalized to facilitate comparisons between the curves.

To try to understand the effects of cyclic AMP in the dependent strain, some effects of deprivation on various classes of RNA have been studied. The formation and breakdown of pulse-labelled RNA in S107 is compared in Fig. 3, and the parental strain GPI growing in presence and absence of cyclic AMP. In each case, rifampicin is added to block further initiation of RNA chains [12], and the

Table 1

Distribution of Pulse-labelled RNA in Cultures Grown With or Without cAMP

Strain	< 10 S		~ 10 S–50 S		70 S & Polyribosomes	
	cts/min	% of total	cts/min	% of total	cts/min	% of total
Expt. 1 S107 +cAMP	54,000	27	60,100	30	84,900	43
−cAMP	36,600	43	10,000	12	39,400	46
Expt. 2 S107 +cAMP	25,800	18	51,500	36	65,300	46
−cAMP	18,500	32	4,900	9	33,900	59
Expt. 3 S107 +cAMP	67,500	27	99,000	39	84,300	34
−cAMP	21,900	43	7,550	15	21,400	42
Expt. 4 S106 +cAMP	82,500	33	85,000	34	83,500	33
−cAMP	22,600	35	5,900	9	35,600	56

Strains were first grown in presence of cAMP. Then portions of culture were centrifuged and washed with minimal medium to remove cAMP. Equal numbers of cells were then reinoculated with or without cAMP, incubated 4 to 5 hours at $30°C$, and then pulse-labelled. 5 ml cultures of each strain were labelled at about 3×10^8 cells/ml with 5 μC ^3H uracil/ml (17 C/mmole) for 2 min. Cells were then harvested on ice, lysed [13], and analysed in sucrose gradients. Samples were precipitated with acid and counted to locate soluble RNA, ribosomal precursors and 30 S and 50 S ribosomes, and 70 S monosomes and polyribosomes [14]. The fraction of newly-formed ^3H RNA in each region was then computed.

breakdown of unstable pulse-labelled RNA is then followed. Less RNA is unstable in the culture growing in absence of cAMP, and the shape of the synthesis-breakdown curve indicates a slightly sluggish response in the deprived cells. In some experiments less than 50% of the degradation of pulse-labelled RNA occurs in deprived compared to control cultures.

Additional information about RNA metabolism was obtained by lysing pulse-labelled cells [13] and looking at the distribution of newly-formed RNA in sucrose gradients. The fraction of pulse-labelled RNA in polyribosomes is equated with mRNA, since all mRNA is in polyribosomes, and little other RNA enters polyribosomes during a short pulse [14]. The labelled RNA sedimenting in sucrose gradients with the 4 S peak provides an estimate of soluble RNA, while the new ribosomal RNA appears predominantly in ribosome precursors moving between 4 S and 50 S [14].

Table 1 summarizes the results of these experiments. For S107 and S106, the cAMP requiring (*car*) mutants, the distribution of RNA shows a decrease in the relative amount of mRNA and an increase in ribosomal RNA formation when the cells are growing in the presence of cAMP.

The result is not in agreement with the results in Fig. 3. Judged by the sucrose gradient analyses, the relative amount of mRNA is, if anything, higher in the cells starved of cAMP (Table 1); but a decreased fraction of the RNA is unstable (Fig. 3). Combined, the two results hint that some mRNA is considerably more stable in the cells deprived of cAMP—that is, there are apparently effects on mRNA that are not limited to transcription. However, these effects can be indirect and subordinate to the major event that freezes RNA and protein formation at linear rates in absence of cAMP.

The nature of car *mutants*
Thus far, the evidence is fragmentary, and falls far short of defining any specific role for cAMP in *car* mutants. However, we have not found any trivial explanation for cAMP dependence, and the type of mutant represented in S107 offers one of the strongest arguments to date, that cyclic AMP is, or can be, a metabolite essential for the growth of *E. coli*. While the precise lesion is not clear, it seems to be related to transcription—perhaps of a universally indispensible messenger RNA (rather than of mRNA for an inducible enzyme like β-galactosidase).

Analysis of such an imputed 'regulatory mutation' is especially difficult. A known case of a mutation involved in the regulation of RNA synthesis, the 'relaxed' mutation [15], remains poorly understood more than 15 years after its discovery.

Are there major effects of cAMP at translation?

From the first evidence with the cAMP-requiring mutants, as well as the work with other systems, there is no compelling argument for effects of cyclic AMP directly at translation. Perlman and Pastan have reported an apparent effect of cyclic AMP on the translation yield of the messenger RNA for tryptophanase [16], and Aboud and Berger [17], and independently Yudkin and Moses [18] have even found that it may affect translation as well as transcription of the *lac* operon. We have also reported a partial inhibition of mRNA breakdown and G translocation factor activity by cyclic AMP in cell extracts [19]. But none of these effects is as extensive or dramatic as those demonstrated at transcription [1-5].

The experiment of Fig. 3 is of interest in this regard. As Fig. 3 (left) shows, cAMP leads to no change of the rate or extent of mRNA breakdown in a cyclase-less strain. However, labile RNA does seem to be affected in the cyclic AMP-dependent mutants (see above). It is impossible to know at this point whether such an effect is a direct or indirect result of the lesion in the cell. DNA : RNA hybridization tests should show whether a specific class of messenger RNA is stabilized in the mutant.

One line of evidence which we had followed—a GTP-dependent binding of cyclic AMP detected on millipore filters [19]—proves to have been at least partly misleading. The binding activity followed the G translocation factor through considerable purification in some trials, and would therefore have been expected to affect translation processes. However, most binding activity proved to be supported by a complex of several proteins that were separable from G factor [20]. These proteins might affect G factor function, or the effects of cAMP on G factor might again be indirect or non-specific.

In summary, the existence of *car* mutants suggests that minimal cAMP levels may be required to permit exponential growth of *E. coli.* Furthermore, there is apparently protein (other than CRP protein [5]) with which cAMP must interact—conceivably one of the proteins that show GTP-dependent cAMP binding. The mutants may provide a way to analyse features of the synthesis and degradation of mRNA, but like other studies in *E. coli,* have given only a few tentative hints of any effects on messenger RNA function.

Perhaps the only major effects of cAMP in *E. coli* will prove to be at transcription. This might be a measure of the fact that nearly all *E. coli* mRNA species seem to have a comparable lifetime [14, 21, 22]. In contrast, in higher cells, mRNA lifetimes and the repertoire of means to regulate mRNA expression—including the use of cyclic AMP—seem to be much more extensive. In other words, *E. coli* may truly fail to provide adequate models for some processes that were only invented for organisms later in evolution.

Acknowledgements

These studies were supported by grants from the American Cancer Society (P-477C) and the National Science Foundation (GB 23052). D.S. receives additional support of RCDA GM-11710 of the National Institutes of Health, and Y.O., of the Naito research grant for 1970.

Discussion

Cohen (Open University)

Couldn't *car* mutants be lacking a nuclease resulting in build-up of more stable RNA, and hence feedback on to less RNA synthesis?

Schlessinger (St Louis)

While *car* mutants might lack a nuclease, it is difficult to see how this would render the cells either cyclic AMP-requiring or temperature-sensitive. In particular, if the temperature-sensitive lesion were in a nuclease, then the stable RNA should accumulate relatively more at 42°C; instead, we have observed less stabilization of pulse-labelled mRNA at the higher temperature. However, the analysis of the strains is still at an early stage of phenomenology, and it is probably too soon to exclude any model.

Monard (Friedrich Miescher Institute)

1. Did you measure the cyclic AMP level in your *car* mutants grown at different temperatures?

2. Did you test for protein kinase activity in these mutants under the different conditions?

Schlessinger (St Louis)

We have not yet measured cyclic AMP or protein kinase levels in *car* mutants. As an indirect assay of cyclic AMP levels, we have looked at the inducibility of β-galactosidase in cells washed free of c-AMP. The levels of β-galactosidase induced in absence of c-AMP are comparable to those observed in the parental strain (GP1; see text above); however, it is very hard to be sure that all traces of c-AMP have been washed away from the cells before the experiment starts.

References

1. Perlman, R. L. and Pastan, I.; *J. biol. Chem.*; **243**, (1968) 5420.
2. Perlman, R. L., de Crombrugghe, B. and Pastan, I.; *Nature Lond.*; **223**, (1969) 810.
3. Pastan, I. and Perlman, R.; *Science*; **169**, (1970) 340.
4. Pastan, I. and Perlman, R.; *Nature New Biology*; **1**, (1971) 5.
5. de Crombrugghe, B., Chen, B., Gottesman, M., Pastan, I., Varmus, H. E., Emmer, M. and Perlman, R. L.; *Nature Lond.*; (1971) in press.
6. Zubay, G., Schwartz, D. and Beckwith, J.; *Proc. Nat. Acad. Sci. U.S.A.*; **66**, (1970) 104.
7. Schwartz, D. and Beckwith, J.; In: 'The Lac Operon', Eds D. Zipser and J. Beckwith. *Cold Spring Harbor Lab. quant. Biol.*; (1970).
8. Yokota, T. and Gots, G. S.; *J. Bact.*; **103**, (1970) 513.
9. Perlman, R. and Pastan, I.; *Biochem. biophys. Res. Commun.*; **37**, (1969) 151.
10. Barman, T. E.; In: 'Enzyme Handbook'; Springer-Verlag, New York, (1969).
11. Crane, R. K.; In: 'The Enzymes'; **6**, (1969) 52.
12. DiMauro, E., Snyder, L., Marino, P., Lambert, A., Coppo, A. and Tocchini-Valentini, G. P.; *Nature Lond.*; **222**, (1969) 533.
13. Godson, G. N.; In: 'Methods in Enzymology, Nucleic Acids', Eds L. Grossman and K. Moldave. New York: Academic Press, (1967), Vol. **12A**, p. 503.
14. Mangiarotti, G and Schlessinger, D.; *J. molec. Biol.*; **29**, (1967) 395.
15. Edlin, G. and Broda, P.; *Bact. Rev.*; **32**, (1968) 206.
16. Perlman, R. and Pastan, I.; *Biochem. biophys. Res. Commun.*; **30**, (1968) 656.

17. Aboud, M. and Berger, M.; *Biochem. biophys. Res. Commun.*; **38**, (1970) 1023.
18. Yudkin, M. D. and Moses, V.; *Biochem. J.*; **113**, (1969) 423.
19. Kuwano, M. and Schlessinger, D.; *Proc. Nat. Acad. Sci. U.S.A.*; **66**, (1970) 146.
20. Ohnishi, Y., Kuwano, M. and Schlessinger, D.; in preparation.
21. Kennell, D.; *J. molec. Biol.*; **34**, (1968) 85.
22. Geiduschek, E. P. and Haselkorn, R.; *Ann. Rev. Biochem.*; **38**, (1969) 647.
23. Lennox, E. S.; *Virology*; **1**, (1955) 190.
24. Schwartz, T., Craig, E. and Kennell, D.; *J. molec. Biol.*; **54**, (1971) 299.

INTERACTION OF PROSTAGLANDINS AND CYCLIC AMP

Peter W. Ramwell and I. Rabinowitz

Alza Corporation, Palo Alto, California
and
Stanford University, Stanford, California

A. Introduction

There are only a few large classes of naturally occurring compounds which possess high biological activity, and the discovery of a new family is an event of major significance to the biomedical community. It is against this background that one must view the discovery of prostaglandins by von Euler [1], Goldblatt [2], and Bergström and Sjövall [3]. The promise of these substances in therapeutics is already great [4], but perhaps greater is their significance in cell biology.

The formation of such active substances as the prostaglandins is not restricted, as with other highly active substances like the hormones, to certain critical cells. Synthesis of prostaglandins, like cyclic AMP synthesis, occurs in most tissues. Although definitive indentification of prostaglandins by mass spectrometry has only been demonstrated in a few mammalian tissues [5] and also coral [6], there is good evidence, based on either bioassay or use of radioactive precursors and chromatography [7], that indicates there are very few cells and possibly few, if any, animal species where prostaglandins are absent.

The list of tissues from which prostaglandin release may be detected is rapidly increasing; such increased release may be detected following neural and humoral stimulation as well as by the effect of phospholipases, foreign bodies, ischaemia, etc. (Table 1).

It is now clear that many of the effects of prostaglandins may be mediated either directly or indirectly through cyclic nucleotide systems. Most of the emphasis, in proposals on the mechanism of action of prostaglandins [8] has been on the interaction between the

Table 1
Stimulated Release of Prostaglandins from Various Tissues

Species	Tissue	Stimulus	Reference
Rabbit	Eye (ant. chamber)	Mechanical	1.
	Spleen	Catecholamines	2.
		Serotonin	2.
	Epigastric fat pad	Hormones	3.
	Somatosensory cortex	Neural	4.
		Analeptics, etc.	4.
		Reticular formation	5.
	Spleen	Catecholamines	6.
	Adrenal	Acetylcholine	7.
Dog	Spleen	Neural	8.
		Neural Catecholamines	9.
		Neural Colloids	10.
		Colloids	
	Bladder	Distension	11.
	Cerebral ventricles	Serotonin	12.
Rat	Phrenic diaphragm	Neural	13.
		Biogenic amines	14.
	Epididymal fat pad	Neural	
		Biogenic amines	15.
	Stomach	Neural Stretch	16.
		Neural	17.
		Neural Secretagogues	18.
	Skin	Inflammation	19.
	Liver	Glucagon	20.
	Lung	Air embolus	21.
		Infusion of particles	22.
Guinea-pig	Lung (whole, perfused)	Anaphylaxis	23, 24.
		Particles	22, 25, 26.
		Histamine	27.
		Tryptamine Serotonin	21.
		Massage Air embolus	26.
		Distension	28.
	Lung (chopped)	Stirring	29.
Human	Thyroid	Medullary Carcinoma	30.
	Uterus	Parturition	31.
		Distension	32.
	Platelets	Thrombin	33.
Frog	Intestine	Distilled water	34.
	Skin	Isoproterenol	35.
	Spinal cord	Neural Analeptics	36.

Reproduced from Ref. *26.*

1. Ambache, N., Kavanagh, L. and Whiting, J.; *J. Physiol.*; **176,** (1965) 378. *2.* Vane, J. R. and Willis, A. L.; Ph.D. Thesis in the University of London (1971). *3.* Lewis, G. P. and Matthews, J.; *J. Physiol.*; **202,** (1969) 95. *4.* Ramwell, P. W. and Shaw, J. E.; *Amer. J. Physiol.*; **211,** (1966) 125. *5.* Bradley, P. B., Samuels, G. M. R. and Shaw, J. E.; *Brit. J. Pharmacol.*; **37,** (1969) 151. *6.* Vane, J. R., Willis, A. L. and Pojda; Private communication. *7.* Ramwell, P. W., Shaw, J. E., Douglas, W. W. and Poisner, A. M.; *Nature, Lond.*; **210,** (1966) 273. *8.* Davies, B. N. and Withrington, B. N.; *Brit. J. Pharmac. Chemother.*; **32,** (1968) 136. *9.* Ferreira, S. H. and Vane, J. R.; *Nature, Lond.*; **216,** (1967) 868. *10.* Gilmore, N. Vane, J. R. and Wyllie, J. H.; *Nature, Lond.*; **218,** (1968) 1135. *11.* Gilmore, N.; Ph.D. thesis in the University of London (1968). *12.* Holmes, S. W.; *Brit. J. Pharmacol.*; **38,** (1970) 653. *13.* Ramwell, P. W., Shaw, J. E. and Kucharski, J.; *Science*; **149,** (1965) 1390. *14.* Laity, J. L. H.; *Brit, J. Pharmacol.*; **37,** (1969) 698. *15.* Shaw, J. E. and Ramwell, P. W.; *J. Biol. Chem.*; **243,** (1968) 1498. *16.* Bennett, A., Friedmann, C. A. and Vane, J. R.; *Nature, Lond.*; **216,** (1967) 873. *17.* Coceani, F., Pace-Asciak, C., Volta, F. and Wolfe, L. S.; *Amer. J. Physiol.*; **213,** (1967) 1056. *18.* Shaw, J. E. and Ramwell, P. W.; *Prostaglandin symposium of the Worcester Foundation for Exp. Biol.*; Eds P. W. Ramwell and J. E. Shaw, New York, (1968) p. 55. *19.* Willis, A. L.; *J. Pharm. Pharmacol.*; **21,** (1969) 126. *20.* Dawson and Ramwell P. W. (1970). *21.* Alabaster, V. A. and Bakhle, Y. S.; *Brit. J. Pharmacol.*; (1971) in press. *21.* Lindsey, H. E. and Wyllie, J. H.; *Brit. J. Surg.*; **57,** (1970) 738. *23.* Piper, P. J. and Vane, J. R.; *Nature, Lond.*; **223,** (1969) 29. *24.* Piper, P. J. and Vane, J. R.; In: 'Prostaglandins, Peptides and Amines'. Eds P. Mantegazza and E. W. Horton. Academic Press, London, (1969) p. 15. *25.* Palmer, M. A., Piper, P. J. and Vane, J. R.; *Brit. J. Pharmacol.*; **40,** (1970) 547. *26.* Piper, P. and Vane, J.; *Proc. New York Academy of Sciences Conference on Prostaglandins*; 17-19 September, 1970, Vol. 180, p. 363 (1971). *27.* Alabaster, V. A. and Bakhle, Y. S.; *private communication.* *28.* Berry, E. M., Edmonds, J. F. and Wyllie, J. H.; *Brit. J. Surgery*; **58,** (1971) 189. *29.* Palmer, M. A., Piper, P. J. and Vane, J. R.; *Brit. J. Pharmacol*; **40,** (1970) 581. *30.* Williams, E. D., Karim, S. M. M. and Sandler, M.; *Lancet*; **1,** (1968) 22. *31.* Karim, S. M. M.; *Brit. Med. J.*; **4,** (1968) 618. *32.* Horton, E., Jones, R., Thompson, C. and Poyser, N.; *Proc. New York Academy of Sciences Conference on Prostaglandins*; 17-19 September, 1970, Vol. 180, p. 351 (1971). *33.* Smith, J. B. and Willis, A. L.; *Brit. J. Pharmacol.*; (1971) in press. *34.* Vogt, W. and Distelkotter, B.; *Nobel Symposium 2, Prostaglandins*; Eds S. Bergström and B. Samuelsson. Almqvist and Wiksell, Stockholm, (1967) p. 29. *35.* Ramwell, P. W. and Shaw, J. E.; *Rec. Prog. Horm. Res*; **26,** (1970) 139. *36.* Ramwell, P. W., Shaw, J. E. and Jessup, R.; *Amer. J. Physiol.*; **211,** (1966) 998.

catalytic site of the adenyl cyclase enzyme and the substrate, or on the catabolizing enzyme, phosphodiesterase. For example, Stock *et al.* [9] have suggested that in rat epididymal fat pads, prostaglandins interfere with the binding of ATP and Mg^{2+} ions to the enzyme. Paoletti and his colleagues [10] believe that the competitive effects of PGE_1 on lipolysis induced by theophylline, is evidence that PGE_1

activates phosphodiesterase. However, not all actions of prosta-glandins are necessarily mediated through the adenyl cyclase system (Section E). Earlier we have discussed the role of prostaglandins in initiating a change in the cell membrane, to cause cation fluxes which in turn modify adenyl cyclase activity [11]. In this paper we wish to give more consideration to the possibility that prostaglandins have an effect on cooperative membranes and that prostaglandins may therefore exert many of their effects by indirectly influencing membrane-bound enzymes, including adenyl cyclase, which are likely to be susceptible to structural changes as well as ionic changes in their environment.

B. Prostaglandin Specificity

There are two contrasting points which can be made immediately with respect to prostaglandin specificity:

1. *Generality of pharmacological effects*

In studying the prostaglandins, one is always impressed by their remarkably wide spectrum of pharmacological activity which is unrivalled in biology by any other major group of naturally occurring compounds. This most unusual lack of specificity of prostaglandins (Table 2) is associated with high pharmacological activity, the half maximal concentrations of PGE_1 and PGE_2 being 4×10^{-9} M, for inhibition of epinephrine-stimulated cyclic AMP formation in adipo-cytes [12, 13]. This is in contrast to the situation with cyclic AMP, where notoriously high doses have to be used or where a more soluble derivative, such as dibutyryl cyclic AMP, is employed to elicit a response. The contrast may reflect the marked differences in cell permeability to prostaglandins and cyclic AMP or perhaps that the site of action of prostaglandins is more superficial than that of cyclic AMP, which is believed to be intracellular.

2. *Structure–activity relationships*

The second point is that in spite of the generality of prostaglandin effects, the individual compounds themselves exhibit strict structure-activity specificity in individual cell types. It will be helpful to consider the molecules in detail with respect to their conformation.

(a) *Conformation*   The crystal structure of one prostaglandin, $PGF_{1\beta}$, has been determined [14]. A computer drawing of the $PGF_{1\beta}$ molecule (using the published atomic position coordinates) is depicted in slight perspective in Fig. 1. Only carbon and oxygen atoms are shown; the heavy atom groups used in the structure determination are excluded. Since the structure was reported as the incorrect enantiomorph, we are now presenting the mirror image in order to view the correct antipode. In Fig. 1 the plane of the zig-zag

Table 2
Pharmacological Spectrum of Prostaglandin Actions

1. Behaviour
   Individual neurones: cerebellar and reticular formation
   Hypothalamus–Pituitary
   Special centres, vasomotor, temperature regulation
   Autonomic and neuromuscular junctions

2. Trophic hormone target tissues
        e.g. testes, ovary, thyroid, adrenal
   Exocrine hormone target tissues
        e.g. gastric mucosa, pancreas
   Endocrine target tissues
        e.g. adipoctyes, renal tubules, bone

3. Smooth muscle
        e.g. reproductive, alimentary, respiratory, cardiovascular

4. Blood
        e.g. red cells, leucocytes, platelets

of carbon atoms 1 to 7 is perpendicular to the plane of the zig-zag of carbon atoms 15 to 20. This mode of packing of hydrocarbon chains in the crystalline state is characteristic of long-chain fatty acids such as stearic acid, and also of polyethylene. In Fig. 2 the molecule has been rotated to get an edge-on view which emphasizes the essential coplanarity of the side chains with each other and with the ring. Evidence has been presented elsewhere [15] that this aligned or hairpin conformation may be the most favoured conformation of the molecule, certainly in a lipophilic environment. Briefly, the argument turns on the fact that both $PGF_{1\beta}$ and PGE_1 crystallize in space group $P_{2_1 2_1 2_1}$, and that this symmetry imposes close packing of hairpins in the crystalline state. This minimum-energy conformation should also be present in less ordered states since there are considerable London-van der Waals forces of attraction between the two chains which act in concert with steric forces in the ring to produce approximately -38 J mole^{-1} (-9 cal/mole) of conformation stabilization energy. Small changes in conformational potential energy can be correlated with biological activity. Gross changes in

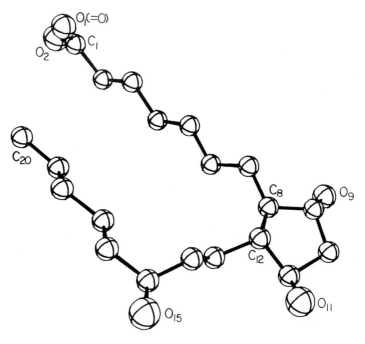

Fig. 1. Computer drawing of corrected x-ray crystallographic data to show PGF$_{1\beta}$ in slight perspective.

the hairpin conformation can only be induced by supplying energy, for example, through cation chelation or interphase reactions.

Using this basic conformation as a tenable starting point, space-filling CPK models have been prepared of some of the isomers of E and F prostaglandins. The importance of the 11 and 15 positions for activity has been established [16]. From Fig. 3 it will be seen that the active prostaglandins are those which have a right-hand wedge where the 9, 11 and 15 positions form the top and right side of the wedge, and the carboxylic group is at the thin end.

11, 15 epi E_1 is not active, and although it presents us with three oxygen functions at the 9, 11 and 15 positions when turned through 180° (Fig. 3) it then becomes a left-hand wedge. In contrast, ent 11,

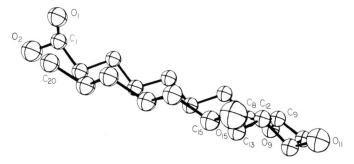

Fig. 2. Edge-on view to show puckering of the ring.

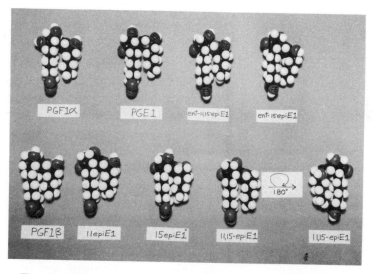

Fig. 3. CPK models of prostaglandins to show hairpin conformation and steric relationships at the 9, 11 and 15 positions.

15 epi PGE_1 exhibits the right-hand wedge appearance and is active.

Thus the biologically active prostaglandins appear to be amphipathic molecules of novel design in that their hydrophilic groups lie on one *side* of the molecule and the other *side* is hydrophobic, while both ends are hydrophilic.

(b) *Postulated membrane interaction*   These molecules in fact possess many of the requisites set out by Onsager [17] for cation-transporting molecules at a pore: they are (i) partially lipid soluble, (ii) can hold a stable conformation as the calculations indicate, and (iii) may relieve internal electrostatic repulsive forces by forming a cation complex. More attractive to us, in the light of our considerations of the conformational energies of these molecules, is a view of the prostaglandins as effector molecules in a cooperative membrane. The general scheme would involve (i) a change in the molecular environment of the prostaglandin, (ii) succeeded by a conformational change of the prostaglandin, (iii) followed by an interphase action of the prostaglandin to (iv) act on an enzyme system, ion channel, etc.

3. *Qualitative actions of prostaglandins*

Prostaglandins appear in some cells to have different qualitative actions, such as in the vascular pressor and depressor responses to the intravenous administration of the PGF and PGE compounds in both rat and dog. However, these apparent contradictory effects of prostaglandins may be mediated via an action on different cell types. Thus the arterioles and capillaries are sensitive to the PGE series [18, 19]. The venules, in contrast, are more sensitive, directly or indirectly, to the PGF compounds which induce vasoconstriction and so indirectly increase blood pressure.

There are certain important exceptions which are of considerable interest. One of these is the rat platelet system where PGE_1 prevents ADP-induced platelet aggregation and PGE_2 stimulates aggregation. This exception has been analysed in detail by Dr Hideo Shio and will be described elsewhere. Careful analysis of these exceptions indicate that the different prostaglandins exert their apparent contradictory effects by acting on *different* cellular mechanisms and not by antagonizing each other on the same mechanism.

4. *Prostaglandin antagonists*

A number of relatively specific antagonists for prostaglandins discovered recently encourages the idea that prostaglandins may interact specifically with membranes. Eakins [20] has shown that polyphloretin phosphate has a reversible effect on PGE_2 and $PGF_{2\alpha}$

in a number of smooth-muscle preparations, and Sanner [21] has shown similar effects against PGE_1 and PGE_2 with SC19220. Fried *et al.* [22] have observed specific antagonism with 7-oxa-13-prostynoic acid and other analogues. In all three cases the concentration of antagonist to agonist is high, being in the order of approximately 1000:1. Differences in degree of antagonism to the PGE and PGF compounds also encourage the idea of a high degree of specificity between the individual prostaglandins and their initial site of cellular action.

5. *Tachyphylaxis*

It is interesting that specific tachyphylaxis to the individual prostaglandins can be obtained on the rat uterus and on brain-stem neurone [23]. The effect is more marked with the monoenoic prostaglandins than the dienoic [24]. These results are important in that they substantiate the suggestion that the different prostaglandins may have different sites of action.

C. Effect of Hormones and Cyclic AMP on Prostaglandin Release

1. *Hormonal and other effects*

It is now well established that hormonal stimulation of many tissues and organs is associated with increased efflux of prostaglandins both *in vivo* and *in vitro* (Table 1). In some cases, as in the rat stomach, prostaglandin release into the stomach lumen has been demonstrated following vagal, gastrin, histamine and acetyl choline stimulation [25]. In others, such as the rat fat pad, those hormones causing increased lipolysis stimulated prostaglandin efflux significantly, and it is noteworthy that insulin, a known antilipolytic agent, decreased prostaglandin efflux [26]. This result suggests that stimulation of prostaglandin synthesis and release is specific.

From work performed on the perfused cat's adrenal, we concluded that more prostaglandin was released than could be initially extracted [27], i.e. that increased release of prostaglandin reflects activation of a biosynthetic process rather than release from a preformed store. This has proved to be true for the rat stomach [28], frog skin [29], spleen [30, 31], and other tissues. Further evidence to substantiate this possibility is that the release of prostaglandin may also be enhanced by infusing prostaglandin precursors, i.e. the C20ω polyenoic precursors from phospholipid. Bee and snake venom also release prostaglandin, and it is known that they contain phospholipase A [32]. Moreover, the free acid is known to be required before cyclization may occur since homo-γ-linolenyl and arachidonyl phosphatidylcholine are not effective substrates for prostaglandin biosynthesis [33]. The general belief, therefore, is that prostaglandin release is preceded by activation of an acid hydrolase which leads to increased synthesis [34, 35].

2. *Qualitative differences in prostaglandin release*

An early problem associated with determination of prostaglandins released from various structures following nerve stimulation was caused by change in the type of prostaglandins released. Indentification of the prostaglandins depended upon use of two thin-layer systems, and frequently the losses on the silica gel were such as to make quantitation difficult. However, qualitative changes were observed, for example, in the perfused frog spinal cord which were confirmed recently by Coceani *et al.* [36]; in both studies stimulation elicited release of $PGF_{1\alpha}$. In contrast, in the perfused dog spleen both Davies and Withrington [37] and Gilmore *et al.* [38] observed increased release of PGE_2 on stimulation. A similar increase in PGE_2 was also observed in rabbit spleen [39]. To date no consistent pattern in the changes occurring on stimulation of different tissues can be discerned.

There were two possible explanations for these qualitative changes in prostaglandin release. The first was that different neurone pools or cells were activated on stimulation, especially if different afferent pathways were employed, and different cells contained different prostaglandins. The second explanation was based on the possibility that the direction of biosynthesis may be changed on stimulation, since it is known that different cofactors have appreciable effects in directing the biosynthesis from a common precursor to either the PGE or PGF derivative. Recently Foss *et al.* [40] have shown that epinephrine, when added directly to washed microsomes obtained from bovine seminal vesicles, increased the yield of $PGF_{2\alpha}$ (1.5 to 19%). Moreover, certain prostaglandin synthetase inhibitors are now being found to have a differential inhibitory action [41]. Work on single-cell types and better and more sensitive analytical methods are required before the two hypotheses can be evaluated.

These results indicate quite clearly that changes in the direction of the biosynthesis may provide a means of cell regulation and raise the possibility that such changes may be responsible in part for some of the symptomatology of asthma. For example, the PGE compounds cause bronchodilation, but the PGF series induce bronchoconstriction and may be preferentially synthesized in asthma.

3. *Cyclic AMP experiments on prostaglandin release*

A number of hormones, including isoproterenol, stimulate the short-circuit current across frog ventral-skin preparations. This effect is known to be associated with activation of adenyl cyclase and an increase in intracellular cyclic AMP [42], which is believed to mediate the effect of the hormone since both exogenous cyclic AMP and theophylline also stimulate short-circuit current. Recently PGE_1 has been shown to have a dose-dependent effect on short-circuit current [11, 43]. We have found both this prostaglandin and its congener, PGE_2, to be present in frog skin, and we investigated whether isoproterenol would stimulate prostaglandin release and whether such an effect was mediated through cyclic AMP.

Isoproterenol (10^{-8} M) applied to the inside surface of frog skin significantly stimulated release of prostaglandin-like material into superfusates of the outer skin surface [29]. Thin-layer chromatography of acidic diethyl ether extracts of the superfusate indicated that this smooth muscle stimulating material was a mixture of PGE_1 and PGE_2. In contrast, dibutyryl cyclic AMP (2.4×10^{-3} M) and theophylline (10^{-4} M) applied to the inside surface, failed to increase prostaglandin efflux significantly.

A similar result was observed using rat epididymal fat pads and rat diaphragm. Treatment with both cyclic AMP and dibutyryl cyclic AMP failed to elicit a significantly increased release of material capable of stimulating smooth muscle. Some evidence was obtained to indicate that dibutyryl cyclic AMP, which can have qualitatively different effects from cyclic AMP, may stimulate efflux of prostaglandin-like substances from the rat gastric mucosa *in vivo* [44]. These preliminary results indicate that prostaglandin formation and release on hormonal stimulation may well result from an action of the hormone which is not necessarily mediated via cyclic AMP.

4. *Prostaglandin-deficient cells*

Human red cells which are deficient in adenyl cyclase do not synthesize or metabolize prostaglandins. Moreover, tissues which contain a hormone-sensitive adenyl cyclase system may not necessarily synthesise and metabolise the parent prostaglandins. The turkey erythrocyte contains no detectable pharmacologically-active prostaglandins nor is there significant prostaglandin metabolism or synthesis. The findings indicate that prostaglandins are not a prerequisite for a functional adenyl cyclase system in some cell types (see later).

Where cells have been deprived of the prostaglandin precursors by rearing animals on a diet deficient in essential fatty acids, the lipolysis rate is known to be high, which can be interpreted as indicating decreased endogenous prostaglandin formation. Decreased prostaglandin content does indeed occur under these conditions [35].

D. Effects of Prostaglandins on Adenyl Cyclase systems

1. *Introduction*

The relation of prostaglandins to cyclic AMP concentrations was derived firstly from the work of Steinberg *et al.* [45] who demonstrated that PGE_1 inhibited lipolysis and also phosphorylase activation in rat epididymal fat pads. Butcher *et al.* [46] then showed that PGE_1 inhibited the effect of epinephrine in increasing intracellular cyclic AMP in the same tissue. As will be seen later, Orloff *et al.* [47] provided evidence in the toad bladder that the antihormonal effects of PGE_1 may indeed be mediated through an action on the adenyl cyclase mechanism. Finally, Butcher *et al.* [48, 49] showed that other tissues responded to PGE_1 stimulation by increased intracellular cyclic AMP concentrations. Other workers have established that a wide range of tissues are affected by prostaglandins. It is convenient to summarize the data in two Tables (3 and 4) showing the opposite effects of PGE_1 although a number of adenyl cyclase systems such as in frog and turkey erythrocytes, are known to be unresponsive (see later).

2. *Adipose tissue*

Butcher *et al.* [48] originally obtained results which suggested that PGE_1 was acting as a partial agonist on fat pads, in that by itself PGE_1 elicited a small increase in cyclic AMP but antagonized the stimulating effect of epinephrine. By separating the fat cells with collagenase, Butcher and Baird [12] showed that this partial agonist

Table 3
Some Stimulatory Effects of Prostaglandins on Cyclic AMP

Tissues where prostaglandins increase accumulation of cyclic 3'5'-AMP

Tissue	Species	Prostaglandin (μM) most active		Reference
Lung	rat	PGE_1	2.8	a
Spleen	rat	PGE_1	2.8	a
Diaphragm	rat	PGE_1	2·8	a
Adipose	rat	PGE_1	2.8	a
Leucocytes	human	PGE_1	—	a
Platelets†	human	PGE_1	0.28	b
Platelets†	human	PGE_1	0.01	c
Platelets†	human	PGE_1	0.1	d
Platelets†	human	PGE_1	0.1	e
Platelets†	rabbit	PGE_1	0.1	e
Platelets†	rabbit	PGE_1	0.15	f
Anterior pituitary†	rat	PGE_1	2.8	g
Aorta	rat	PGE_1	2.8	h
Bone	rat	PGE_1		i
Gastric mucosa†	guinea-pig	PGE_1		j
Kidney	dog, rat	PGE_1		k
Heart	guinea-pig	PGE_1	0·01	l
		$PGF_{1\alpha}$	0.01	
Corpus luteum†	bovine	PGE_2	28	m
Thyroid†	dog	PGE_2		n
Erythrocytes†	rat	PGE_2	0.03	o

† Indicates those tissues where prostaglandins increase adenyl cyclase activity.
• Reproduced from Ref. [64].

a Butcher, R. W. and Baird, C. E.; *J. Biol. Chem.*; **243**, (1968) 1713. b Robison, G. A., Arnold, A. and Hartmann, R. C.; *Pharmac. Res. Commun.*; **1**, (1969) 325. c Wolfe, S. M. and Shulman, N. R., *Biochem. Biophys. Res. Commun.*; **35**, (1969) 265. d Vigdahl, R. L., and Tavormina, P. A.; *Biochem. Biophys. Res. Commun.*; **37**, (1969) 409. e Moskowitz, J., Harwood, J. P., Reid, W. D. and Krishna, G.; *Fed. Proc.*; **29**, (1970) 602. f. Shio, H.; private communication. g Zor, U., Kaneko, T., Schneider, H. P. G., McCann, S. M., Lowe, I. P., Bloom, G., Borland, B. and Field, J. B.; *Proc. Nat. Acad. Sci.*; **63**, (1969) 918. h LaRaia, P. J. and Reddy, W. J.; *Circulation*; **38**, suppl. VI, VI-122 (1968). i Chase, L. R. and Aurbach, G. D.; *Clin. Res.*; **17**, (1969) 380. j Perrier, C. V. and Laster, L.; *J. Clin. Invest.*; **49**, (1970) 73a. k Davis, B., Zor, U., Kaneko, T., Mintz, D. H. and Field, J. F.; *Clin. Res.*; **17**, (1969) 458. l Sobel, B. E. and Robison, A. K.; *Circulation*; **40**, Suppl. III, p. 189 (1969). m Marsh, J. M.; *Fed. Proc.*; **29**, (1970) 387. n Field, J. B., Zor, U. and Kaneko, T.; *Abst. 51st Meeting Endocr. Soc.*; New York, (1969) p. 98. o Sheppard, H. and Burghardt, C. R.; *Molecular Pharmacol.*; **6**, (1970) 425.

effect was due to a stimulant action of PGE_1 on the vascular stroma of the fat pad on the one hand and an inhibitory effect on the adipocytes on the other. These studies have served as a useful warning not to confuse the cyclic AMP values obtained from

Table 4
Tissues where Prostaglandins* Inhibit Hormonally-Induced Responses

Tissue	Hormone	Response	Reference
Toad bladder	vasopressin	water transport	*a*
Toad Bladder†	vasopressin	water transport	*b*
Rabbit kidney tubules	vasopressin	water transport	*c*
Hamster renal medulla†	vasopressin	water transport	*d*
Rat adipose†	epinephrine ACTH TSH glucagon growth hormone	lipolysis	*e* *f*
Cerebellar Purkinje cells	norepinephrine	inhibition of discharge frequency	*g*
Renal cortex†	PTH	^{32}P phospholipids	*h*

* PGE_1 most effective, at < 0.28 μM.
† Inhibition associated with decreased cyclic AMP accumulation.

a Orloff, J., Handler, J. S. and Bergström, S.; *Nature, Lond.*; **205**, (1965) 397. *b* Lipson, L., Hynie, S. and Sharp, G.; *Proc. New York Academy of Sciences Conference on Prostaglandins*; 17-19 September, 1970, Vol. 180, p. 261 (1971). *c* Grantham, J. J. and Orloff, J.; *J. Lab. Clin. Invest.*; **47**, (1968) 1154. *d* Marumo, F. and Edelman, I.; *J. Clin. Invest.*; in press. *e* Steinberg, D., Vaughan, M., Nestel, P. and Bergström, S.; *Biochem. Pharmacol.*; **12**, (1963) 764. *f* Butcher, R. W. and Baird, C. E.; *J. Biol. Chem.*; **243**, (1968) 1713. *g* Siggins, G. R., Hoffer, B. J. and Bloom, F. E.; *Science*; **165**, (1969) 1018. *h* Beck, N. P., DeRubertis, F., Michelis, M. F., Fusco, R. D., Field, J. B. and Davis, B. B.; *J. Lab. Clin. Med.*; **76**, (1970) 1005.

nonhomogeneous tissues as being characteristic for a particular cell type.

In contrast to their effects on basal lipolysis, prostaglandins were found not to modify the basal concentrations of cyclic AMP in adipocytes. Their order of effectiveness in reducing epinephrine-elevated cyclic AMP levels was $PGE_1 > PGE_2 > PGA_1 > PGF_{1\alpha}$ and $PGF_{1\beta}$ had no effect; this sequence is the same as for inhibition of lipolysis [50]. After epinephrine stimulation, PGE_1 rapidly reduces cyclic AMP concentrations within two minutes, and no effects were observed in cell-free systems. In contrast, Frank and Braun [51] in Hechter's group found that prostaglandins were effective in fat-cell ghosts of rabbits, and moreover, in this species prostaglandins increased adenyl cyclase activity. Species differences in the action of prostaglandins are known to occur for several tissues, including heart [52], vas deferens and renal transporting epithelia [53,54]. Support for a species difference can also be obtained from a recent observation that in rabbit epididymal fat pads both PGE_1 and PGE_2 failed to inhibit ACTH-induced lipolysis [55].

Such a marked qualitative difference in fat tissue may reflect the difference between intact cells and cell-free systems. In rat adipose tissue several groups have failed to find any effect of PGE_1 on cell-free systems [12, 13, 56, 57]. However, in another tissue where PGE_1 has an inhibitory effect on intact cells, namely the hamster renal papilla, this effect has been observed in a broken-cell preparation [58].

As indicated earlier, prostaglandins inhibit lipolysis induced by methylxanthines [10, 50, 59, 60]. Two groups [10, 59] found that PGE_1 had a noncompetitive effect on norepinephrine-induced lipolysis but a competitive effect for theophylline-induced lipolysis, and they concluded that PGE_1 reduced cyclic AMP by a direct intracellular action, the blocking of phosphodiesterase inhibition. The action of hormones and prostaglandins on phosphodiesterase activity is still an open question.

3. *Rat platelets*

The qualitative differences in prostaglandin action are perhaps best exemplified by studying the aggregation of rat platelets where PGE_1 is an extremely potent inhibitor of aggregation [61]. In parallel with the response of many other tissues, PGE_1 and cyclic AMP have similar effects, both cyclic AMP itself and the dibutyryl form inhibiting the aggregation of platelets. Indeed, PGE_1 has been shown to stimulate the adenyl cyclase activity of platelets in intact-cell preparations [48], homogenates and membrane fractions. This suggests that the PGE_1 effect may be mediated through cyclic AMP accumulation. The synergistic effects of methylxanthines and PGE_1 on both aggregation and adenyl cyclase stimulation support this hypothesis. Moreover, the ability of several prostaglandins to inhibit aggregation correlates well with the degree to which they stimulate adenyl cyclase activity, at least when human platelets are considered [62].

In the rat, PGE_2 enhances rather than inhibits ADP-induced aggregation of platelets [61, 63]. Using intact-cell preparations, the formation of cyclic AMP from incorporated ^{14}C-adenosine has been determined. As shown in Fig. 4, exposure of platelets to PGE_2 evokes only a small enhancement of adenyl cyclase activity. Thus

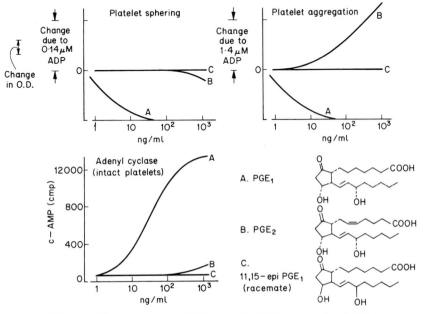

Fig. 4. The action of PGE_1 and PGE_2 on rat platelet aggregation.

PGE_2 has the same qualitative action as PGE_1 on platelet adenyl cyclase, but in contrast, it has an opposite effect on aggregation, which suggests that PGE_2 at low doses is having an effect which may not necessarily be mediated via cyclic AMP. At high concentrations of PGE_2, inhibition of platelet aggregation is clearly seen, and this action of PGE_2 is likely to be mediated via cyclic AMP.

The aggregating effect of PGE_2 is surprisingly specific since it was mimicked by ent-15-epi-PGE_2 and not by 15-epi-PGE_2 which was inactive (see Fig. 5). Further analysis has revealed that the two effects of PGE_2 are on two distinct and separate platelet mechanisms.

4. *Turkey erythrocytes*

Not all tissues which contain hormone sensitive adenyl cyclase systems synthesize and metabolize prostaglandins, for the turkey erythrocyte was found not to contain prostaglandins. This situation

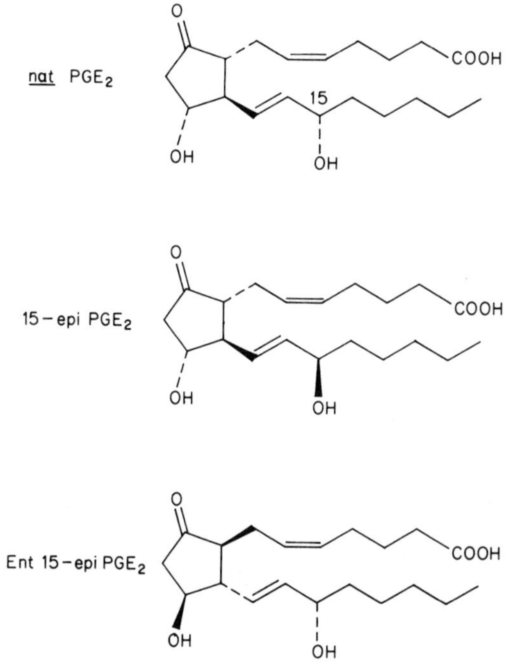

Fig. 5. Specificity of PGE_2 isomers on stimulation of rat platelet aggregation. *Top*: Naturally occurring PGE_2 which enhances rat platelet aggregation. *Middle*: One of chemically synthesized 15-epi PGE_2 compounds which has a structure similar to above *nat* PGE_2 except 15 OH. This compound has no effect on rat platelet aggregation. *Bottom*; Another chemically synthesized 15-epi PGE_2 compound, which is structurally a mirror image of above *nat* 15-epi PGE_2. This compound is equipotent to *nat* PGE_2 in the stimulation of rat platelet aggregation.

was not due to absence of an acid hydrolase since there was no prostaglandin synthesis from exogenous ^{3}H-arachidonic acid. Nor was the absence of prostaglandins due to rapid metabolism, for no β-oxidation of ^{14}C-PGE_1 was detected, and moreover, exogenous PGE_1 incubated with homogenates suffered no loss of biological activity [64].

The turkey erythrocyte adenyl cyclase system, which is readily stimulated by epinephrine, cannot be affected by exogenous prostaglandins except in the presence of caffeine where PGE_1 (2.8×10^{-6} M) significantly inhibited the cyclic AMP response evoked by epinephrine. PGE_1 alone, within one minute, stimulated calcium release from the lipid-bound calcium-containing fractions of the cell. In contrast, in frog erythrocyte lysates, PGE_1, PGE_2, PGA_1, PGB_1 and $PGF_{1\alpha}$ (0.1-25 μg/ml) did not stimulate adenyl cyclase activity [65].

These results indicate that intracellular prostaglandin formation is not in all instances associated with adenyl cyclase activity.

5. *Thyroid*

The interaction of prostaglandins and cyclic AMP in the thyroid gland is of particular interest in view of the number of parameters studied, which far exceeds that in any other preparation. Most of the work has been performed in a single species, namely dog. The results indicate that although prostaglandins are less potent stimulators of adenyl cyclase than TSH, they might effectively compete with TSH for receptor sites and serve to modulate the intracellular effects of TSH.

Field *et al.* [66] have recently reviewed their data and also those of other workers [67-70]. They emphasized that although there are many similarities between effects of prostaglandins and those of TSH, the effects of prostaglandins may be more complicated than simple activation of adenyl cyclase and generation of cyclic AMP. The different prostaglandins had widely variable effects on adenyl cyclase activation in dog thyroid homogenates. The results in slices were more consistent, and dose-dependent effects were observed (Table 5).

The effect of PGE_1 is to stimulate glucose oxidation, but Burke [70] and Field *et al.* [66] differ markedly in their results with other prostaglandins. For example, Burke finds $PGF_{1\alpha}$ inhibits TSH stimulation of glucose oxidation without inhibiting adenyl cyclase.

PGE_1 (1 μg cm^{-3}) increases colloid droplet formation, but not as effectively as TSH (10 mg cm^{-3}). High doses (100 μg cm^{-3}) of prostaglandins were required to mimic the effect of TSH in stimulating ^{32}P incorporation into phospholipid, and PGA_1 caused inhibition. To attempt to correlate effects at these concentrations with other parameters may not be fruitful.

A summary of Field's results is shown in Table 5. The difficulty once more is that of working with mixed-cell populations. In addition, it should be understood that while TSH is a blood-borne humour, it is likely that prostaglandins, if they are to have a physiological role in this tissue, may exert their effects from the target cells themselves.

6. *Transporting epithelia*

As indicated earlier, one of the first clues to prostaglandin action came from the studies of Orloff *et al.* [47] in water transport in the

Table 5
**Summary of the Effects of Prostaglandins on Different
Parameters of Thyroid Function**

Parameter	PGA_1	PGB_1	PGE_1	$PGF_{1\alpha}$	TSH
Adenyl cyclase	↑ 0.2	↑ 0.2	↑ 0.02	↑ 0.2	↑
^{3}H Cyclic AMP	↑ 10	↑100	↑ 1	↑ 10	↑
Cyclic AMP	↑100	○100	↑ 1	○100	↑
$^{14}CO_2$	↑100	↑100	↑ 1	↑ 10	↑
^{32}Phospholipid	↓100	○100	↑100	↑100	↑
Colloid droplets	↑100	↑100	↑ 1	↑100	↑

Reproduced from Ref. [66].

toad bladder where water and sodium transport are believed to be mediated by separate adenyl cyclase systems [71].

As shown by several groups [11, 43, 72], PGE_1 increases sodium transport and short-circuit current in frog skin. Orloff *et al.* [47] showed that PGE_1 by itself had no effect on water transport in the toad bladder but that it inhibited the effect of ADH. In the rabbit collecting tubule, Grantham and Orloff [53] found that PGE_1 inhibited the effect of ADH on water transport but also enhanced the effect of theophylline, i.e. PGE_1 acted as a partial agonist. Eggena *et al.* [73] do not aggree with Orloff [74] that PGE_1 competes with ADH for a common receptor site. Their findings indicate that PGE_1 behaves as a non-competitive inhibitor of neuro-hypophyseal hormones and theophylline. They also find that PGE_1 inhibition of oxytocin is similarly non-competitive.

In the toad bladder Lipson *et al.* [75] have shown that PGE_1 stimulates both adenyl cyclase and cyclic AMP accumulation. However, the degree of inhibition by PGE_1 of ADH-induced changes in adenyl cyclase was slight.

There have been a number of studies of the effect of PGE_1 on kidney adenyl cyclase, but the problem of interpreting the results from a mixed-cell population is formidable; moreover, interpretation is rendered more hazardous by species differences [76]. Recently Edelman [58], using hamster renal papilla, has succeeded in obtaining an inhibitory effect of PGE_1 on ADH-stimulated adenyl cyclase in a broken-cell preparation; this is the first time that PGE_1 has been observed to have an inhibitory effect in a cell-free system.

An interesting example of where PGE_1 and another agent have similar effects in one system and antagonistic effects in another is seen with cholera exotoxin where both stimulate intestinal mucosal adenyl cyclase and inhibit water transport [75, 77], but in adipose tissue exotoxin is lipolytic and PGE_1 is antilipolytic [78]. Moreover, this lipolytic effect of exotoxin was inhibited by PGE_1 itself.

E. Other Effects of Prostaglandins

1. *Muscle*

The effects of spasmogenic agents on rat uterus and fundus are unlikely to be mediated through increased intracellular concentration of cyclic AMP since this nucleotide, dibutyryl cyclic AMP, and the methylxanthines cause relaxation. The spasmogenic response of the rat uterus has not been associated with an increase in cyclic AMP [79]. Moreover, the response to prostaglandins of both fundus and uterus is more susceptible to calcium deprivation than to other agonists [80, 81] which indicates a requirement for an ion which has been widely shown to inhibit adenyl cyclase [11].

In other areas, such as the heart, where both prostaglandins and cyclic AMP have inotropic effects, and where epinephrine induces very rapid changes in cyclic AMP, it is of interest that Oye and Asbjorn [82] have obtained conditions in which the effect of epinephrine was not related to phosphorylase activation. It may be argued that phosphorylase activation is not necessary for contractile activity and that cyclic AMP may be acting at another site. However, when cyclic AMP was applied at low temperatures (16°C) to facilitate diffusion, it was clear that penetration occurred since phosphorylase was activated, but under these conditions only epinephrine stimulated contractile activity. The authors concluded that cyclic AMP was not an obligatory mediator of the inotropic and chronotropic action of epinephrine in the rat heart.

No studies have been performed on the effect of prostaglandins on heart adenyl cyclase; however, a direct effect of PGE_1 and $PGF_{2\alpha}$ has been observed on isolated cardiac sarcoplasmic reticulum by Sabatini-Smith [83] who observed significant uptake of calcium. Unfortunately, this effect was not studied in relation to adenyl cyclase.

2. *Human erythrocytes*

Human erythrocytes which are devoid of adenyl cyclase [84] respond to PGE_1 in two ways. Firstly, PGE_1 (2.8×10^{-8} M) significantly modified the distribution of plasma and erythrocyte sodium when blood was incubated at $37°C$ for 15 min [11]. Subsequently Allen and Rasmussen [85] found that at even smaller doses (10^{-10} M) PGE_2 decreased the deformation capacity of the erythrocyte membrane. The effect was dose-dependent and occurred in several species [85].

F. Conclusions

It is clear that many of the effects of prostaglandins are associated with changes in intracellular cyclic AMP. The similarity of the effects of these two agents also indicate that a causal relationship exists. Experiments to show that cyclic AMP stimulates prostaglandin formation have been equivocal in contrast to the effects of prostaglandins on cyclic AMP formation. From these results and those of the action of PGE_1 on systems where cyclic AMP does not appear to be implicated, it is likely that prostaglandins may exert their effects on the cell membrane prior to cyclic AMP formation. The site of action of the prostaglandins exhibits considerable structural specificity. The unique physico-chemical properties of the prostaglandins suggest that they may have substantial interactions with lipid-protein membranes and that their orientation at interphases may be the basis of their mechanism of action.

Acknowledgement

We are most grateful to Dr Neils Andersen, University of Washington, Seattle, for his comments and Dr Hideo Shio of the Alza Corp. The work was supported in part by ONR N00014-67-A-0122-0055 and NIH 2 RO1 NS 09585-02 grants to Stanford University.

Discussion

Graham (Welsh National School of Medicine)

I would like to show you the results of a small experiment which may be relevant to what Dr Ramwell has been saying.

My colleague Mrs S. Altai and I have used the isolated rabbit ear vascular bed, perfused at $37°C$ with gassed Krebs' solution containing noradrenaline (NA) 10^7 g/ml at a constant flow of 2 ml/min in which the peripheral resistance is recorded (Fig. 6). An upward deflection of the record indicates vasoconstriction and a downward one dilatation. In this preparation injections of prostaglandins PGE_1 or $PGF_2\alpha$ are dilator; infusions of PGE_1 have a small and variable effect, and infusions of $F_2\alpha$ are moderately constrictor. If the rabbits are pretreated with intramuscular injections of stilboestrol 0.5 mg stat and 0.1 mg daily for 14 days the dilator effect of injection of PGE_1 is abolished and may be reversed and the effect of the infusion is markedly constrictor, as also is the effect of $PGF_2\alpha$. If theophylline or the nucleotides ATP or $3'5'$AMP are added to the perfusate or ears of untreated rabbits, a similar reversal of the response to PG is found, especially $PGF_2\alpha$ (see Figure).

Stilboestrol treatment activates adenylcyclase [86] and potentiates the vasoconstrictor effect of catecholamine in NA-perfused rabbit ear [87]. Theophylline inhibits the diesterase. We suggest that the above evidence links the vascular response to PG in the rabbit ear vessels to the adenylcyclase-phosphodiesterase system and speculate that its presence or absence may act as a balance, determining the affinity of NA, the level of $3'5'$AMP and thus the response (constriction for high $3'5'$AMP, relaxation for low).

We gratefully acknowledge temporary laboratory facilities given to one of us (Suhaila Altai) by Professor V. R. Pickles and supplies of PG from Professor Van Dorp.

Pickles (Cardiff)

Dr Ramwell has mentioned the complex inter-relations of cyclic AMP, prostaglandins and calcium ions. My group at Cardiff is interested in the function of these substances in the myometrium.

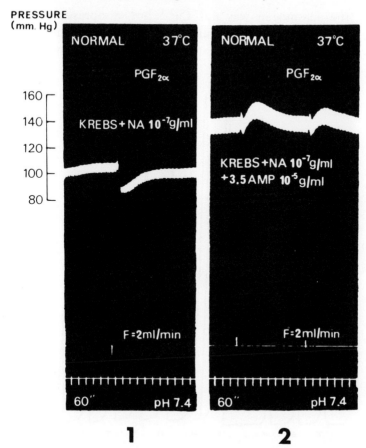

Fig. 6. Isolated rabbit ear perfused with gassed Krebs' solution containing NA 10^{-7} g/ml at 37°C and 2 ml/min. Record of the resistance in mm.Hg. Panel 1: vasodilator response to injection of 1 μg of $PGF_2\alpha$ in 0.1 ml saline. Panel 2: addition of 10^{-5} g/ml of 3'5' AMP to the perfusate results in constrictor responses to same injection.

Fig. 7, from an experiment by Jacqueline M. Wynne, shows the responses of guinea-pig uterus *in vitro* in a low-Ca medium with α- and β-blockers present. The contractions are caused by constant doses of additional Ca^{2+}. A dose of PGE_1, too small to cause a contraction response itself, increases the responses to the Ca^{+2} for at least 40 min after the PG is washed out. This effect seems to be identical with the rather specific form of potentiation or 'enhancement' described by Clegg, Hall and Pickles [88], in experiments in which the spasmogen was not Ca^{2+} but vasopressin. It was then suggested that the PGE might be improving the excitation-contraction coupling by facilitating intracellular Ca^{2+} movements.

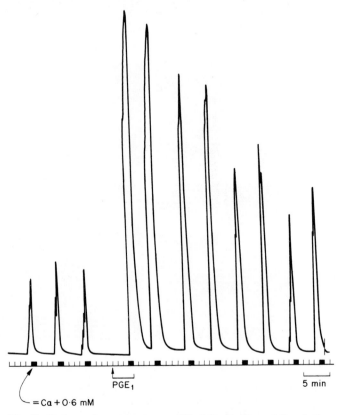

Fig. 7. Guinea-pig uterus in modified Krebs-Henseleit solution containing Ca 0.2 mM, Mg 3 mM, phentolamine and pro-pranolol 10^{-6} g/ml each. The responses to the addition of 0.6 mM Ca^{2+} are markedly enhanced following brief application of PGE_1 0.1 ng/ml.

Fig. 8 is from a further study of this possibility [89] and it shows that the effect of PGE_1 on Ca^{2+} responses can be mimicked by a much larger dose of dibutyryl cyclic AMP. Among the possible explanations of the similarity shown by these two Figs. are the following: (1) PGE_1 may increase the intracellular cyclic AMP concentration, which in turn facilitates Ca influx as does the exogenous dibutyryl derivative; (2) the dibutyryl-c-AMP releases an endogenous PGE, which itself facilitates Ca^{2+} influx by forming a readily-dissociable complex such as has been described by D. A. van Dorp and I. Heertje (personal communication).

Matthews (Boots)

Would you like to comment a little more on an apparent difference between rabbit and rat adipose tissue? Whereas we detected a prostaglandin in the epigastric tissue of rabbits during lipolysis [90, 91], did you say none was found in isolated rat fat pads?

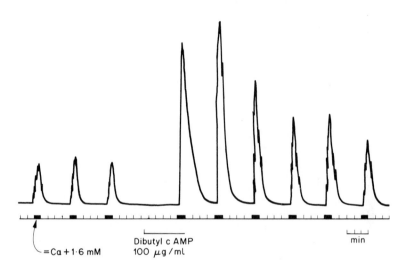

Fig. 8. Essentially as Fig. 7 (another preparation), but dibutyryl c-AMP 100 μg/ml has been applied instead of PGE_1.

Ramwell (Alza Corporation)

Rat epididymal fat pads contain and moreover synthesise prostaglandins [92]. This work was confirmed recently by Christ (see van Dorp [93]).

Bennett (King's College Hospital)

Do copper bracelets popularly worn for rheumatism act by altering prostaglandin synthesis?

Ramwell (Alza Corporation)

Some phlogistic action of prostaglandins have been observed [94] and it seems likely that inhibitors of prostaglandin synthetase may reduce inflammatory responses. Certain non-steroidal anti-inflammatory agents may act in part by inhibition of prostaglandin synthesis [95-97]. Certain metal ions have indeed been reported either to inhibit PGE_1 synthesis [98] or to change the direction of synthesis from the more inflammatory E compounds to the relatively inactive F compounds [99]. Thus there may be a very real basis for this question.

References

1. von Euler; *J. Physiol.*; **88**, (1936) 213.
2. Goldblatt, M. W.; *J. Soc. chem. Ind., Lond.*; **52**, (1933) 1056.
3. Bergström, S. and Sjövall, J.; *Acta chem. scand.*; **14**, (1960) 1693.
4. Hinman, J. W.; *Postgraduate Medical J.*; **46**, (1970) 562.
5. Bergström, S., Carlson, L. A. and Weeks, J. R.; *Pharmac. Rev.*; **20**, (1968) 1.
6. Weinheimer, A. J. and Spraggins, R. L.; *Tetrahedron Lett.*; No. 59 (1969) 5185.
7. van Dorp, D. A.; *Prog. Biochem. Pharmac.*; **3**, (1967) 71.
8. Butcher, R. W.; In: 'Role of Cyclic AMP in Cell Function. Advances in Biochemical Psychopharmacology'; Eds P. Greengard and E. Costa. Raven Press, New York, (1970) p. 173.
9. Stock, K., Aulich, A. and Westermann, E.; *Life Sci.*; **7**, (1968) 113.
10. Paoletti, R., Lentati, R. L. and Korlkiewicz, Z.; *Nobel Symposium 2, Prostaglandins*; Eds S. Bergström and B. Samuelsson. Almqvist and Wiksell, Stockholm, (1967) p. 147.
11. Ramwell, P. W. and Shaw, J. E.; *Rec. Prog. Horm. Res.*; **26**, (1970) 139.
12. Butcher, R. W. and Baird, C. E.; *J. biol. Chem.*; **243**, (1968) 1713.
13. Butcher, R. W. and Baird, C. E.; *Proc. 4th Int. Congr. Pharmac.*; Basle, 14-18 July, 1969, Vol. 4, p. 42, Schwabe, Basle (1970).
14. Abrahamsson, S.; *Acta Crystallogr.*; **16**, (1963) 409.
15. Rabinowitz, I., Ramwell, P. and Davison, P.; *Biochim. biophys. Acta*; in press.
16. Ramwell, P. W., Shaw, J. E., Corey, E. J. and Andersen, N.; *Nature, Lond.*; **221**, (1969) 1251.
17. Onsager, L.; In: 'The Physical Principles of Biological Membranes'; Eds F. Snell, J. Wolken, G. Iverson, and G. Lam. Gordon and Breach, New York, (1970) p. 137.
18. Hedwall, P. R., Abdel-Sayed, W. A., Schmid, P. G. and Abboud, F. M.; *Proc. Soc. exp. Biol. Med.*; **135**, (1970) 757.
19. Kaley, G. and Weiner, R.; *Proc. New York Academy of Sciences Conference on Prostaglandins*; 17-19 September, 1970, Vol. 180, p. 338 (1971).
20. Eakins, K.; *Proc. New York Academy of Sciences Conference on Prostaglandins*; 17-19 September, 1970, Vol 180, p. 386 (1971).
21. Sanner, J.; *Proc. New York Academy of Sciences Conference on Prostaglandins*; 17-19 September, 1970, Vol. 180, p. 396 (1971).
22. Fried, J., Mehra, M., Lin, C., Kao, W. and Dalven, P.; *Proc. New York Academy of Sciences Conference on Prostaglandins*; 17-19 September, 1970, Vol. 180, p. 38 (1971).
23. Avanzino, G. L., Bradley, P. B. and Wolstencroft, J. H.; *Br. J. Pharmac. Chemother.*; **27**, (1966) 157.
24. Eliasson, R. and Brzdekiewicz, Z.; *Life Sci.*; **9**, part 1, (1970) 925.

25. Ramwell, P. W. and Shaw, Jane E.; *Proc. Intern. Union Physiol. Sci.*; Vol. VII, Abstr. 1077. (1968).
26. Shaw, Jane E. and Ramwell, P. W.; *J. biol. Chem.*; **243**, (1968) 1498.
27. Ramwell, P. W., Shaw, Jane E., Douglas, W. W. and Poisner, A. M.; *Nature, Lond.*; **210**, (1966) 273.
28. Coceani, F., Pace-Asciak, C. and Wolfe, L. W.; *Prostaglandin Symposium of the Worcester Foundation for exp. Biol.*; Eds P. W. Ramwell and J. E. Shaw. Interscience, New York, (1968) p. 39.
29. Jessup, Sheila J., McDonald-Gibson, W. J., Ramwell, P. W. and Shaw, Jane E.; *Fed. Proc.*; **29**, (1970) 804.
30. Davies, B. N., Horton, E. W. and Withrington, P. G.; *Br. J. Pharmac. chemother.*; **32**, (1968) 127.
31. Gilmore, N., Vane, J. R. and Wyllie, J. H.; *Nature, Lond.*; **218**, (1968) 1135.
32. Kunze, H. and Vogt, W.; *Proc. New York Academy of Sciences Conference on Prostaglandins*; 17-19 September, 1970, Vol. 180, p. 123 (1971).
33. Lands, W. E. M. and Samuelsson, B.; *Biochim. biophys. Acta*; **164**, (1968) 426.
34. Änggård, E.; *Proc. 4th Int. Congr. Pharmac., Basle*; 14-18 July, 1969, p. 1, Schwabe, Basle (1970).
35. Dorp, D. van; *Proc. New York Academy of Sciences Conference on Prostaglandins*; 17-19 September, 1970, Vol. 180, p. 181 (1971)
36. Coceani, F., Puglisi, L. and Lavers, B.; *Proc. New York Academy of Sciences Conference on Prostaglandins*; 17-19 September, 1970, Vol. 180, p. 289 (1971).
37. Davies, B. N. and Withrington, P. G.; *Br. J. Pharmac. Chemother.*; **32**, (1968) 136.
38. Gilmore, N., Vane, J. R. and Wyllie, J. H.; In: 'Prostaglandins, Peptides and Amines.' Eds P. Mantegazza and E. W. Horton. Academic Press, London, (1969) p. 21.
39. Willis, A. L.; Ph.d. thesis in the University of London (1971).
40. Foss, P., Takeguchi, C., Tai, H. and Sih, C.; *Proc. New York Academy of Sciences Conference on Prostaglandins*; 17-19 September, 1970, Vol. 180, p. 126 (1971).
41. Wlodawer, P., Sammuelsson, B., Albonico, S. M. and Corey, E. J.; *J. Am. chem. Soc.*; **93**, (1971) 2815.
42. Bastide, F. and Jard, S.; *Proc. 24th Intern. Congr. physiol. Sci., Washington, D.C.*; Abstr. 97 (1968).
43. Fassina, G., Carpenedo, F. and Santi, R.; *Life Sci.*; **8**, part 1, p. 181 (1969).
44. Shaw, J. E. and Ramwell, P. W.; *Prostaglandin Symposium of the Worcester Foundation for exp. Biol.*; Eds P. W. Ramwell and J. E. Shaw. New York, (1968) p. 55.
45. Steinberg, D., Vaughan, M., Nestel, P. J., Strand, O. and Bergström, S.; *J. clin. Invest.*; **43**, (1964) 1533.
46. Butcher, R. W., Ho, R. J., Meng, H. C. and Sutherland, Earl W.; *J. biol. Chem.*; **240**, (1965) 4515.
47. Orloff, J., Handler, J. S. and Bergström, S.; *Nature, Lond.*; **205**, (1965) 397.
48. Butcher, R. W., Pike, J. E. and Sutherland, E. W.; *Nobel Symposium 2, Prostaglandins*; Eds S. Bergström and B. Samuelsson. Almqvist and Wiksell, Stockholm, (1967) p. 133.
49. Butcher, R. W., Baird, C. E. and Sutherland, E. W.; *Prostaglandin Symposium of the Worcester Foundation for exp. Biol.* Ed. P. W. Ramwell and J. E. Shaw, Interscience, New York (1968) p. 109.

50. Steinberg, D. and Vaughan, M.; *Nobel Symposium 2, Prostaglandins.* Eds S. Bergström and B. Samuelsson. Almqvist and Wiksell, Stockholm, (1967) p. 109.
51. Frank, H. and Braun, T.; *Fed. Proc.*; **30**, (1971) 625.
52. Berti, F., Naimzada, M. K., Lentati, R., Mategazza, P. and Paoletti, R.; *Prog. Biochem. Pharmac.*; **3**, (1967) 110.
53. Grantham, J. J. and Orloff, J.; *J. Lab. clin. Invest.*; **47**, (1968) 1154.
54. Orloff, J. and Handler, J.; *Am. J. Med.*; **42**, (1967) 757.
55. Bowery, N. G., Lewis, G. P. and Matthews, J.; *Br. J. Pharmac.*; **40**, (1970) 437.
56. Vaughan, M. and Murad, F.; *Biochem.*; **8**, (1969) 3092.
57. Bär, H. P. and Hechter, O.; *Biochem. biophys. Res. Commun.*; **35**, (1969) 681.
58. Marumo, F. and Edelman, I.; *J. clin. Invest.*; in press.
59. Mühlbachová, E., Sólyom, A. and Puglisi, L.; *Eur. J. Pharmac.*; **1**, (1967) 321.
60 Humes, J. L., Mandel, L. R. and Kuehl, F. A., Jr.; *Prostaglandin Symposium of the Worcester Foundation for exp. Biol.*; Eds P. W. Ramwell and J. E. Shaw. Interscience, New York, (1968) p. 79.
61. Kloeze, J.; *Nobel Symposium 2, Prostaglandins*; Eds S. Bergström and B. Samuelsson. Almqvist and Wiksell, Stockholm, (1967) p. 241.
62. Robison, G. A., Arnold, A. and Hatmann, R. C.; *Pharmac. Res. Commun.*; **1**, (1969) 325.
63. Shio, Hideo, Plasse, Anne Marie and Ramwell, Peter W.; *Microvascular Res.*; **2**, (1970) 294.
64, Shaw, J., Gibson, W., Jessup, S. and Ramwell, P.; *Proc. New York Academy of Sciences Conference on Prostaglandins*; 17-19 September, 1970, Vol. 180, p. 241 (1971).
65. Rosen, Ora M., Goren, Elihu N., Erlichman, Jack and Rosen, Samuel M.; In: 'Role of Cyclic AMP in Cell Function. Advances in Biochemical Psychopharmacology.' Eds P. Greengard and E. Costa. Raven Press, New York, (1970). p. 31.
66. Field, J., Dekker, A., Zor, U. and Kaneko, T.; *Proc. New York Academy of Sciences Conference on Prostaglandins*; 17-19 September, 1970, Vol. 180, p. 278 (1971).
67. Rodesch, F., Neve, P., Willems, C. and Dumont, J. E.. *Eur. J. Biochem.*; **8**, (1969) 26.
68. Onaya, T. and Solomon, D. H.; *Endocrinology*; **86**, (1970) 423.
69. Ahn, C. S. and Rosenberg, I. N.; *Endocrinology*; **86**, (1970) 396.
70. Burke, G.; *Am. J. Physiol.*; **281**, (1970) 1445.
71. Petersen, M. J. and Edelman, I. S.; *J. clin. Invest.*; **43**, (1964) 583.
72. Barry, E. and Hall, W. J.; *J. Physiol.*; **200**, (1969) 83P.
73. Eggena, P., Schwartz, I. L. and Walter, R.; *J. gen. Physiol.*; **56**, (1970) 250.
74. Orloff, J. and Grantham, J.; *Nobel Symposium 2, Prostaglandins*; Eds S. Bergström and B. Samuelsson. Almqvist and Wiksell, Stockholm, (1967) p. 143.
75. Lipson, L., Hynie, S. and Sharp, G.; *Proc. New York Academy of Sciences Conference on Prostaglandins*; 17-19 September, 1970, Vol. 180, p. 261 (1971).
76. Davis, B., Zor, U., Kaneko, T., Mintz, D. H. and Field, J. B.; *Clin. Res.*; **17**, (1969) 458.
77. Sharp, G. W. and Hynie, S.; *Nature, Lond.*; **229**, (1971) 266.

78. Vaughan, M., Pierce, N. F. and Greenough, W. B.; *Nature, Lond.*; **266**, (1970) 658.
79. Dobbs, J. W. and Robison, G. A.; *Fed. Proc.*; **27**, (1968) 352.
80. Paton, D. M. and Daniel, E. E.; *Can. J. Physiol. Pharmac.*; **45**, (1967) 795.
81. Wolfe, L. S., Coceani, F. and Pace-Asciak, C.; *Nobel Symposium 2, Prostaglandins*; Eds S. Bergström and B. Samuelsson. Almqvist and Wiksell, Stockholm, (1967) p. 265.
82. Oye, Ivar and Langslet, Asbjorn; *Acta Pharmacol.*; Supp. 1, p. 93 (1970).
83. Sabatini-Smith, S.; *Pharmacologist*; **12**, (1970) 239.
84. Wolfe, S. M. and Shulman, N. R.; *Biochem. biophys. Res. Commun.*; **35**, (1969) 265.
85. Allen, J. and Rasmussen, H.; in press.
86. Butcher, R. W., Robison, G. A. and Sutherland, E. W.; In: 'Control Processes in Multicellular Organisms', *Ciba Foundation Symp.*; ed. Wostenholme, G. E. W. and Knight, J., (1970) p. 64-85.
87. Altai, Suhaila A. and Graham, J. D. P., *J. Physiol. (Lond.)*; **212P**, (1971) *in press*.
88. Clegg, P. C., Hall, W. J., and Pickles, V. R.; *J. Physiol.*; **183**, (1966) 123.
89. Eagling, E. M., Lovell, H. G. and Pickles, V. R.; unpublished work.
90. Lewis, G. P. and Matthews, J.; *J. Physiol. Lond.*; **202**, (1969) 95.
91. Bowery, N. G., Lewis, G. P. and Matthews, J.; *Br. J. Pharmac.*; **40**, (1970) 437-445.
92. Shaw, Jane E. and Ramwell, P. W.; *J. biol. Chem.*; **243**, (1968) 1498.
93. Dorp, D. van.; Proc. New York Academy of Sciences Conference on Prostaglandins; 17-19 Sept., New York, (1971) p. 181.
94. Kaley, G. and Weinder, R.; Proc. New York Academy of Sciences Conference on Prostaglandins; 17-19 Sept. 1970., New York (1971) p. 338.
95. Ferreira, S. H., Moncada, S., and Vane, J. R.; *Nature, new Biol.*; **231**, (1971) 237.
96. Smith, J. B., and Willis, A. L.; *Nature, new Biol.*; **231**, (1971) 235.
97. Vane, J. R.; *Nature, new Biol.*; **231**, (1971) 232.
98. Nugteren, D. H., Beerthuis, R. K., and Dorp, D. A. van.; *Recl. Trav. Chim. Pays-Bas. Belg.*; **85**, (1966) 405.
99. Lands, W., Lee, R., and Smith, W.; Proc. New York Academy of Sciences Conference on Prostaglandins; 17-19 Sept.; New York, (1971) p. 107.

PLATELET AGGREGATION
AND CYCLIC AMP

G. V. R. Born

*Department of Pharmacology, Royal College of Surgeons
of England, Lincoln's Inn Fields, London, W.C.2*

Non-standard abbreviations: cyclic AMP = adenosine $3',5'$-(cyclic)-monophosphate; PGE_1 = prostaglandin E_1.

The only certain physiological function of blood platelets is in haemostasis [1]. Normal haemostasis depends on (i) contraction of the injured blood vessels; (ii) adhesion and aggregation of platelets which form a haemostatic plug; and (iii) coagulation of the plasma around the plug. The contribution of each of these processes to the overall haemostatic effect varies in different types of blood vessel and under different physiological conditions. The platelets contribute to normal coagulation by making available a phospholipid accelerator substance. Whether they also contribute to vascular contraction is less certain; they could do so through the release of vasoconstrictor substances such as 5-hydroxytryptamine or through the mechanism by which they cause clot retraction. The contribution of platelet plugs to haemostasis is greatest in small vessels, i.e. in arterioles and venules.

The formation of haemostatic plug of platelets depends on their rapid transformation from a non-adhesive to an adhesive state; this permits them to adhere to the walls of injured blood vessels and to each other so that millions of platelets aggregate in a few seconds (Fig. 1: from ref. [2]). The ease with which this change can be induced makes it more astonishing that blood is normally free of platelet aggregates than that they should tend to form also in diseased vessels, particularly in arteries, as thrombi. The involvement of platelets in acute thromboses, the incidence of which is still increasing rapidly, is an important reason for efforts to elucidate the biochemical mechanism of platelet aggregation as a rational basis for the discovery of effective antithrombotic drugs.

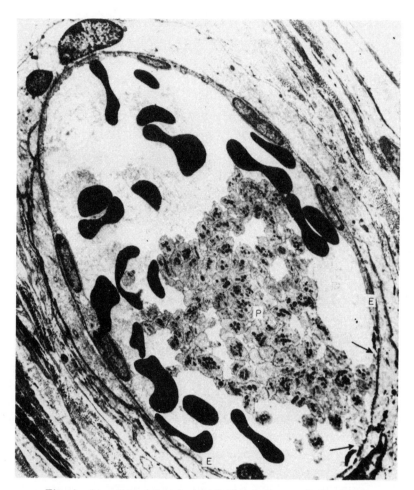

Fig. 1. An artery injured electrically. A mass of platelets is attached to the wall at the point (arrows) where the endothelium (E) has been destroyed. x 3600. (From ref. [1a].)

Platelet aggregation in vivo

An unsolved problem is the nature of the signal which causes circulating platelets to adhere to a vascular injury site. The injury may be very slight; indeed it is not known what constitutes the least abnormality required for adhesion to begin. Platelets do not adhere to normal endothelial cells but when these cells are made to contract, e.g. by histamine, intercellular gaps appear in which platelets tend to adhere to exposed basement membrane [3]. When vessels are exposed experimentally and remain uninjured, platelets do not adhere in them unless substances, e.g. adenosine diphosphate (ADP) or thrombin, are applied which cause platelet aggregation *in vitro.* ADP can be applied iontophoretically to the outside of small venules in the hamster cheek pouch by currents so small (10-100 nA) that they leave the endothelial lining intact [4]: this causes platelets to form aggregates in the lumen opposite the micropipette tip in a few seconds (Fig. 2). Amongst nucleotides, this effect is specific for ADP and rapidly disappears when the current is switched off.

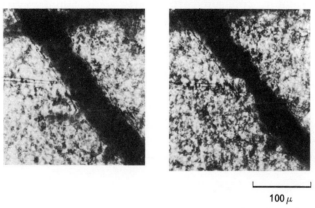

100 μ

Fig. 2. Normal venule before (left) and after (right) the application of a negative potential to the microelectrode shown, which was filled with 10^{-2} M ADP. The iontophoretic current was 150 nA. The photograph on the right was taken when the white body had grown for 50 sec. Scale, 100 μm. (From ref. [4].)

The details of the mechanism of platelet *adhesion* in living vessels are difficult to investigate experimentally. Platelet *aggregation,* on the other hand, can be investigated *in vitro* so that much more is known about it. Elucidation of the haemostatic function of platelets will involve finding out how far the *in vitro* findings apply *in vivo.*

Platelet aggregation in vitro
Most information has been obtained by a simple turbidimetric

technique [5, 6, 7] in which optical density changes of rapidly stirred suspensions of platelets in plasma or physiological saline solutions are continuously recorded. Platelet aggregation is associated with an increase and disaggregation with a decrease in light transmittance. The velocities of these optical changes provide a measure of aggregation or disaggregation and can be used to quantitate the effects of agents that promote or inhibit either process.

There are two classes of aggregating agent. One class consists of susbstances which do not occur naturally, such as polylysine; it seems that such positively charged molecules cause aggregation by bridge formation between negatively charged platelet surfaces. Whether such non-physiological aggregation is associated with effects on platelet cyclic AMP is not known.

The other class consists of naturally occurring substances which include thrombin, collagen, certain fatty acids, 5-hydroxytryptamine catecholamines, and ADP (for review see [8]). There is evidence that aggregation by all these different agents depends on the formation and/or release of ADP in the platelet membrane; it is convenient, therefore, to summarise the effects produced by added ADP.

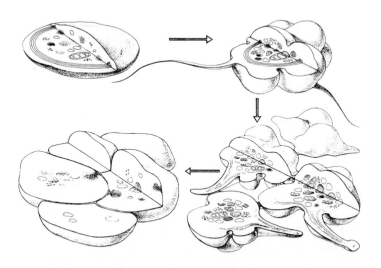

Fig. 3. Morphological changes of platelets during their aggregation. Top left, normal platelet; top right, after shape change; bottom right, during first phase of aggregation; and bottom left, during second phase of aggregation.

In human citrated platelet-rich plasma, ADP first causes a rapid morphological change of the platelets so that from being disc-shaped they become more spherical and extend irregular pseudopodia (Fig. 3); in the optical system this is associated with a small decrease in light transmittance through the plasma. Within 3 sec or so this is overtaken by a large increase in light transmittance associated with the formation of platelet aggregates of increasing sizes. If the ADP concentration is low (less than about 10^{-6} M) the aggregates rapidly disperse. Higher concentrations cause a further increase in light transmittance [9] associated with an increase in the closeness with which the platelets are packed together in the aggregates [10]. This second phase of aggregation is associated with the release from cytoplasmic granules of 5-hydroxytryptamine and adenine nucleotides, in man predominantly ADP [11].

Effect of catecholamines

Several years ago it was first shown [12] that adrenaline causes human platelets to aggregate. Our interest in the role of cyclic AMP in platelet aggregation can be traced back to continuing investigations of the effects of adrenaline and other catecholamines on platelets. Adrenaline greatly potentiates the aggregating effects of other agents including ADP [13], thrombin [14] and 5-hydroxytryptamine [15]. Noradrenaline is less active than adrenaline and isopropyl noradrenaline (isoprenaline) inhibits aggregation by ADP [16]. This suggested that the catecholamines can initiate aggregation by acting on an α-receptor and inhibit it by acting on a β-receptor. Indeed, aggregation by adrenaline is blocked by the α-antagonists phentolamine and dihydroergotamine but not by the β-antagonist propranolol except at high concentrations which probably affect the cell membrane non-specifically. It was known that the effects of the catecholamines on other tissues are accompanied by changes in the concentration of cyclic AMP [17, 18]. Ardlie, Glew and Schwartz [13] showed that high concentrations of the methyl xanthines, which inhibit phosphodiesterase, inhibit the aggregation of platelets and on the basis of this observation first suggested that cyclic AMP is involved in platelet aggregation. Much work has been done since then to find out whether this is so. Up to now the evidence indicates that, although increases in the concentration of cyclic ADP cause or contribute to the inhibition of aggregation, aggregation itself does not depend on a decrease in the cell's cyclic AMP.

Effects of added cyclic AMP

Platelet aggregation by AMP is inhibited by added cyclic AMP at high concentrations (10^{-3} M) and by dibutyryl cyclic AMP at somewhat lower concentrations (2×10^{-4} M) [19], presumably because the platelet membrane is almost impermeable to cyclic AMP itself but more permeable to its dibutyryl derivative.

Activation of adenylcyclase

Isoprenaline inhibits aggregation by thrombin or collagen as well as by ADP and this inhibition can be prevented by propranolol (Fig. 4: ref. [20]). Isoprenaline increases the activity of adenyl cyclase in particulate fractions of platelet homogenates [21, 22, 23].

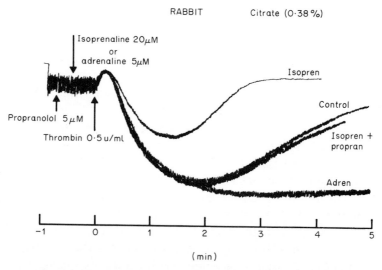

Fig. 4. The inhibition of the aggregation of rabbit platelets by isoprenaline and enhancement by adrenaline. Top trace: isoprenaline (20 μM) added 20 sec before thrombin (0.5 NIH u/ml). Second from top: Control response to thrombin alone. Third: Propranolol (5 μM) given 20 sec before isoprenaline; the response to thrombin was the same as in the control. Bottom trace: Adrenaline (5 μM) added 20 sec before thrombin. Aggregation is represented by a downward deflection of the trace. (From ref. [20].)

The most potent inhibitor of platelet aggregation known so far is prostaglandin E_1 (PGE_1) [24]; it inhibits aggregation by ADP completely at a molar ratio PGE_1 : ADP of 1:4.6. PGE_1 also increases the activity of platelet adenyl cyclase [19, 22, 23].

Inhibition of phosphodiesterase

If cyclic AMP is involved in controlling the aggregability of platelets, inhibitors of phosphodiesterase should enhance the inhibitory effect on aggregation of adenyl cyclase activators. This is indeed so. Aggregation by ADP, as well as platelet phosphodiesterase itself, are inhibited by the methyl xanthines, theophylline and caffeine alone in high concentrations [13, 21]. Furthermore, theophylline, in concentrations which have no effect by themselves, greatly increases the inhibitory potency of isoprenaline or of PGE_1; this combined effect is a true potentiation.

PGE_1 by itself causes small increases in the concentration of cyclic AMP in platelets but much larger increases in the presence of theophylline; this can be shown by increases in cyclic AMP radioactivity in platelets labelled either with radioactive adenosine [20, 25] or with radioactive adenine [36].

Effects of adenosine and 2-chloroadenosine

Next to PGE_1 the most potent inhibitors of platelet aggregation are adenosine and some of its analogues, notably 2-chloroadenosine [26, 27, 28]. There has been particular interest in efforts to establish the mechanism of inhibition by these substances. When they are used to inhibit aggregation produced by *low* concentrations of ADP, double reciprocal plots suggest that the inhibition is competitive [29, 30]. However, this does not explain the following observations: (i) the inhibition increases with time [26, 27]; (ii) the nucleosides inhibit much more than adenosine monophosphate (AMP) does which is closer in structure to ADP; and (iii) the inhibition is non-competitive against high concentrations (100-500 μM) of ADP [20].

It had been proposed that the inhibition results from the uptake of adenosine into the platelets which proceeds via the adenosine kinase reaction in which the nucleoside is phosphorylated [31]. This explanation was made unlikely by the demonstration [20, 32] that the drugs dipyridamole and papaverine, which block the uptake of adenosine by platelets [20, 33], actually potentiate the inhibitory effect of adenosine on aggregation.

The uncertainty about the mechanism of adenosine inhibition of platelet aggregation made two recent observations particularly interesting. First, adenosine, as well as the adenine nucleotides, increases the concentration of cyclic AMP in guinea-pig brain preparations [34]. Secondly, papaverine and dipyridamole inhibit ox heart phosphodiesterase [35]. These observations suggested that inhibition of aggregation by adenosine might depend also on an increase in the cyclic AMP content of platelets. Recently, Mills and Smith [36] have indeed demonstrated essential similarities in the inhibitory effects of isoprenaline, PGE_1, and adenosine or 2-chloroadenosine on platelet aggregation by ADP. Furthermore, the degree of inhibition by the nucleosides in the presence of phosphodiesterase inhibitors has been correlated under the same conditions with increases in the formation of cyclic AMP.

Methods for determining Cyclic AMP [36]

Human citrated platelet-rich plasma was incubated with $[U-^{14}C]$ adenine of high specific activity until about 90% of the radioactivity had been taken up by the platelets by incorporation into their adenine nucleotides including cyclic AMP. Aggregation was measured photometrically [6, 16] as the maximum rate of change of light transmission 10-30 sec after the addition of ADP. High concentrations of ADP (more than 100 μM) were used at which the inhibition by adenosine is no longer competitive.

One ml samples of platelet-rich plasma were incubated at 37° with drugs in the aggregometer and successive samples were used for measuring platelet aggregation and for determining radioactive cyclic AMP. For this, the sample was removed from the aggregometer and mixed with perchloric acid containing carrier as well as radioactive cyclic AMP as internal marker to control for variations in recovery in the subsequent stages. After centrifuging down the proteins a sample of supernatant was passed through Dowex 50W (X4) resin in a small column which was washed and eluted with water. The eluates were treated twice with zinc sulphate and barium hydroxide [37]. The radioactivity of the final supernatant was determined by scintillation counting. In a control experiment the recovered radioactivity was identified as cyclic AMP by isolation using paper electrophoresis.

Results are shown as radioactivity of cyclic AMP, expressed as a percent of the total adenine nucleotide radioactivity extracted from platelets in 1 ml plasma.

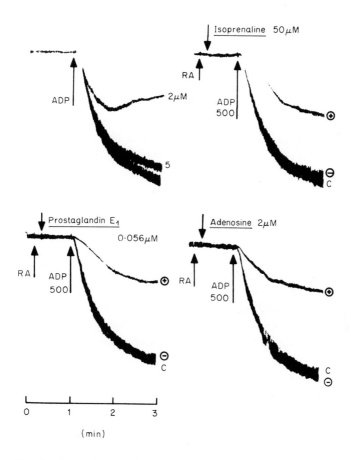

Fig. 5. Records of platelet aggregation in stirred human citrated platelet-rich plasma at 37°C, induced by ADP in the presence of an inhibitor of platelet $3':5'$-cyclic AMP phosphodiesterase (compound RA 233) and of isoprenaline, PGE_1 and adenosine. Aggregation is represented by a downward deflection of the trace. The top-left diagram shows ADP added alone to give final concentrations of 2, 5 and 500 μM (superimposed tracings). In each of the remaining three diagrams, line C represents response to ADP (500 μM) in presence of RA 233, line — represents responses to ADP in presence of isoprenaline, prostaglandin E_1 and adrenaline respectively, and line + represents response to ADP in presence of RA 233 *and* the additional drug. (From ref. [36].)

Synergism between adenyl cyclase activators and phosphodiesterase inhibitors

It was shown [36] first that several drugs inhibit platelet phosphodiesterase more potently than theophylline does. Phosphodiesterase activity in dialysed extracts of human platelets was measured with radioactive cyclic AMP as substrate by determining the unchanged cyclic AMP. The inhibiting drugs included papaverine and an analogue of dipyridamole (Persantin) known as compound RA 233 (2,6-bis-(diethanolamino)-4-piperidinopyrimido, [5,4d]-pyrimidine).

The phosphodiesterase inhibitors potentiated the inhibitory effect on aggregation of isoprenaline, PGE_1 and adenosine in a very similar manner (Fig. 5; ref. [36]). This effect was investigated further with compound RA 233. Increasing concentrations of PGE_1 alone caused increasing inhibition of aggregation. In the presence of compound RA 233 in concentrations which by themselves had little effect, the log-dose-response curve with PGE_1 was shifted to the left to an extent equivalent to an approximately ten-fold increase in its effectiveness. Determinations of cyclic AMP in the same experiment showed that the increasing inhibitory effect of PGE_1 was correlated with increasing concentrations of cyclic AMP which were somewhat greater in the presence of compound RA 233. Furthermore, compound RA 233 alone, in increasing concentrations (50-500 μM), also increased both cyclic AMP and inhibition of aggregation. However, these correlations differed in the three cases: the inhibition of aggregation associated with a given cyclic AMP concentration was greater in the presence of compound RA 233. This indicated that the rate of aggregation is not related directly to the concentration of cyclic AMP *when that was measured at the time of the addition of the aggregating agent.* The difference may be explained by the finding that during inhibition by PGE_1 [38] after an initial peak the concentration of cyclic AMP decreases again [39] and that, for a given peak, this fall is smaller in the presence of a phosphodiesterase inhibitor.

Adenosine inhibition in relation to cyclic AMP

Adenosine or 2-chloroadenosine, when added before ADP, produced a dose-dependent inhibition of aggregation (Fig. 6; ref. [36]). Only 2-chloroadenosine inhibited aggregation more or less completely; adenosine even at the highest concentrations used (5×10^{-4} M) did not inhibit more than about 50%. In the presence of the phosphodiesterase inhibitor compound RA 233 (50 μM), the

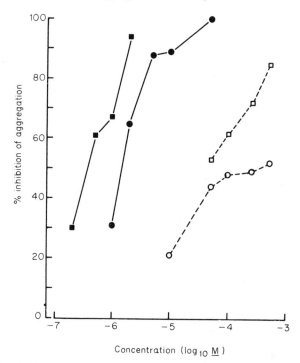

Fig. 6. Potentiation of the inhibition of platelet aggregation caused by adenosine and by 2-chloroadenosine by compound RA 233. ○, Adenosine alone; ●, adenosine added 10 sec after compound RA 233 (50 μM); □, 2-chloroadenosine alone; ■, 2-chloroadenosine added 10 sec after compound RA 233 (50 μM). Platelet-rich plasma was incubated for 40s with the nucleoside before the initiation of aggregation by ADP (100 μM).

log-dose response curves were displaced to the left to an extent indicating an approximately 100-fold increase in the effectiveness of the nucleosides; furthermore, inhibition by adenosine also became total with increasing concentrations. As for cyclic AMP under these conditions, adenosine or 2-chloroadenosine by themselves caused only small increases over the controls and without any demonstrable dose-dependence, probably because the increases were transient. In the presence of compound RA 233, however, the increases were larger and proportional to the concentrations of adenosine (Fig. 7; ref. [36]) or 2-chloroadenosine. Furthermore, there were correlations between the increases in the concentration of cyclic AMP and the percentage inhibition of aggregation which depended on the concentrations of RA 233.

If PGE_1 and adenosine were acting solely through activation of adenyl cyclase, and theophylline and compound RA 233 solely through inhibition of phosphodiesterase, then the relative potentia-

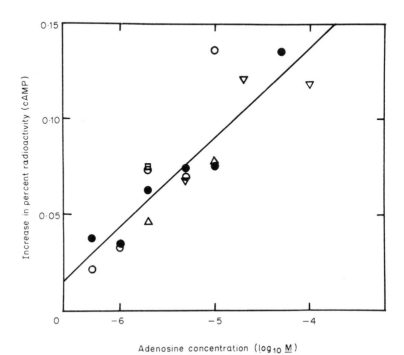

Fig. 7. Correlation between adenosine concentration and increased incorporation of radioactivity into $3':5'$-cyclic AMP in platelets prelabelled with $[^{14}C]$ adenine. Results from five experiments are given. The diagonal line is the regression of increase in % radioactivity as $3':5'$-cyclic AMP on the logarithm of the adenosine concentration; the correlation coefficient was calculated as $r = 0.88$.

tion of PGE_1 and of adenosine by compound RA 233 should be the same as that produced by theophylline. However, compound RA 233 potentiated adenosine much more than theophylline did at concentrations in which both caused similar potentiation of PGE_1. This suggested that there must be some other difference in these inhibitory mechanisms.

What this difference is is not yet clear. One possibility was suggested by the difference in the effect of compound RA 233 and theophylline on the uptake of adenosine by platelets. Compound RA 233 inhibited this uptake almost as effectively as dipyridamole [20,

33] whereas theophylline had no such effect. However, although the inhibitory effect of adenosine on aggregation (produced by 100 μM ADP) was potentiated somewhat by compound RA 233, it was potentiated little or not at all by dipyridamole, nor by dipyridamole together with theophylline. This showed that the difference between compound RA 233 and theophylline as potentiators of the inhibition of aggregation by adenosine cannot be attributed to the difference in their effect on adenosine uptake.

In slices of guinea-pig cerebral cortex the cyclic AMP concentration is greatly increased in the presence of low concentrations (50 μM) of adenosine and this effect is antagonised by theophylline [34]. The reason for this antagonism is not yet known. However, a similar antagonism in platelets could at least explain why theophylline increases the effects of PGE_1 on their cyclic AMP and aggregation but not those of adenosine.

Another possible explanation of the inhibitory effect of adenosine and 2-chloroadenosine would be by inhibition of platelet phosphodiesterase. However, the enzyme is inhibited by the nucleosides only at comparatively high concentrations, i.e. mM rather than μM [36]. In any case, adenosine is phosphorylated as rapidly as it is taken up into platelets [40] so that its concentration in them is probably never high enough to cause significant inhibition of intracellular phosphodiesterase. It is not known whether the uptake and metabolism of 2-chloroadenosine by platelets is similar to that of adenosine but the similarities in their effect suggest that this is so. These considerations make it unlikely that these nucleosides inhibit by diminishing the breakdown of cyclic AMP.

This leaves as their most likely mode of action an activating effect on adenylate cyclase in the platelet membrane whereby the concentration of cyclic AMP is increased.

By how much would the cyclic AMP concentration in platelets have to increase to produce significant inhibition of aggregation? When complete inhibition is produced by compound RA 233 alone, the associated increase in cyclic AMP is only from about 0.09 to 0.1% of the total radioactivity. This difference represents an increase of about 5×10^{-10} mole/10^{11} platelets or about 3000 molecules per platelet; this is a remarkably small number of molecules to have such a profound effect.

From what has gone before it might be expected that aggregation itself is associated with a *decrease* in platelet cyclic AMP. Careful experiments by Mills and Smith, with techniques which should have permitted such a decrease to be observed, provide no evidence for it.

Possible connections between increased cyclic AMP and inhibition of aggregation

How could increases in cyclic AMP concentration cause inhibition of platelet aggregation? The answer is not known but some possibilities may be considered.

First, in at least one type of cell, viz. the cellular slime mould *Dictyostelium discoideum*, cyclic AMP diffuses out of the single cells to cause their aggregation at a certain stage of their physiological life cycle [41]. As the physiological aggregating agent for platelets appears to be ADP, one possibility would be that increased cyclic AMP antagonises ADP directly at a site of action in the platelet membrane; for this there is no evidence.

A more likely possibility is that inhibition of aggregation is associated with a reaction which is specifically promoted by cyclic AMP. This would presumably be a side reaction which normally either does not proceed in platelets, or proceeds only slowly. One reaction that can apparently be excluded is the formation of active phosphorylase. Neither cyclic AMP itself nor activators of adenyl cyclase have any effect on the phosphorylase activity in intact platelets or in subcellular fractions [43]. Indeed, in contrast to many other tissues, platelet phosphorylase activity does not appear to be regulated by a direct effect of cyclic AMP.

Phosphorylations of platelet proteins

Cyclic AMP mediates the enzymic phosphorylations of many different proteins [44]. We are, therefore, engaged in exploring the phosphoproteins (and incidentally also the phospholipids) of platelets both during aggregation and under conditions in which inhibition of aggregation is associated with increases in cyclic AMP. Several years ago evidence was provided [42] that during clotting of human platelet-rich plasma, some of the platelet ATP phosphorylates protein (Fig. 8) and that, at the same time, some phospholipids become less extractable. The time courses of these changes were similar to those of the appearance of plasma thrombokinase [1] and it was suggested that the formation of this clotting factor might depend on platelet ATP.

Recently, the formation and turnover of platelet phosphoprotein (and phospholipids) have been followed with the help of radioactive phosphorus. Human citrated platelet-rich plasma was incubated at 37° with ^{32}P in the absence and presence of ADP as aggregating agent and/or a mixture of PGE_1 and RA 233 as augmentors of cyclic AMP in the platelets. Platelets were separated from plasma by centrifugation and fully extracted successively with trichloracetic acid, water, and a mixture of ethanol and ether which removed the

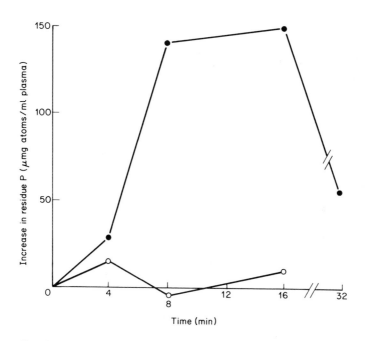

Fig. 8. Changes in concentration of phosphorus in the protein residues of platelet-rich (●) and platelet-free (○) plasma on clotting. Abscissa: time in minutes. Ordinate: increase in P (μmg atom/ml of plasma). (Modified from ref. [42].)

phospholipids; the residue consisted almost entirely of protein because platelets contain no DNA and only very little RNA. The protein and lipid fractions were dissolved in perchloric acid and the P and its radioactivity determined in the solutions.

In the absence of drugs, ^{32}P was incorporated into the phosphoprotein (and phospholipid) fractions of normal platelets with the time course shown in Fig. 9. On the assumption that these platelets were under steady-state conditions and that there was no change in the amount of protein-bound phosphorus, it was clear that this phosphorus has a turnover. When aggregation was induced by the addition of ADP (10 μM) there was a rapid increase in the rate of ^{32}P incorporation into the protein fraction (and a smaller increase in the lipid fraction). This increase occurred whether the ADP was added immediately after the ^{32}P or later when the specific activity of the platelet phosphoprotein fraction approached that of the P in the plasma. This indicated that the aggregating effect of ADP is associated with phosphorylation of platelet protein.

Such an increase could be due to the net new formation of phosphoprotein or to increases in the turnover rates of existing phosphoproteins or to both. To decide this, platelet-rich plasma was incubated at 37° with enough ADP (10 μM) to cause aggregation at a

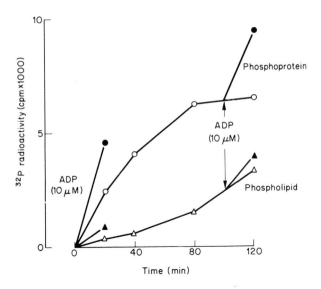

Fig. 9. Incorporation of phosphorus radioactivity into the phosphoproteins (circles) and into the phospholipids (triangles) of normal human platelets in citrated plasma at 37°. Open symbols controls, closed symbols after addition of ADP (10 μM) to induce aggregation.

maximal velocity. After 3 and 10 min intervals (Fig. 10), when aggregation was still maximal, there was an increase in total phosphoproteins as well as a closely corresponding increase in radioactivity. This indicated that aggregation by ADP is associated with a net increase in protein-bound P. After 30 min, by which time secondary processes produce alterations in aggregated platelets, there was a decrease in the phosphoprotein phosphorus but a great increase in its radioactivity, indicating that there was by now a much increased rate of turnover of protein-bound P. To relate these observations to effects of increased cyclic AMP on proteins, other samples of platelet-rich plasma were incubated with PGE_1 (1 μM) and compound RA 233 (50 μM) in concentrations known to cause

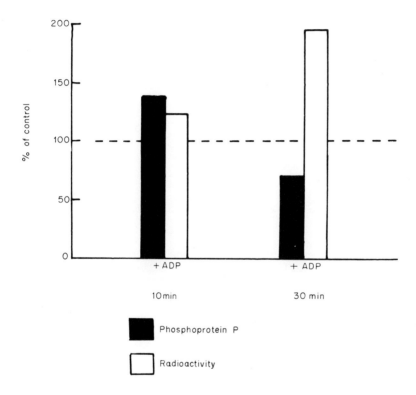

Fig. 10. Percentage change in phosphorus (black columns) and in phosphorus radioactivity (open columns) in the proteins of human platelets in citrated plasma at 37°, 10 min and 30 min after the addition of ADP (10 μM) to cause aggregation.

large increases in cyclic AMP. This caused considerable increases in the radioactivity of the protein fraction which appeared to be due to increased turnover rather than to net P incorporation. When ADP was added after the mixture of PGE_1 and RA 233 there was no further increase in radioactivity of the protein fraction (Fig. 11). From these results it seems that platelet aggregation by ADP is associated with a *net* increase in phosphoprotein. On the other hand,

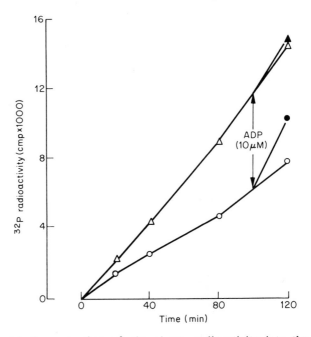

Fig. 11. Incorporation of phosphorus radioactivity into the phosphoprotein fraction of human platelets in citrated plasma at 37°: open circles, control; and closed circle, after addition of ADP (10 μM); open triangles, in presence of PGE_1 (1 μM) plus compound RA 233 (50 μM) to increase the intracellular cyclic AMP. Closed triangle was after addition of ADP (10 μM).

increases in cyclic AMP that are associated with inhibition of aggregation raise the turnover rate of phosphoprotein P.

Conclusions

On the basis of the observations made so far it seems reasonable to suggest that the aggregating effect of ADP depends on the protein phosphorylation which has now been demonstrated. Inhibition of aggregation by cyclic AMP could then be explained by assuming that the increased turnover of protein-bound P which it causes represents an acceleration in the phosphorylation of other proteins at the expense of the phosphoprotein involved in the aggregation process. Now, as ATP is necessary for the phosphorylations caused by both ADP and cyclic AMP, their opposing effect on aggregation could be accounted for by assuming competition for a limited pool of ATP.

The idea of such a competition can be shown as follows:

(1) Either, to produce aggregation:

ATP + membrane protein in conformation *a* $\xrightarrow[\text{dependent on cyclic AMP}]{\text{protein kinase not}}$ ADP + phosphorylated membrane protein in conformation *b*

(2) Or, to produce inhibition:

ATP + other protein(s) $\xrightarrow[\text{activated by cyclic AMP}]{\text{protein kinase(s)}}$ ADP + other phosphorylated proteins

It has to be assumed that any regeneration of the ATP used in these reactions, presumably from the main metabolic pool of ATP [45], is rate determining.

It has already been suggested that the rapid shape change reaction to ADP and to other aggregating agents depends on a conformational change in membrane protein [46]. It now seems likely that such a change is caused by a phosphorylation reaction. The results indicate that the phosphoprotein formed during aggregation is stable at least for several minutes; it should, therefore, be possible to isolate it. Further understanding of aggregation and of its cyclic AMP-dependent inhibition will require identification of the phosphorylated proteins and conclusive tests of the idea of competition for ATP or, conceivably, for another cofactor such as Ca^{2+}. Experimental work is continuing with these aims in mind.

Discussion

Haslam (I.C.I.)

By measuring [^{14}C]-cyclic AMP after pre-incubation of platelet-rich plasma with [^{14}C]-adenine we have recently found three pieces of evidence which suggest that platelet aggregation induced by adrenaline or any other agent is not mediated by a decrease in the level of cellular cyclic-AMP. Firstly, aggregating agents caused no significant changes in basal [^{14}C]-cyclic AMP levels in platelets even when these were measured by a more refined technique (including a chromato-graphic step) than used by Professor Born and his colleagues. Secondly, the inhibitions of PGE-induced formation of $[^{14}C]$-cyclic AMP by *different* aggregating agents were not related to the rates of aggregation they caused in the absense of PGE. Thirdly, in the presence of PGE_1 considerable aggregation was observed at $[^{14}C]$-cycle AMP levels well above the basal value. We reported these results at a recent meeting in Paris, which will shortly appear in book form [47].

Born (Royal College of Surgeons)

I knew that we were in agreement with Dr Haslam and I am happy about that.

Mitchell (Birmingham)

You have shown stimulation of phospholipid turnover, as well as turnover of phosphoprotein, during platelet aggregation. Have you any information on the cellular site of this reaction or of the types of phospholipid which are involved?

Born (Royal College of Surgeons)

Not yet.

References

1. Born, G. V. R.; In: 'Platelets in haemostasis and blood coagulation'. Ed. R. Biggs. Blackwell, Oxford, (1971) in press.
2. French, J. E., Macfarlane, R. G. and Sanders, A. G.; *Br. J. Exp. Path.*; **45**, (1964) 467.
3. Tranzier, J. P. and Baumgartner, H.; *Nature, Lond.*; **216**, (1967) 1126.
4. Begent, N. and Born, G. V. R.; *Nature, Lond.*; **227**, (1970) 926.
5. Born, G. V. R.; *J. Physiol.*; **162**, (1962) 67.
6. Born, G. V. R.; *Nature, Lond.*; **194**, (1962) 927.
7. Mills, D. C. B. and Roberts, G. C. K.; *J. Physiol.*; **193**, (1967) 443.
8. Mustard, J. G. and Packham, M. A.; *Pharm. Rev.*; **22**, (1970) 97.
9. Macmillan, D. C.; *Nature, Lond.*; **211**, (1966) 140.
10. Born, G. V. R. and Hume, M.; *Nature, Lond.*; **215**, (1967) 1927.
11. Mills, D. C. B., Robb, J. A. and Roberts, G. C. K.; *J. Physiol.*; **195**, (1968) 715.
12. Clayton, S. and Cross, M. J.; *J. Physiol.*; **1969**, (1963) 82.
13. Ardlie, N. G., Glew, G. and Schwartz, C. J.; *Thromb. Diathes. Haem.*; **18**, (1967) 670.
14. Thomas, D. P.; *Nature, Lond.*; **215**, (1967) 298.
15. Baumgartner, H. R. and Born, G. V. R.; *J. Physiol.*; **201**, (1969) 39.
16. Mills, D. C. B. and Roberts, G. C. K.; *J. Physiol.*; **193**, (1967) 443.
17. Sutherland, E. W., Oye, I. and Butcher, R. W.; *Recent Prog. Horm. Res.*; **21**, (1965) 623.

18. Sutherland, E. W., Robison, A. and Butcher, R. W.; *Circulation*; **37**, (1968) 27.
19. Marquis, N. R., Vigdahl, R. L. and Tavormina, P. A.; *Biochem. biophys. Res. Comm.*; **35**, (1969) 265.
20. Mills, D. C. B., Smith, J. B. and Born, G. V. R.; *Proc. 18th Annual Symp. on Blood*; Detroit, in press.
21. Abdulla, Y. H.; *J. Atheroscler. Res.*; **9**, (1969) 171.
22. Wolfe, S. M. and Shulman, N. R.; *Biochem. biophys. Res. Comm.*; **35**, (1969) 265.
23. Zieve, P. D. and Greenough, W. B.; *Biochem. biophys. Res. Comm.*; **35**, (1969) 462.
24. Kloeze, J.; In: 'Prostaglandins'; Eds S. Bergstrom, and S. A. Samuelson. Interscience Publishers, London, (1967) p. 241.
25. Vigdahl, R. L., Marquis, N. R. and Tavormina, P. A.; *Biochem. biophys. Res. Comm.*; **37**, (1969) 409.
26. Born, G. V. R. and Cross, M. J.; *J. Physiol.*; **168**, (1963) 178.
27. Born, G. V. R.; *Nature, Lond.*; **202**, (1964) 95.
28. Maguire, H. M. and Michal, F.; *Nature, Lond.*; **217**, (1968) 571.
29. Skoza, L., Zucker, M. Jerushalmy, Z. and Grant, R.; *Thromb. Diathes. Haem.*; **18**, (1967) 713.
30. Michal, F. and Born, G. V. R.; *Nature, Lond.*; **(1971) in press**.
31. Rozenberg, M. C. and Holmsen, H.; *Biochim. biophys. Acta.*; **155**, (1968) 342.
32. Born, G. V. R. and Mills, D. C. B.; *J. Physiol.*; **202**, (1969) 41.
33. Markwardt, F., Barthel, W., Glusa, E. and Hoffman, A.; *Arch. exp. Path. Pharmak.*; **257**, (1967) 420.
34. Sattin, A. and Rall, T. W.; *Molec. Pharmac.*; **6**, (1970) 13.
35. Poch, G., Juan, H. and Kukovetz, W. R.; *Arch. exp. Path. Pharmak*; **264**, (1969) 293.
36. Mills, D. C. B. and Smith, J. B.; *Biochem. J.*; **121**, (1971) 185.
37. Krishna, G., Weiss, B. and Brodie, B. B.; *J. Pharmac. exp. Ther.*; **163**, (1968) 379.
38. Ball, G., Brereton, G. G., Fulwood, M., Ireland, D. M. and Yates, P.; *Biochem. J.*; **114**, (1969) 669.
39. Salzman, E. W. and Neri, L. L.; *Nature, Lond.*; **224**, (1969) 609.
40. Ireland, D. M. and Mills, D. C. B.; *Biochem. J.*; **99**, (1966) 283.
41. Konijn, T. M., Barkley, D. S., Chang, Y. Y. and Bonner, J. T.; *The American Naturalist*; **102**, (1968) 225.
42. Born, G. V. R.; *Biochem. J.*; **68**, (1958) 695.
43. Deisseroth, A., Wolfe, S. M. and Shulman, N. R.; *Biochem. biophys. Res. Comm.*; **39**, (1970) 551.
44. Rodnight, R. B.; This Symposium.
45. Holmsen, H.; 'Adenine Nucleotide Metabolism of Blood Platelets'; Oslo; Universitetsforlaget. (1969).
46. Born, G. V. R.; *J. Physiol.*; **209**, (1970) 487.
47. Haslam, R. J. and Taylor, A. In 'Platelet Aggregation' Ed. Caen, J. P.; Masson, Paris (1971).

CYCLIC 3', 5'- ADENOSINE MONOPHOSPHATE AND THE ANAPHYLACTIC REACTION

E. S. K. Assem

Department of Pharmacology, University College London, and Medical Unit, University College Hospital Medical School

Non-standard abbreviations: Cyclic AMP = Adenosine 3',5'-cyclic monophosphate. DB-CAMP = Dibutyryl-adenosine 3',5'-cyclic monophosphate. SRS-A = slow reacting substance of anaphylaxis [16].

Mechanism of Anaphylaxis

Anaphylactic antibodies

The anaphylactic reaction (immediate-type allergy) is the reaction mediated by certain classes of antibodies known collectively as anaphylactic (tissue-sensitising) antibodies. Various species produce their own characteristic anaphylactic antibodies [1, 2, 3].

Various classifications are applied to these antibodies. The term 'homocytotropic' antibody was introduced by Becker and Austen [4] to describe a specialised class of anaphylactic antibodies capable of attaching to certain target cells of the same species. Homocytotropic antibodies may further be classified into 'reaginic' and non-reaginic. Antibodies mediating the anaphylactic reaction in man are of the reaginic type. They belong mainly to the recently discovered γE (IgE) class of immunoglobulins [5, 6].

The anaphylactic reaction

The interaction between cell-bound anaphylactic antibody and specific antigen (allergen) triggers a chain of reactions leading to the release of pharmacological mediators of the anaphylactic reaction. The diagrammatic representation of the main steps of this process

259

which is initiated at the cell surface (e.g. on the surface of mast cells or polymorphonuclear leucocytes) is shown in Fig. 1. The Fc region of the antibody molecule is the part involved in cell fixation. The other end of the antibody molecule is the part involved in antigen-binding (fragment antigen binding, Fab). It has been suggested that the combination of cell-bound antibody with the specific allergen induces a conformational change within the Fc region of the antibody molecule which initiates a critical reaction at the cell surface. This is thought to activate a series of enzyme reactions which finally end in the release of the pharmacological mediators of

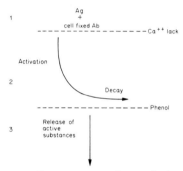

Fig. 1. Diagrammatic representation of the anaphylactic mechanism. Inhibitors (like phenol) may prevent mediator release without interference with activation and decay of the anaphylactic mechanism, i.e. they inhibit mediator release without inhibiting desensitisation. Calcium may not be essential for the 'activation' of the enzyme system but is necessary for the mediator release process [39].

the reaction [7, 8, 9]. The activated system becomes rapidly inactivated again. Activation of the anaphylactic system requires calcium and seems to involve a normal component of tissue which is heat labile. This factor is inactivated at 43° to 45°C [10]. All anaphylactic systems seem to require calcium and in the absence of calcium, mediators such as histamine are not released. Under experimental conditions the effects of calcium and pH are interdependent, e.g. calcium lack can be partially counteracted by increasing pH [10, 11]. The system behaves as if a calcium–protein complex were formed, dissociation occurring at an acid pH. The nature of this cellular response and the identity of the activation system has not been established. Becker [12] suggested that the reaction involves direct or indirect activation of serine esterases.

Most investigators consider that the interaction between cell-bound antibody and antigen is a non-cytotoxic mechanism. It leads to selective rather than generalised loss of cell constituents, and the integrity of the cell membrane is maintained. The release of pharmacological mediators has been considered a sort of secretion, or a form of reverse phagocytosis, when granules containing stored mediators are extruded. Although oxidative metabolic processes do not seem to be required in most of the anaphylactic models, like the isolated rat peritoneal mast cells [13] and the human leucocyte preparation, the glycolytic pathways are essential [14]. Further support for the secretory nature of the antigen-induced histamine release was obtained from the effect of colchicine. Colchicine, which distorts the microtubular structure of a variety of cell types, has been shown to inhibit allergic histamine release [15]. Studies with other inhibitors, as discussed later, are compatible with the postulated secretory nature of anaphylactic histamine release in a variety of test systems.

Pharmacological mediators

Several pharmacologically active substances may be released or formed in the anaphylactic reaction, but only a few fulfil the criteria of a 'mediator'. The nature of the released mediators depends on the species and tissue involved in the reaction. An ever-extending list includes histamine, slow-reacting substance of anaphylaxis (SRS-A) [16], 5-hydroxytryptamine (serotonin), kinins e.g. bradykinin [17], prostaglandins e.g. $PGF_{2\alpha}$, and a recently discovered substance, one of the main characteristics of which is the ability to produce contraction of rabbit aorta [18]. Other suggested mediators include substances released from the lysosomes of polymorphonuclear leucocytes, platelets [19] and macrophages [20]. The factors responsible for the chemotactic response of polymorphonuclear leucocytes may be added to this list.

The manifestations of the anaphylactic reaction can, in general terms, be explained by the effect of the released pharmacological mediators on various 'shock' organs or tissues. Examples of these manifestations are bronchospasm, as in allergic bronchial asthma, and increased vascular permeability.

Inhibition of the anaphylactic reaction

Studies of the possible ways of inhibiting this reaction are of great value for two main reasons. Firstly, they help us to understand the fundamental mechanism of the anaphylactic reaction. Secondly, they are essential for the development of new remedies for allergic conditions, such as bronchial asthma.

From the pharmacological point of view at present, there are three main approaches: (1) the use of drugs which interfere specifically with action of the released mediator on its specific receptor; (2) physiological antagonism of the effect of mediators e.g. production of bronchodilation by sympathomimetics in asthma; (3) interference with the cellular processes which lead to mediator release. A

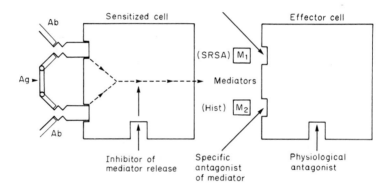

Fig. 2. Schematic representation of the anaphylactic reaction (e.g. in asthma). Inhibition of this reaction can be produced in three different ways, two of which (inhibition of mediator release and physiological antagonism of mediators) are probably mediated by cyclic AMP.

schematic representation of these three different approaches is shown in Fig. 2.

The role of cyclic AMP in the anaphylactic reaction is related to two of these; interference with the mediator release mechanism [21-25] (referred to as the anti-anaphylactic effect), and the physiological antagonism of mediator effects.

Cyclic AMP and Inhibition of the Anaphylactic Reaction

Evidence of the role of cyclic AMP in the suppression of the anaphylactic mechanism is mainly circumstantial at present. However it is supported by the following observations.

Inhibition of the anaphylactic mediator release by sympatho-mimetics

Until recently, the effectiveness of sympathomimetics in bronchial asthma was attributed entirely to their direct relaxation of bronchial smooth muscle. Their additional effect as inhibitors of mediator release has escaped attention for many years, although Schild, in 1936 [26], observed that adrenaline produced significant inhibition of histamine release from isolated perfused guinea-pig lung. This was completely forgotten until recently, when interest in inhibitors of the anaphylactic mechanism was revived.

The effect of sympathomimetics as inhibitors of mediator release in allergic bronchial asthma cannot be distinguished from the direct effect on bronchial smooth muscle. It is not surprising, therefore,

Table 1
Anaphylactic Models used for the Study of Inhibition of Mediator Release

---

In vitro
　　Actively sensitised human leucocytes [21,22]
　　Passively sensitised human and monkey lung [22,25]
　　Actively and passively sensitised guinea-pig lung [23,46]
　　Isolated rat peritoneal mast cells.[28] Histamine release by;
　　　　a. Antigen
　　　　b. Compound 48/80

*In vivo**
　　Passive intraperitoneal anaphylaxis (rat)[24]
　　Passive cutaneous anaphylaxis (rat, guinea pig) [27,28]
　　Dextran-induced anaphylactoid reaction in rats [28]
　　Bronchial, nasal and skin tests in man[28]

---

* In all but intraperitoneal anaphylaxis, inhibition of mediator release has to be ascertained by other methods.

that the evidence was first obtained from *in vitro* anaphylactic models and then from certain *in vivo* models, which are listed in Table 1. In all these models sympathomimetics produced inhibition of mediator release, though to a variable extent.

The catecholamine concentrations required for inhibition of antigen-induced histamine release from isolated human leucocytes were high; for example, 50% inhibition was obtained with 2-6 x 10^{-4} M isoprenaline [21, 22]. These results were rather discouraging as the effective catecholamine levels seemed too high to be of any therapeutic or physiological value. However, we have obtained further evidence which has changed the outlook. This has been brought about in two ways: firstly, using other anaphylactic models, since in our experience the human leucocyte preparation is one of the most resistant to various inhibitors; secondly, using suboptimal antigen concentrations. This is of particular importance in actively sensitised preparations where inhibition is particularly dependent on antigen concentration.

Figure 3 shows the inhibition of histamine release from sensitised human leucocytes when optimal (20 μg/ml) and suboptimal (4

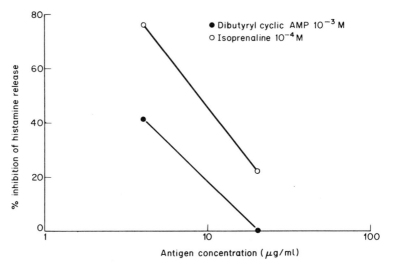

Fig. 3. Inhibition of antigen-induced histamine release from isolated human leucocytes (Antigen: *Dermatophagoides pteronyssinus*). Note: (1) the high concentration of isoprenaline required to produce inhibition; (2) marked inhibition was obtained only in the presence of low (sub-optimal) antigen concentration (4 μg/ml). Uninhibited histamine release in the latter case was 63% of total cell content, while in the presence of optimum antigen concentration (20 μg/ml) it was 94%.

μg/ml) antigen concentrations were applied. In both instances, histamine release was high (94% and 63%, respectively). Even with 10^{-4} M, isoprenaline inhibition of histamine release could be obtained only in the presence of suboptimal antigen concentration.

Figure 4 shows the inhibition, by various sympathomimetics of the antigen-induced histamine release, from passively sensitised human lung [22]. Histamine release by antigen in this preparation is very sensitive to inhibition by these agents. Isoprenaline in concentrations of 5 x 10^{-9} M or even much smaller concentrations, as shown in the experiment illustrated in Fig. 4, produced almost complete inhibition of the antigen-induced histamine release. The inhibition of mediator release by sympathomimetics is not restricted to histamine, since it has been shown by Ishizaka *et al.* [25] that in monkey lung passively sensitised with human IgE, isoprenaline inhibited the release of both histamine and SRS-A. Sympatho-

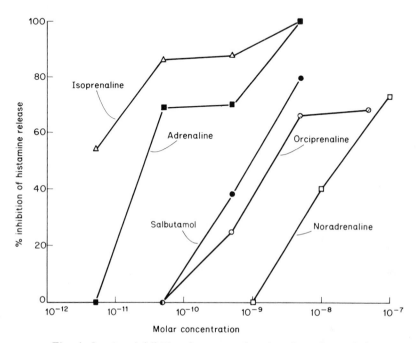

Fig. 4. *In vitro* inhibition by sympathomimetic amines of the antigen-induced histamine release from human lung passively sensitised to the house-dust mite *Dermatophagoides pteronyssinus*. Uninhibited histamine release 36.6% of total tissue content. (From ref. [22].)

mimetics were also shown to be active in *in vivo* anaphylactic models such as passive intraperitoneal anaphylaxis [24], and passive cutaneous anaphylaxis in the rat [27, 28].

Correlation of anti-anaphylactic effect of sympathomimetic amines with their β-adrenoceptor stimulating activity

The rank order of the relative anti-anaphylactic activity (inhibition of antigen-induced mediator release) of catecholamines, isoprenaline

> adrenaline > noradrenaline, suggests that this activity may be mediated through stimulation of β-adrenergic receptors. Other β-adrenoceptor stimulating drugs e.g. salbutamol and orciprenaline, were also more potent than noradrenaline [22]. The rank order of the anti-anaphylactic activity of various β-adrenoceptor stimulants e.g. isoprenaline > salbutamol > orciprenaline, in various *in vitro* anaphylactic models [29] was correlated with β-activity in certain non-anaphylactic *in vitro* preparations, e.g. on isolated guinea-pig trachea [30].

β-Adrenergic catecholamines promote the formation of cyclic AMP by a direct action on adenyl cyclase [31]. Since the anti-anaphylactic activity of various sympathomimetics was correlated with their β- rather than α-activity, it seems that this effect is likewise mediated through the adenyl cyclase system. It may seem that the inhibitory effect of sympathomimetics is too quick to be explained by the accumulation of cyclic AMP, since a large part of the histamine-releasing effect of antigen occurs within seconds of its application. It is known, however, that the promoting effect of catecholamines on the accumulation of cyclic AMP is likewise fast [32].

It has been suggested that α-adrenergic stimulants may increase rather than decrease SRS-A release in passive intraperitoneal anaphylaxis in the rat [24]. It was thought that this finding was compatible with the concept that stimulation of α-receptors may be mediated by a decrease in cyclic AMP in certain preparations [33]. This concept is yet to be established.

Table 2, which is based on material collected mainly from the literature, shows the comparison between the anti-anaphylactic activity of sympathomimetics and their effect on accumulation of cyclic AMP [34], lipolysis [35, 36] relaxation of guinea-pig trachea, and cardiac stimulation [37, 38]. The anti-anaphylactic activity seems to be best correlated with the relaxation of tracheal smooth muscle. The ability to promote accumulation of cyclic AMP seems to correlate well with the lipolytic, but not the anti-anaphylactic activity. However, this does not refute the hypothesis that the anti-anaphylactic activity is mediated by cyclic AMP.

Effect of NaF on the anaphylactic histamine release

The effect of fluoride on mediator release is a complex one since, in addition to stimulation of adenyl cyclase, it produces inhibition of glycolytic pathways which seem to be essential for the anaphylactic mechanism.

Lichtenstein [14] and his collaborators, while studying the influence of interference with the glycolytic pathway on the anaphylactic histamine release from isolated human leucocytes reported that 50% inhibition could be obtained with 10^{-2} M fluoride. Again using intact homogenised tissues, we obtained very little inhibition of histamine release, e.g. in chopped guinea-pig lung. Fluoride in a concentration of 10^{-3} M produced a small inhibition of

Table 2
Comparison of Anti-anaphylactic Effect of Sympathomimetics with other Activities

	Isoprenaline	Adrenaline	Salbutamol	Noradrenaline
receptor	$\beta_1 + \beta_2$	$\alpha + \beta_1$ and β_2	$\beta_2 > \beta_1$	$\alpha > \beta$
Accumulation of cyclic AMP (rat epid. fat pad)[34]	++++	+++	N.R.	+++
Anti-anaphylaxis (man, rat, guinea-pig)[22,23,28]	++++	+++	++	+
Lipolysis (rat, rabbit)[35,36]	++++	+++	++	+++
Relaxation of tracheal chain (guinea-pig)[30]	++++	+++	+++	+
Cardiac stimulation (rabbit, dog)[36]	++++	+++	+	++

N.R. = not reported.

about 10% (Fig. 9). In the isolated human leucocyte preparation, a very small inhibition (5%) was obtained with 10^{-4}-10^{-3} M NaF, even when it was added to leucocytes 15 min prior to challenge with antigen (Fig. 8). On the whole, fluoride has little effect on adenyl cyclase activity when applied to intact cells. Therefore, the small inhibition of histamine release was not surprising.

Adenyl cyclase in anaphylactic models

Apart from the evidence so far presented, there is little to support the direct implication of adenyl cyclase in the anti-anaphylactic effect of β-stimulants. Using intact human leucocytes without stimulation, we obtained little or no measurable activity of adenyl cyclase, but a measurable response was obtained on stimulation with isoprenaline (Fig. 5). Scott [40] reported that mixed human leucocyte homogenates did not produce any assayable amounts of cyclic AMP without the addition of stimulatory agents. So far, information about adenyl cyclase in the other anaphylactic models is scanty. Martin [27] could not obtain any stimulation of this enzyme system by the β-adrenergic agents in rat peritoneal mast cells,

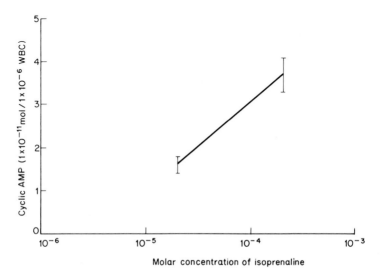

Fig. 5. Stimulation by isoprenaline of ^{3}H-cyclic AMP formation in the leucocytes of an allergic patient. Unstimulated level less than 1×10^{-11} mol/l $\times 10^6$ WBC. Incubation performed at 37°C for 15 min in Tyrode solution (pH 7.4-7.6), 0.3 mg/ml human serum albumin, Ca^{++} 0.9 mM, Mg^{++} 0.7 mM, theophylline 10^{-3} M. Final addition of ATP and unlabelled cyclic AMP to 10^{-3} M concentrations.

although these agents produced strong inhibition of SRS-A release in passive intraperitoneal (*in vivo*) rat anaphylaxis and relatively small inhibition of histamine release from mast cells *in vitro* [28].

Antagonism of the anti-anaphylactic effect of sympathomimetics by β-adrenergic blocking agents

β-Adrenergic blocking drugs like propranolol antagonised the anti-anaphylactic effects of β-adrenergic agents both *in vitro* (Fig. 6)

[22, 41] and *in vivo* [24, 27]. The anti-anaphylactic effect of isoprenaline was also inhibited by the 'selective' β-blockers, practolol and butoxamine, a response similar to some of the metabolic activities [42, 43]. Inhibition of adenyl cyclase by β-blocking agents has also been reported [34, 44].

Inhibition of mediator release by phosphodiesterase inhibitors
  The methylxanthines theophylline, theobromine and caffeine, which promote cellular levels of cyclic AMP through the inhibition

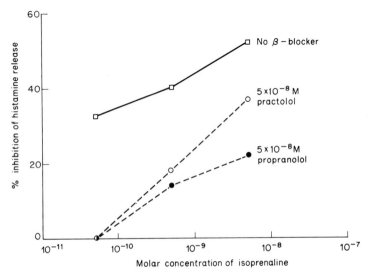

Fig. 6. Antagonism by propranolol and practolol of the inhibition by isoprenaline of the antigen-induced histamine release from passively sensitised human lung (antigen; *Dermatophagoides pteronyssinus*). Uninhibited histamine release 11.0 ± 1.0%. (From ref. [41].)

of nucleotide phosphodiesterase [45], also inhibit the antigen-induced histamine release from sensitised human leucocytes, from human, monkey and guinea-pig lung [21, 23, 25, 46], and SRS-A release in rat intraperitoneal anaphylaxis [24]. Although significant inhibition may be produced by low concentrations of theophylline (10^{-7}-10^{-6} M) in human and guinea-pig lung preparations, this effect is not consistent. Furthermore, the shape of the inhibitor dose-reponse curve was not clearly progressive with concentration (Fig. 7).

Two new phosphodiesterase inhibitors (ICI 30,966 and 58,301) were also found to produce a degree of inhibition of histamine release from human leucocytes (unpublished). One of these compounds (ICI 30,966) has been found to be about ten times more potent than theophylline, as an inhibitor of human lung phosphodiesterase [27]. Both theophylline and ICI 30,966 enhanced the inhibitory activity of low doses of β-adrenergic stimulants.

All the previously mentioned findings suggest that the inhibition of anaphylactic mediator release is mediated by cyclic AMP, since

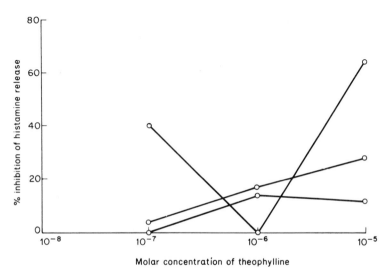

Fig. 7. Inhibition by theophylline of histamine release by antigen (*D. pteronyssinus*) from passively sensitised human lung. Results obtained from three experiments. (Uninhibited histamine release 11.1-47.7%). (From ref. [46].)

both β-adrenergic agents and phosphodiesterase inhibitors promote cellular levels of this nucleotide. This hypothesis is reinforced by the specific action mechanism of these various agents. For example, disodium cromoglycate, while it is also an inhibitor of anaphylactic mediator release [47, 48] was not antagonised by β-adrenergic blocking agents [29] nor was it potentiated by phosphodiesterase inhibitors [27].

Effect of exogenous cyclic AMP

The dibutyryl derivative of cyclic AMP (DB-CAMP) inhibits mediator release to different degrees in various anaphylactic models

[21, 24, 25]. Significant inhibition, however, required high concentration (10^{-4}-10^{-3} M) (Fig. 3). Cyclic AMP itself produces little or no inhibition of mediator release. The great potency of the dibutyryl derivative has been attributed to its greater lipid solubility and ease of penetration of cell membrane. However, one of the unexplained findings was that cyclic AMP occasionally enhanced rather than inhibited immunologic histamine release (unpublished).

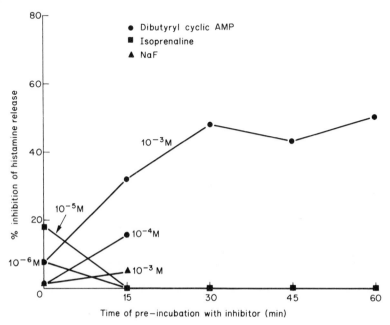

Fig. 8. Effect of prior incubation of sensitised leucocytes (before addition of antigen) with isoprenaline, dibutyryl cyclic AMP and NaF, on the histamine release by antigen (*D. pteronyssinus*).

Dibutyryl cyclic AMP, unlike catecholamines and methylxanthines, produced greater inhibition when applied before the antigen. Maximum inhibition requires at least 30 min of prior incubation with DB-CAMP (Fig. 8) while β-adrenergic stimulants produced maximal inhibition when they were applied either immediately before, or together with antigen. The apparently slow action of DB-CAMP may again be explained by limitation in access into cells. But one cannot exclude the possibility that this compound may have a different mode of action.

Differential response to catecholamines and cyclic AMP

The evidence implicating cyclic AMP as an important inhibitor of the anaphylactic mechanism is based mainly on the hypothesis that β-adrenergic catecholamines act on discrete and specific receptors that in turn affect the activity of an adenyl cyclase system, and on the inhibition of mediator release by exogenous DB-CAMP. However, the relative responsiveness to catecholamines and DB-CAMP shows great variation from one tissue to another. The best example is the difference between lung tissue and leucocytes. The first indication of

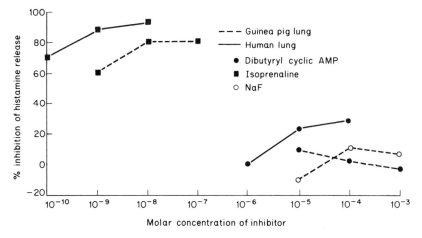

Fig. 9. Comparison of the inhibition by isoprenaline and dibutyryl cyclic AMP of antigen-induced histamine release from passively sensitised human and guinea-pig lung. Human lung sensitised by homologous reaginic serum (Antigen: *D. pteronyssinus*). Guinea-pig lung sensitised by purified anti-dinitrophenyl antibodies.

this difference was the relatively high concentrations of β-adrenergic stimulants required to produce inhibition of histamine release from human leucocytes, which has been mentioned previously. Even with sub-optimal antigen concentrations, inhibition of histamine release from leucocytes required at least 1000 higher concentrations than either human or guinea-pig lung. In lung preparations, isoprenaline is very highly potent when compared with DB-CAMP, e.g., the potency ratio in the experiments illustrated in Fig. 9 is of the order of 10^6. By contrast with the relative insensitivity of human leucocytes to the action of β-adrenergic stimulants, they seem to be nearly as sensitive (if not more sensitive) to inhibition by phosphodiesterase inhibitors and DB-CAMP (Figs 9 and 10). This suggests that the difference between lung and leucocytes regarding the inhibition of histamine release by β-adrenergic stimulants lies either in the receptor or the adenyl cyclase system. This possibility still exists, despite the detectable activity of adenyl cyclase in leucocytes, particularly in cell homogenate, and despite the response to stimulation by isoprenaline in some patients. Another possibility, which is currently being investigated in our laboratory, is that the leucocytes of allergic patients might be abnormal in this respect.

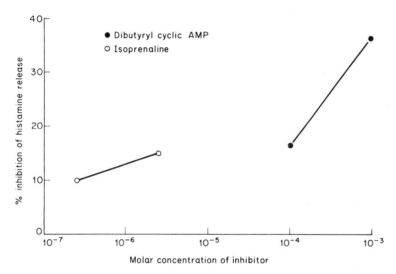

Fig. 10. Comparison of the inhibition by isoprenaline and dibutyryl cyclic AMP of the histamine release by antigen (*D. pteronyssinus*) from isolated human leucocytes. Note that the relative potency of these two inhibitors in this preparation is different from that in the lung preparations (Fig. 9).

Further evidence of the difference in receptor mechanism in lung and leucocyte preparations was obtained from studies with β-adrenoceptor blocking drugs. They failed to antagonise the anti-anaphylactic effect of isoprenaline on human leucocytes, and in some cases potentiated it [41].

It is of interest to make a comparison between the effect of inhibitory concentrations of catecholamines on histamine release from leucocytes, which are high, and the effect of similar concentrations on lipolysis. Allen, Hillman and Ashmore [49] reported a biphasic lipolytic response to catecholamines in isolated fat cells. The first phase of lipolysis (Lipolysis I) occurred with concentration of the catecholamines from 3.3×10^{-8} M to 10^{-5} M. This was inhibited competitively by β-adrenergic blocking agents. The second phase of lipolysis (Lipolysis II) occurred with concentrations of catechol-amines from 10^{-5}-10^{-3} M and was not inhibited by β-adrenergic blocking agents.

Isolated rat peritoneal mast cells seem to behave like blood leucocytes since they are also resistant to the anti-anaphylactic action of β-adrenergic stimulants. Cyclic AMP in mast cells did not increase after stimulation with isoprenaline and salbutamol [27], but a rise was obtained with fluoride (Martin, personal communication).

Physiological and Therapeutic Implications

Physiological auto-regulatory mechanism

Low concentrations of catecholamines, particularly those with β-activity, can inhibit histamine release from lung. It seems, therefore, that circulating adrenaline (of the order of 10^{-8} M) [50] may well exert a modulating influence on allergic reactivity in preventing particularly the effects of exposure to small amounts of antigen. This may explain why there are fewer people who are clinically allergic than one would expect from the results of highly sensitive *in vitro* tests like those in isolated leucocytes. Common antigens such as the house-dust mite *D. pteronyssinus,* produce low but significant histamine release from the leucocytes of nearly one-third of clinically non-allergic subjects.

Another possibility, which at present is only speculative, is that this autoregulatory mechanism may be defective in allergic patients. This possibility may be related to another type of suggested abnormality in asthmatics. Several authors [51, 52, 53] believe that asthmatic subjects (usually used without specifying whether they were allergic or not) may have malfunction of adrenoceptive mechanisms, which was thought to explain, at least in part, the abnormal reactivity of bronchial smooth muscle in asthmatics. This abnormal reactivity involves the response of bronchial smooth muscle to various stimuli, including the pharmacological mediators of anaphylaxis [54, 55]. In support of this hypothesis was the observation that the mouse, said to be normally resistant to histamine, becomes markedly sensitive to this substance following injection of *Bordetella pertussis* vaccine, or by the injection of β-adrenoceptor blocking agents [56, 57].

One of the best evidences of malfunction of adrenoceptive mechanisms was obtained by Middleton and Finke [53]. They compared the elevation of free fatty acids, lactate, pyruvate and glucose after the injection of adrenaline in severely asthmatic, mildly asthmatic and non-asthmatic subjects. The group of severe asthmatics had significantly less elevation of lactate, pyruvate and glucose, than the other groups. The elevation of free fatty acids and glucose was also lower in the severely asthmatic patients, but the difference from other groups was not significant.

Therapeutic implications

According to the evidence so far available, β-adrenergic stimulants have a dual mechanism of action in allergic bronchial asthma: (1) relief of bronchospasm by direct relaxation of bronchial smooth muscle; (2) protective anti-anaphylactic effect due to inhibition of release of pharmacological mediators of the anaphylactic reaction. Though these compounds are therapeutically effective, they have some limitations such as side effects, and development of resistance to their bronchodilator action, which may be caused by a multitude of factors, the discussion of which is beyond the scope of this review. There is, however, an important question which requires careful consideration. If cyclic AMP was the mediator of the various activities of β-adrenergic stimulants, then the lack of response to these agents in absence of obvious causes, would be to suggest an attempt to overcome this 'blockade' through the restoration of adequate levels of cyclic AMP in the right place. There have been reports on the effect of exogenous cyclic AMP and its dibutyryl derivative in man [58]. It remains to be seen if the use of these compounds or related derivatives would be of value in the control of symptoms of allergic conditions.

Acknowledgements

I wish to thank the Wellcome Trust for financial support, Professor J. L. Mongar for providing Fig. 1, Miss Kay Folkard and Miss Susan Brown for excellent technical assistance.

Discussion

Bennett (King's College Hospital)
Have you used actively sensitized human lung?

Assem (London)
Human lung specimens obtained from surgical operations are the only suitable material for this type of study. During the past five years we have obtained lung specimens from more than one hundred patients from different hospitals. All these patients had operations for removal of lung cancer. Only one patient was pre-operatively known to us as suffering from asthma, but skin tests with various antigens were negative and *in vitro* challenge of lung tissue also gave negative results.

Smith (Beecham)
  1. Could not the difference in sensitivities between the leucocytes and the chopped human lung preparations be due to the fact that the former are actively sensitized whilst the latter are passively sensitized?
  2. How did you measure the histamine concentrations released from the leucocyte system in the presence of 10^{-4} M concentration of catecholamines?

Assem (London)
  1. I at first thought that this was the possible explanation. Therefore we made a comparison between the response of actively and passively sensitized guinea-pig lung, which showed a significant difference between the two modes of sensitization [46]. However, the difference was not as great as that between passively sensitized human lung and actively sensitized human leucocytes. We have not been successful in getting reasonably strong passive sensitization of human leucocytes, and comparison of the latter with active sensitization would not be valid under these circumstances. The comparison between actively and passively sensitized guinea-pig lung was further pursued (unpublished work) in order to investigate one of the main possible explanations of these differences, namely a cellular change other than fixation of anaphylactic antibodies occurring during the process of active sensitization, which might lead to the development of resistance to the action of β-adrenergic stimulants. Such a possibility would have a great clinical implication.

For this study lung tissue from guinea-pigs actively sensitized against ovalbumin were passively sensitized against another antigen (dinitro-phenyl-bovine gamma globulin, DNP BGG). This 'doubly-sensitized' (both actively and passively) tissue was challenged with DNP BGG and inhibition of histamine release by isoprenaline was compared with the inhibition of histamine release from normal guinea-pig lung sensitized to the same antigen. To my disappointment there were no differences in the inhibition of histamine release in these two preparations, thus this possibility was eliminated in experimentally-induced active sensitization. However, these findings cannot exclude this possibility in naturally-developed active sensitization as occurring in allergic patients.

2. Isoprenaline used in final concentrations exceeding 4×10^{-7} M under our experimental conditions (which include incubation with leucocytes for 30 min, followed by boiling for 10 min and then freezing over night before histamine assay is carried out) usually interfered with histamine assay by the biological method [46]. The biological assay can be used to estimate concentrations of histamine as low as 1 ng or even smaller. I assume that your question was in connection with the leucocyte experiment shown in Fig. 3 which is one of a few experiments where relatively high concentrations of isoprenaline used in the first step of incubation with antigen did not interfere in the final assay of histamine, mainly because of the unusually high histamine content in the supernatants (100-300 ng/ml). These supernatants were therefore diluted more than fifty fold before the assay was carried out. A blank where 10^{-4} M isoprenaline was incubated with unchallenged leucocytes and pro-cessed in the usual way, when diluted to an equivalent degree, did not interfere with a response of guinea-pig ileum to the histamine standards used in the assay. Further details of this and other experimental details are published elsewhere [46].

References

1. Benacerraf, B.; In: 'Immunopharmacology' (Proceedings of the Third International Pharmacological Meeting, Sao Paulo). Ed. H. O. Schild. Pergamon Press, Oxford, (1968) vol. **11**, p. 3.
2. Becker, E. L. and Austen, K. F.; In: 'Textbook of Immunopathology; Eds P. A. Miescher and H. J. Müller. Eberhard, Grune and Stratton, New York and London, (1968) vol. **1**, p. 76.
3. Bloch, K. J.; In: 'Cellular and Humoral Mechanisms in Anaphylaxis and Allergy'; Ed. H. Z. Movat. S. Karger, Basel, (1969) p. 1.

4. Becker, E. L. and Austen, K. F.; *J. exp. Med.*; **124**, (1966) 379.
5. Ishizaka, K., Ishizaka, T. and Hornbrook, M. M.; *J. Immunol.*; **97**, (1966) 840.
6. Johansson, S. G. O. and Bennich, H.; In: 'Gamma Globulins' (Proceedings of the Third Nobel Symposium). Ed. J. Killander. Almqvist and Wiksell, Stockholm, (1967) p. 193.
7. Mongar, J. L. and Schild, H. O.; *Physiol. Rev.*; **42**, (1962) 226.
8. Stanworth, D. R.; *Clin. exp. Immunol.*; **6**, (1970) 1.
9. Ishizaka, K., Ishizaka, T. and Lee, E. H.; *Immunochemistry*; **7**, (1970) 687.
10. Mongar, J. L. and Schild, H. O.; *J. Physiol.*; **140**, (1958) 272.
11. Schild, H. O.; In: 'Biochemistry of the Acute Allergic Reaction'; Eds K. F. Austen and E. L. Becker. Blackwell, Oxford, (1968) p. 99.
12. Becker, E. L.; *Fed. Proc.*; **28**, (1969) 1704.
13. Mongar, J. L. and Perera, B. A. V.; *Immunology*; **8**, (1965) 511.
14. Lichtenstein, L. M.; In: 'Biochemistry of the Acute Allergic Reaction'; Eds K. F. Austen and E. L. Becker. Blackwell, Oxford, (1968) p. 153.
15. Levy, D. A. and Carlton, J. A.; *Proc. Soc. exp. Biol. (N.Y.)*; **130**, (1969) 1333.
16. Brocklehurst, W. E.; In: 'Histamine'; Eds G. E. W. Wolstenholme and C. M. O'Connor. Churchill, London (1956) p. 175.
17. Brocklehurst, W. E. and Lahiri, S. C.; *J. Physiol.*; **160**, (1962) 15.
18. Piper, P. J. and Vane, J. R.; *Nature, Lond.*; **223**, (1969) 29.
19. Movat, H. E., Taichman, N. S., Uriuhara, T. and Wasi, S.; *Fed. Proc.*; **24**, (1965) 369.
20. Treadwell, P. E.; *J. Immunol.*; **94**, (1965) 692.
21. Lichtenstein, L. M. and Margolis, S.; *Science*; **161**, (1968) 902.
22. Assem, E. S. K. and Schild, H. O.; *Nature, Lond.*; **224**, (1969) 1028.
23. Assem, E. S. K., Pickup, P. M. and Schild, H. O.; *Br. J. Pharmac.*; **39**, (1970) 212.
24. Koopman, W. J., Orange, R. P. and Austen, K. F.; *J. Immun.*; **105**, (1970) 1096.
25. Ishizaka, T., Ishizaka, K., Orange, R. P. and Austen, K. F.; *Fed. Proc.*; **29**, (1970) 575.
26. Schild, H. O.; *Quart. J. exp. Physiol.*; **26**, (1936) 166.
27. Martin, L. E.; *Post-grad. med. J.*; **47**, (1971, March Supplement) 26.
28. Assem, E. S. K. and Richter, A. W.; *Immunology*; in the press.
29. Assem, E. S. K.; *Post-grad. med. J.*; **47**, (1971, Supplement March) 31.
30. Cullum, V. A., Farmer, J. B., Jack, D. and Levy, G. P.; *Br. J. Pharmac.*, **35**, (1969) 141.
31. Sutherland, E. W. and Robison, G. A.; *Pharmacol. Rev.*; **18**, (1966) 145.
32. Bueding, E., Butcher, R. W., Hawkins, J., Timms, A. R. and Sutherland, E. W.; *Biochim. biophys. Acta.*; **115**, (1966) 173.
33. Robison, G. A., Butcher, R. W. and Sutherland, E. W.; *Ann. N.Y. Acad. Sci.*; **139**, (1967) 703.
34. Butcher, R. W. and Sutherland, E. W.; *Ann. N.Y. Acad. Sci.*; **139**, (1967) 849.
35. Fain, J. N.; *Ann. N.Y. Acad. Sci.*; **139**, (1967) 879.
36. Fain, J. N.; *Fed. Proc.*; **29**, (1970) 1402.
37. Furchgott, R. F.; *Ann. N.Y. Acad. Sci.*; **139**, (1967) 553.
38. Lands, A. M., Arnold, A., McAuliff, J. P., Luduena, F. P. and Brown, T. G. Jr.; *Nature, Lond.*; **214**, (1967) 597.
39. Lichtenstein, L. M. and DeBernardo, R.; *Fed. Proc.*; **29**, (1970) 575 abs.

40. Scott, R. E.; *Blood*; **35**, (1970) 514.
41. Assem, E. S. K. and Schild, H. O.; *Br. J. Pharmac.*; **42**, (1971) 620.
42. Burns, J. J. and Lemberger, L.; *Fed. Proc.*; **24**, (1965) 928.
43. Nakano, J., Kusakari, T. and Berry, J. L.; *Arch. Int. Pharmacodyn.*; **164**, (1968) 120.
44. Turtle, J. R. and Kipnis, D. M.; *Biochem. biophys. Res. Commun.*; **28**, (1967) 797.
45. Butcher, R. W. and Sutherland, E. W.; *J. biol. Chem.*; **237**, (1962) 1244.
46. Assem, E. S. K. and Schild, H. O.; *Int. archs. Allergy*; **40**, (1971) 576.
47. Cox, J. S. G.; *Nature, Lond.*; **216**, (1967) 1328.
48. Assem, E. S. K. and Mongar, J. L.; *Int. archs. Allergy appl. immun.*; **38**, (1970) 68.
49. Allen, D. O., Hillman, C. C. and Ashmore, J.; *Biochemical Pharmacology*; **18**, (1969) 2233.
50. Anton, A. H.; *Science*; **151**, (1966) 709.
51. Cookson, D. U. and Reed, C. E.; *Am. Rev. resp. Dis.*; **88**, (1963) 636.
52. Szentivanyi, A.; *J. Allergy*; **42**, (1968) 203.
53. Middleton, E. and Finke, S. R.; *J. Allergy*; **42**, (1968) 288.
54. Curry, J. J.; *J. Clin. Invest.*; **26**, (1947) 430.
55. Herxheimer, H.; *Internat. Arch. Allergy*; **2**, (1951) 27.
56. Fishel, C. W., Szentivanyi, A. and Talmage, D. W.; *J. Immunol.*; **89**, (1962) 8.
57. Townley, R. G., Trapani, I. L. and Szentivanyi, A.; *J. Allergy*; **39**, (1967) 177.
58. Levine, R. A.; *Clin. Pharmac. and Therap.*; **11**, (1970) 238.

CYCLIC AMP AND TISSUES
OF THE BRAIN

H. McIlwain

Department of Biochemistry, Institute of Psychiatry,
British Postgraduate Medical Federation, University of London

List of enzymes: Adenosine kinase, EC 2.7.1.20. Adenyl cyclase (EC not defined). Adenylate kinase, EC 2.7.4.3. Adenine phosphoribosyl-transferase, EC 2.4.2.7. Cyclic 3′,5′-nucleotide phosphodiesterase (EC not defined). 5′-Nucleotidase EC 3.1.3.5.
Non-standard abbreviation: cyclic AMP = 3′,5′-cyclic adenosine monophosphate.

This contribution concerns tissues prepared from the mammalian brain, with minimal damage to cell-structure. Such tissues constitute the simplest level at which the multiplicity of control mechanisms which operate between the cells of neural systems, are exhibited directly: That is, without a transformation of category. A major method of exhibiting control mechanisms is to cause a system to alter its level of activity. In the brain this can readily be caused by some form of excitation. Impinging on a portion of cerebral tissue *in situ* are two types of input to which the tissue reacts; (i) electrical, by the ion movements of the nerve impulse; and (ii) humoral, from adjacent cells or more distant parts of the body but arriving finally as a chemical substance and by diffusion. Input of each of these types can be brought to bear on the isolated tissue, by electrical stimulation and by chemical additions to the fluid environment of the tissue. This is the order in which responses by the tissue are now to be described.

Electrical stimulation and cyclic AMP
Stimulation caused (Fig. 1) a large increase in the cyclic AMP of isolated cerebral tissues maintained under normal conditions of incubation. The increase showed the following characteristics [1],

some of which were quite unexpected when first observed: (i) the increase could be 10-fold, and commenced promptly; (ii) it was inhibited by theophylline; and (iii) noradrenaline and some other neurohumoral agents acted synergistically with the electrical stimuli so that the cyclic AMP of the tissue could rise to 30 times its initial value.

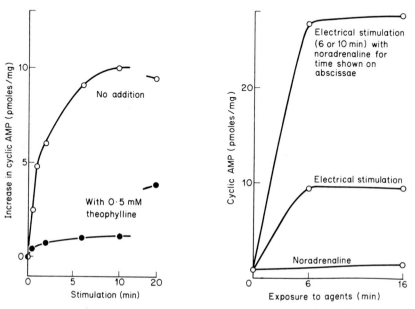

Fig. 1. The cyclic AMP of guinea-pig neocortical tissue incubated for 50 min prior to electrical stimulation (100 pulses/sec) for the duration given by abscissae [1]. Theophylline was present throughout incubation in the instances indicated. The cyclic AMP of unstimulated control tissues was 0.9 nmoles/g. Noradrenaline, 50 μM, was also added after the 50 min (or 60 min) preincubation.

Changes of this magnitude prompt consideration of the precursors of cyclic AMP, that is, of the ATP and other adenine derivatives of the brain. Electrical excitation, indeed, brings about large alterations in the cerebral content of such compounds [2] (Fig. 2) which collectively are plentiful in the brain. Thus ATP, initially at 2-3 μmoles/g tissue is amply available as precursor for the increase of 20-30 nmoles of cyclic AMP/g tissue. The less phosphorylated compounds are however present in smaller amounts. They take part in multiple control processes of intermediary metabolism [2] and under some circumstances their average cerebral concentrations can be not remote from those of cyclic AMP.

The alterations induced by stimulation in most of the cerebral adenine derivatives can be seen from Fig. 2 to be much prompter than is the rise in cyclic AMP (Fig. 1); they are, however, relatively prolonged after a brief stimulus, as is also shown in the figure. Further, ATP, the known precursor of cyclic AMP, decreases on

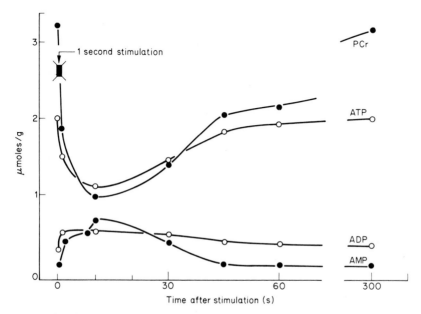

Fig. 2. Adenosine derivatives and phosphocreatine (PCr) of the brain of rats after 1 sec electrical stimulation [20]. Tissues were fixed by rapid freezing at the times indicated after the stimulation.

stimulation, and it is the less phosphorylated adenine derivatives which increase. Another line of investigation also brought attention to these compounds in connection with cerebral cyclic AMP.

Adenosine as precursor of cyclic AMP

This was a search [1, 3] for endogenous cerebral components which might reproduce the actions, (i) to (iii), brought about by electrical excitation. Intriguingly, acid extracts of cerebral tissues brought about these effects, and the properties resided especially in adenosine itself. Thus (Fig. 3) adenosine could cause a 30- to 40-fold increase in the cyclic AMP of cerebral tissues incubated in a simple glucose salines. This increase was inhibited by theophylline and (see later) could be augmented by noradrenaline and cognate compounds. The other adenine nucleotides approached adenosine in potency in yielding cyclic AMP (Fig. 3); possible interconversions are considered in a later section.

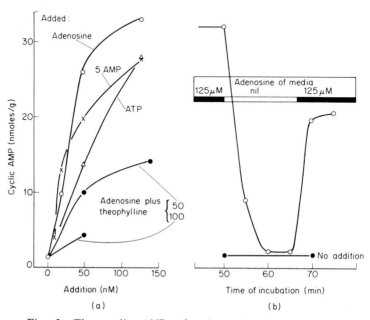

Fig. 3. The cyclic AMP of guinea-pig neocortical tissue preincubated for 50 min before addition of the adenine derivatives stated, and for a further 5 min in their presence [3]. (*a*) In the experiments indicated, the initial preincubation with adenosine was followed by rinsing and transferring the tissues to fresh, adenosine-free media; (*b*) adenosine was subsequently added to some of these media and incubation continued as shown.

The cyclic AMP of incubated tissues responded to added adenosine in a few minutes, that is, with time course similar to that of the change in cyclic AMP during electrical excitation. Rates of formation and breakdown of cyclic AMP can be derived from the data of Fig. 3b in order to judge whether they come within the capacity of the adenyl cyclase and of the cyclic 3′,5′-nucleotide phosphodiesterase of the brain, measuring these enzymes in cerebral dispersions. It is then found that the rapid fall in cyclic AMP occurring when adenosine is removed, corresponds to about 300 nmoles lost/g tissue/hour. The phosphodiesterase of the brain, when examined at maximal activity in enzyme preparations from the cerebral cortex, could degrade cyclic AMP at rates up to 2500 μmoles/g tissue/hour [22]. These activities, however, need relatively high substrate concentrations, and in reaction mixtures 5.5 μM in cyclic AMP [3] rates corresponded to about 10 μmoles/g hour; a K_m of 0.1-0.3 mM is reported for the abundant phosphodiesterase of the brain [23]. Moreover, this reaction is susceptible to inhibition by tissue constituents: ATP gave half-maximal inhibition at about 1 mM and other nucleotide triphosphates and inorganic pyrophosphate also inhibited [23]. It is thus notable that a different phosphodiesterase activity, showing K_m of 1 μM for cyclic AMP, has also been observed in rat brain [24], and that an endogenous activator of the abundant phosphodiesterase appears to lower its K_m [25]. Ample enzyme capacity and a multiplicity of regulatory processes thus suggest that the known phosphodiesterase activities can account for the fall in cyclic AMP reported in Fig. 3. Adenosine was examined for effect on the abundant phosphodiesterase and found not to inhibit [3].

Adenyl cyclase, as observed in cerebral dispersions, is similarly related to the synthesis of cyclic AMP as observed in tissues and recorded in Fig. 3b. Here, the increase in cyclic AMP which followed the addition of adenosine to the tissue commenced at about 240 nmoles/g tissue/hour. This is below the rates reported for adenyl cyclase measured under optimal conditions but without the addition of activating hormones, using cerebral dispersions; values of 1-4 μmoles cyclic AMP synthesized/g hour were so found [27]. Assimilation of adenosine may well have been the rate-limiting reaction during the experiments of Fig. 3b. The rate of adenyl cyclase in particulate preparations from guinea-pig brain increased as ATP was increased from 0.1 to 2 mM [3] (cf. a comparable increase in preparations from the liver [26]). Adenyl cyclase in dispersions was not, however, greatly affected by addition of adenosine [3]. The action of adenosine was a property of the cell-containing preparations. Moreover, it showed tissue-specificity and was absent from beef thyroid or rat diaphragm [3]. The cyclic AMP content of either of these tissues was unaffected by adenosine or 5'-AMP, added with or without a further specific stimulus (thyroid-stimulating hormone or adrenaline).

Adenosine as precursor of adenine nucleotides generally

Work from these laboratories many years ago has shown another special relationship between adenosine and tissues from the brain. Adenosine was the most effective of many compounds examined, in maintaining or increasing the total adenine nucleotides of incubated neocortical samples [5]. When tissues are first prepared for *in vitro*

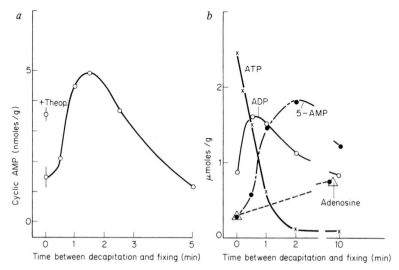

Fig. 4. Changes in the adenine nucleotides of the brain of mice during tissue preparation [8, 9, 10]. Fixation was by rapid freezing. Theophylline, 0.4 mg/g was given intraperitoneally and caused convulsions; the brain was sampled after 0.5 min of convulsive activity. The interrupted line for adenosine refers to guinea-pigs [5]. Note that the ordinate scale *b* is in units 1000 times those of *a*.

incubation, large changes take place in their content of adenine derivatives (Fig. 4). In particular, ATP fell to about 0.1 of its previous value and was largely but not fully restored by incubation in glucose salines. When adenine, adenosine, 5'-AMP and other compounds were examined as potential precursors of the adenine nucleotides of the tissue, adenosine was most effective (Table 1). The methods employed determined adenine nucleotides collectively and to these, ATP and ADP made much the greatest contribution.

Cyclic AMP also undergoes large changes during tissue preparation, but again can regain its initial value (Fig. 4). It increases 3-fold from the original 1-2 nmoles/g tissue, reaching its maximum when ADP and 5′-AMP are also high, and when ATP is minimal. On incubation in oxygenated glucose salines, conditions which restore most of the adenine nucleotides to concentrations close to those of their values in the brain *in situ*, the cyclic AMP levels which were established in the tissues also became close to their original 1-2 nmoles/g. When,

Table 1
Precursors of the Adenine Derivatives of Cerebral Tissues

	Measured		Added compounds *A*		
[Ref.]	(Units)		Adenine	Adenosine	Inosine
1.	Total adenine nucleotides: additional synthesis during 100 min incubation with *A*, guinea-pig cortex				
	[5]	(nmoles/g tissue)	120	380	240
2.	Cyclic AMP: additional net formation during 5 min with *A* at 50-300 μM				
	[3]	(nmoles/g tissue)	0	29	0
3.	Uptake of 5 μM 8-[14]C-*A*: to rat neocortex during 60 min incubation				
	[6]	(% of ^{14}C added)	54	25	7
4.	8-^{14}C-Cyclic AMP: formation from 8-[14]C-*A* on adding 100 μM histamine, guinea-pig cortex				
	[7]	10 min (% of tissue 8-^{14}C-ATP)	5.2	2.7	—
5.	As 4, adding 200 μM histamine and 43 mM K$^+$				
	[19]	10 min (% of tissue 8-^{14}C-ATP)	38	—	—

The protein content of cerebral tissues has been taken as 10% of the fresh. wt. for the calculations of this and of other tables and figures.

now, several purine derivatives were added to incubating neocortical samples and examined as precursors of cyclic AMP, preference to adenosine was again found [3] (Table 1). Some 8 compounds showed little or no activity in this respect, including adenine, inosine and the nicotinamide-adenine nucleotides. Note the apparently greater specificity of adenosine as precursor of cyclic AMP in comparison with it as precursor of adenine nucleotides generally (*1, 2,* Table 1). The deductions to be drawn from this comparison are limited by the derivation of the data from different groups of experiments. The greater specificity was found in briefer experiments (5 min, not 100 min, with the potential precursors). Indeed the rate of increase in cyclic AMP measured in *2,* Table 1, approximates to the rate of increase of total adenine nucleotides in measurements *1,* Table 1.

Neurohumoral agents and cyclic AMP

The properties of adenosine thus appear to confirm that the route to cyclic AMP in cerebral tissues lies through the action of adenyl cyclase on ATP, and attention may be turned to the role of neurohumoral agents whose actions featured also in the experiments first cited (Fig. 1). Cerebral tissues retain noradrenaline and cognate compounds throughout their preparation and incubation, and moreover the compounds are susceptible to release on electrical stimulation of the isolated tissues. The data of Fig. 5 show both the tissue stores, labelled and augmented by added ^{3}H-derivatives assimilated *in vitro,* and their release to extracellular fluids in a superfusion system. The rate of release of noradrenaline, of serotonin and of other neurohumoral agents was increased 5-fold or more by electrical excitation (Fig. 5).

Granted such phenomena, why should added noradrenaline so greatly augment the cyclic AMP formation which occurs on electrical stimulation (Fig. 1)? The answer probably lies in the concentrations involved: 50 nmoles of noradrenaline are added/ml. of fluid, while the tissue contains only about 0.3-3 nmoles/g, and is placed in an experimental system which is designed to dilute with much fluid the proportion of this which is released extracellularly. The *in vitro* arrangements can display the effects of adding, both separately and in various combinations, neurotransmitters and potentiating and blocking agents. Some experiments so based [14, 15] are summarized in Fig. 6.

Taking data from rabbit cerebellar tissues, it is first to be noted that several agents were without action on the cyclic AMP of the tissue, including acetylcholine, γ-aminobutyrate and glutamate despite the importance of some of these to the cerebellum. Noradrenaline, serotonin and histamine gave notable and apparently independent increases in cyclic AMP of the tissue. The almost purely additive relationships between noradrenaline and histamine are shown in Fig. 6a; in Fig. 6b is displayed the fashion in which drugs already known to antagonize either noradrenaline or histamine have their separate actions on cyclic AMP formation induced by one or the other of the amines. Thus diphenhydramine at 5 μM, inhibited the cyclic AMP formation caused by histamine, by more than 60%, while even at 50 μM it caused much smaller antagonism to the action

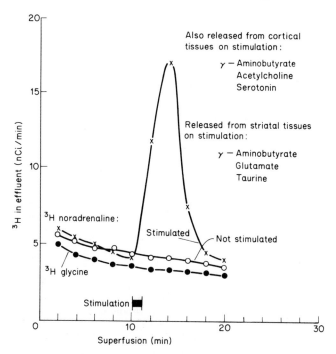

Fig. 5. The time course of release of noradrenaline and glycine from guinea-pig cortical tissues on electrical stimulation [11]. Tissues were first incubated in glucose bicarbonate salines containing ascorbate, nialamide and the ^{3}H-labelled compounds. Excess reagents were removed by a flow of saline without additions, and after 16 min flow (zero time on the diagrams) collection was commenced. For data on the release of the other compounds listed, see [2], [11], [12] and [13].

of noradrenaline on cyclic AMP. These and cognate data are valuable evidence that the action of the neurohumoural agents on cyclic AMP levels is close to their pharmacologically-characterized receptors. Presumably, noradrenaline and histamine when added *in vitro* arrive extracellularly at most parts of the tissue but have their actions at the separate post-synaptic sites close to which the native noradrenaline and histamine are normally released.

Further evidence for highly localized processes in the formation of cyclic AMP has come by further examining the joint action of adenine derivatives and neurohumoural agents.

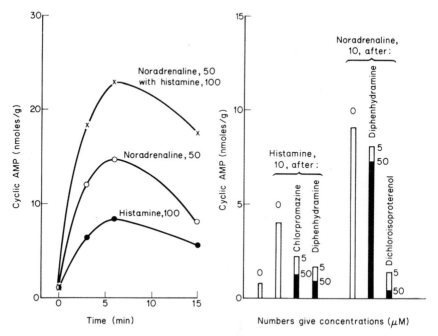

Fig. 6. *a.* Additive actions of noradrenaline and histamine on the cyclic AMP of isolated cerebellar tissues of rabbits [14, 15]. Samples were incubated for 42 min in normal media with 0.5 mM theophylline, and then with the added compounds for the duration indicated. *b.* To tissues incubated as those of *a*, but with the inhibitors specified for the last 12 min, were added histamine or noradrenaline; incubation was continued for a further 6 min before analysis.

Localized sites of cyclic AMP formation

Experiments with isotopically-labelled precursors of cyclic AMP have given important evidence on the localization of cyclic AMP formation in tissues from the brain. Using 8-^{14}C-adenine as precursor at the quite low concentration of 5 μM, the greater part of that added, could be assimilated by rat neocortical tissue during 1 hour incubation (*3,* Table 1). There is a much smaller precursor pool of adenine than of adenosine (Table 2) and possibly for this reason a smaller proportion of the ^{14}C-adenosine added in comparable circumstances, was taken up by the tissue. In the experiments *3,*

Table 1, most of the adenine taken up was found as ^{14}C-ATP. When, now, histamine was added and (see above; *4*, Table 1) augmented the cyclic AMP of the tissue, an appreciable proportion of the assimilated ^{14}C was converted to cyclic AMP. The proportion was greater from ^{14}C-adenine: 5.2% (Table 1) than from ^{14}C-adenosine which yielded 2.7%. When, further, the tissues were treated with high concentrations of potassium salts, the formation of ^{14}C-cyclic AMP

Table 2
Some Adenine Derivatives of Cerebral Tissues under Normal and Modified Conditions

	Compound	[Ref.]	Normal content (nmoles/g)	Treatment of animal	Modified content (nmoles/g)
1.	ATP	[10]	3000	Decapitation, mice; sampled after 4-10 sec	1200
2.	AMP	[10]	210	As *1*	330
3.	Adenosine	[5]	300	Brain removed, cut and sampled after 5 min	750
4.	Adenine	[5]	<50	As *3*	<50
5.	Cyclic AMP	[8,9]	2	As *1*, mice; sampled after 2 min	5

Compounds *1, 2* and *5* were determined in mice and *3* and *4* in guinea-pigs.

rose to suprisingly high proportions, 30-40% of the ^{14}C-adenine which had been taken up by the tissue.

Of the various changes brought about by addition of high concentrations of K^+ salts to isolated cerebral tissues, the relevant effect appears to be the depolarization which it causes and which can be observed using micropipettes for intracellular recordings [16, 17]. This was deduced from the nature of other agents which gave similarly high yields of ^{14}C-cyclic AMP from tissues treated as those of 5. Table 1. These agents were chemically quite diverse, but could each diminish the Na and K gradients normally maintained between the tissue and surrounding fluids. If in place of the 43 mM K^+ added in that experiment, veratridine, ouabain, or batrachotoxin were added, conversion of tissue ^{14}C-adenine derivatives to ^{14}C-cyclic AMP again approached 40% [18].

Adenosine release from superfused tissues

Depolarization of the cells of isolated cerebral tissues results also [17, 21] from the electrical stimulation employed in the experiments of Fig. 5, and thus, possibly, each of the agents named above

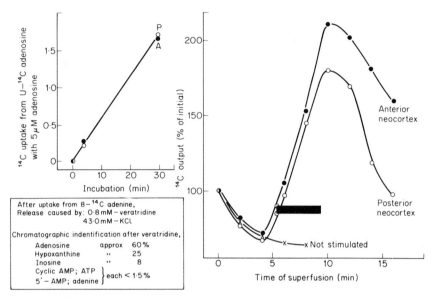

After uptake from 8–[14]C adenine,
Release caused by: 0·8 mM – veratridine
43·0 mM – KCl

Chromatographic indentification after veratridine,

Adenosine	approx	60%
Hypoxanthine	,,	25
Inosine	,,	8
Cyclic AMP; ATP 5′ – AMP; adenine	each < 1·5%	

Fig. 7. The uptake and release of ^{14}C added as adenine derivatives to cerebral tissues [27]. Uptake was measured during incubation in glucose bicarbonate media containing 5 μM added adenosine. The course of release shown occurred during superfusion and electrical stimulation of guinea-pig neocortical tissues which had been incubated for 30 min in media with 5 μM added adenosine containing U-^{14}C-adenosine. The other agents named were added [18] to the tissue previously incubated with 8-^{14}C-adenine. Following veratridine, the ^{14}C-derivatives of the medium were found to be largely adenosine.

liberates the several neurohumoural agents listed in Fig. 5. A further very relevant effect of electrical stimulation has been observed. This is the release of adenine compounds themselves (Fig. 7). It occurred promptly in response to brief stimuli applied at 20/sec, and trebled the output of ^{14}C derivatives to fluids superfusing tissues which had earlier assimilated ^{14}C-adenosine [27]. The ^{14}C-labelled compound released by veratrine and K^+ from tissues which had assimilated ^{14}C as $8^{14}C$-adenine, was found to be preponderantly adenosine [19] (Fig. 7); hypoxanthine and inosine followed in abundance, with only quite small amounts of cyclic AMP, 5′-AMP, and ATP.

These observations of the effective uptake by adenosine from quite dilute solutions, at μM level, and its subsequent release on stimulation, give clues to understanding the remarkably high yield of ^{14}C-cyclic AMP from added ^{14}C-adenine or -adenosine. For conversion of up to 40% of the tissues' ^{14}C-adenine nucleotides to ^{14}C-cyclic AMP cannot reflect a change of 40% of all the tissues' adenine nucleotides to cyclic AMP. These nucleotides total some 3 μmoles/g tissue while the maximal cyclic AMP is some 0.04 μmoles/g. The ^{14}C-nucleotides which yield cyclic AMP in the experiments of 5, Table 1 must have remained a distinct entity constituting no more than 5% of the total adenine nucleotides [19]. If however the uptake and release of adenosine in the experiments of Fig. 7 represent phenomena comparable to the uptake and release of noradrenaline in Fig. 5, then an explanation for the localization of a special fraction of ATP, as a limited precursor pool, is readily available. The uptake and output occur preponderantly at synaptic regions which represent a quite small proportion of the tissue volume. The joint occurrence and release of adenine nucleotides and adrenaline in the adrenal gland is noteworthy here. In the adrenal, the chromaffin granules are rich in both adrenaline and adenine nucleotides, mainly ATP. Secretion of adrenaline is accompanied by secretion of several molar equiv. of adenine derivatives, mainly 5′-AMP [28]. As 5′-AMP is produced by the gland when ATP or ADP are added to solutions which perfuse it, adrenaline is presumed to be liberated together with its associated adenine nucleotides [29].

Synaptic sites of adenosine action?

In the present cerebral systems, adenosine itself has an active role, possibly associated with each of the neurohumours with which it gives enhanced formation of cyclic AMP. Noradrenaline in the brain (or histamine or serotonin) may be liberated together with adenosine (or ATP or adenine) from the same terminals or to a common postsynaptic cell. Pursuing this theme, leads to regarding adenosine as a neurohumour and the increased formation of cyclic AMP as a postsynaptic result of its release. In achieving this result, is adenosine a substrate or a cofactor in the production of cyclic AMP? This question was approached by pre-labelling the adenine nucleotides of cerebral tissues by ^{14}C-adenine, and adding ^{3}H-adenosine as a stimulus to the formation of cyclic AMP ([19]; Table 3). It was then found that the resulting cyclic AMP contained both ^{14}C and [3]H. Accepting adenyl cyclase as the only route to cyclic AMP, it is thus to be concluded that the ^{3}H-adenosine added extracellularly as stimulus has become assimilated to the tissue and converted to ^{3}H-ATP, and that cyclic AMP was yielded from both the [3]H- and ^{14}C-ATP. Veratridine greatly increased the yield of cyclic AMP from both the ^{14}C and ^{3}H precursors (Table 3).

Table 3
Adenine and Adenosine as Precursors of Cyclic AMP

Additions to ^{14}C-adenine labelled tissue (μM)	Incorporation into slice (nmoles/mg N)			Conversion into cyclic AMP (%)		
	[14]C	[3]H	[3]H/[14]C	[14]C	[3]H	[3]H/[14]C
[3]H-Adenosine, 100	7.36	7.56	1.01	3.88	1.91	0.49
[3]H-Adenosine, 100 plus veratridine, 80	6.03	7.21	0.84	22.1	8.25	0.38

Guinea-pig cortical tissues were preincubated for 20 min and then exposed to 13.3 μM ^{14}C-adenine during 40 min further incubation; they were washed, incubation continued for 10 min with the additions specified, and the tissues extracted [19].

Thus extracellularly added adenosine is demonstrated to act, at least in part, as precursor of the cyclic AMP formed by its addition. It is however stated [19] that 'adenosine does stimulate adenyl cyclase and is not merely serving as precursor for cyclic AMP'. To contrast these two propositions may not be entirely valid. If added adenosine sufficiently increases the local concentration of ATP in a range related to the K_m of adenyl cyclase then, as noted above (p. 285), increased formation of cyclic AMP would result. The highly localized entry of added adenosine is again important here. The pool labelled by ^{14}C-adenine was estimated to constitute 5% of the tissue's total adenine nucleotides. The investigation of ^{14}C and ^{3}H-labelling [19] can afford a similar value: labelled precursor pool, 0.11 μmoles/g; total ATP, 2 μmoles/g or a little greater. (The calculation [19] of 0.004-0.012 μmoles/g for the labelled precursor pool appears to be in error.)

The sites at which noradrenaline and cognate neurohumours act and where cyclic AMP is believed to have its major actions, are postsynaptic [4]. In particular, alteration in the firing rate of Purkinje cells in the rat cerebellum was caused by liberation of noradrenaline from micropipettes in the vicinity of the cell body, and this action appeared to involve cyclic AMP [30, 31]. The immediate postsynaptic portions of the Purkinje cells include the perikaryon and spine processes. It would be valuable to have estimates of the proportion of cortical tissue volume contributed by such regions for comparison with the value of 5% quoted in the previous paragraph.

Ten processes related to the formation of cyclic AMP

The statement that the only process yielding cyclic AMP is that catalysed by adenyl cyclase is shown, by the foregoing account, to need much amplification. A scheme based on the data recounted, with some additional features, is given in Fig. 8 and includes some 10 processes or categories of processes. These operate at two cellular regions and an intervening extracellular space; the properties of noradrenaline and cognate compounds which have been recounted, contribute to specifying the regions as pre- or postsynaptic. Comments follow on the individual stages enumerated in the figure.

Added, isotopically-labelled adenine is incorporated very effectively to ATP specifically in the region where cyclic AMP is formed. This is presumably dependent on the localization of selective entry sites for adenine (*1*)*; these may or may not be associated with adenine phosphoribosyltransferase (*3*) which yields 5'-AMP. Added adenosine is incorporated to the tissue in greater amount than is adenine; but when labelled adenosine is added, it reaches the precursor pool for cyclic AMP, less specifically than did adenine. This may be connected with the observation that electrical stimulation or chemical depolarizing agents liberate adenosine in quantities at least 40 times greater than those of the concomitant release of adenine (Fig. 7): the liberation (*2'*) may be from the presynaptic region A from which noradrenaline also is liberated. This presupposes an initial uptake of labelled adenosine to the presynaptic region. The postsynaptic uptake of adenosine (*2*), after its addition or after its liberation by excitation, again may or may not be in association with the adenosine kinase (*5*) which consumes ATP in forming 5'-AMP.

* Numbers in parentheses refer to Fig. 8.

Added ^{14}C-adenine incorporated during preincubation is also liberated as adenosine by depolarizing conditions, including electrical stimulation [18, 27]. Supposing such stimulation to act at presynaptic sites, it must be supposed that adenine has been assimilated presynaptically (*1'*, Fig. 8) and converted there to adenosine,

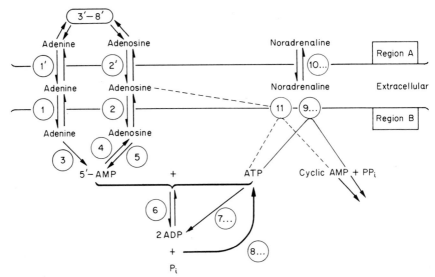

Fig. 8. Processes contributing to the formation of cyclic AMP in cerebral tissues; two cellular regions *A* and *B,* and extracellular fluid, are specified. The numbered processes include:

3, adenine phosphoribosyltransferase; *4*, 5'-nucleotidase; *5*, adenosine kinase; *6*, adenylate kinase; *7*, several adenosine triphosphatases; *8*, several phosphorylating systems and *9*, adenyl cyclases, variously activated.

Processes *3'-8'* in region A refer to similarly-numbered processes in region B. Other numbered processes receive comment in the text.

presumably by the phosphoribosyltransferase and 5'-nucleotidase (*3'* and *4'*, Fig. 8).

Adenylate kinase (*6*) in the postsynaptic region appears likely to ensure effective isotopic mixing of labelled 5'-AMP (derived from adenine or adenosine) with the regional pool of ATP. To this mixing the several processes utilizing (*7*) and reforming (*8*) ATP contribute. The phosphorylating processes have much reserve capacity by augmented respiration, glycolysis, or from phosphocreatine, and on excitation can operate at many times their resting level [2]. Thus there is no problem in phosphorylating incoming adenosine and incorporating it to a common pool of ATP available within the region for formation of cyclic AMP.

The role of noradrenaline, histamine and serotonin in activating the adenyl cyclase or cyclases (9) is discussed more fully by other contributors. Here it may be noted that the additive relationships of Fig. 6 can be interpreted by supposing noradrenaline and histamine to exert their actions at distinct postsynaptic regions. When liberated by neural excitation (10), noradrenaline and histamine would originate from different terminals and this presynaptic specificity contribute to defining the postsynaptic regions at which each augmented cyclic AMP. In the experiments of Fig. 6, noradrenaline and histamine were added to a common extracellular fluid and thus the distinctiveness of their actions must reside more completely in the properties of the receptor sites associated with adenyl cyclase.

The interrupted line from adenosine to cyclic AMP in Fig. 8 (11) expresses the suggestion that adenosine augments the formation of cyclic AMP by factors other than increase in local ATP concentration. To establish whether this is a necessary suggestion requires more detailed investigation of the ATP concentration in immediate postsynaptic regions at different levels of neural activity, and also of the K_m of adenyl cyclase, variously activated. It is to be noted that action at more than one point remains open for the new pharmacological property of methylxanthines which was displayed in Fig. 1: 'blocking that action of adenosine which alters the cyclic 3',5'-AMP of cerebral cortex' [3]. Theophylline may act at process (2', efflux) of Fig. 8, or at (2); action at processes (4) to (8) appears unlikely though this may not have been completely excluded; while action at (11) remains possible.

Comment

In this account little has been said about the utilization of cyclic AMP. This is not because isolated, cell-containing tissues are unsuitable for such studies. A pioneering investigation of mediation by cyclic AMP in ACTH-induced corticosteroid formation, employed such preparations from the adrenal [32]. Comparable examples in cerebral systems may be quoted by other contributors. Cyclic AMP can modify cell-firing in the brain [30, 31]. Excitation of the brain has long-lasting consequences, as well as the short-term actions exemplified by immediate responses in cell-firing. It is in these more lasting actions that a characteristic role can be seen for cyclic AMP, possibly by routes involving histones, or the phosphoproteins which are described in Dr Rodnight's contribution to this Symposium.

Acknowledgements

I am indebted to Mr Ian Pull for permission to quote the unpublished joint work to which reference is made; to the Research Fund of the Bethlem Royal Hospital and the Maudsley Hospital and to the Science Research Council, for support.

Discussion

Smith (Royal College of Surgeons)

In studies on platelets we found that the pyrimidopyridimines (but not theophylline) inhibited the uptake of ^{14}C-adenosine.

McIlwain (Institute of Psychiatry)

Some current findings from our group, and from those quoted in my paper, suggest that movements of adenine or of adenosine at neural tissues can give significant points for drug action, and that it is necessary to differentiate between different cellular regions in a fashion suggested in Fig. 8 (1, 1′ and 2, 2′). Also, efflux from each region may not be by simple reversal of the process of entry. There are thus up to 8 processes to be considered, of which 4 concern a given cell type and could be envisaged in platelets, allowing specificity of the sort which you mention. With cerebral tissues incubated for brief periods with precursors at high dilution, preferential uptake was of adenine, but when tissue so treated was exposed to veratridine, the major labelled compound issuing was adenosine.

Somerville (I.C.I.)

Would you comment on recent work concerning adenine and adenosine with both ^{14}C and ^{3}H labels which shows that adenosine has an additional action over and above increasing the nucleotide pool.

McIlwain (Institute of Psychiatry)

Work of Shimizu, Creveling and Daly [18, 19] with double-labelling techniques showed how small was the pool of ATP which contributed to cyclic AMP. It is this pool which is suggested in Fig. 8 to be post-synaptic, in perikarya or spine processes or both. We do not, however, know at present the concentration of ATP in this pool at the time when cyclic AMP is being formed. My picture is that the concentration at this critical time is rate-limiting in cyclic AMP formation and significant in relation to different possible routes of utilization; this is based on the following considerations.

(i) The concentration at which ATP becomes rate-limiting for cyclic AMP formation is about 1 mM (though this merits more detailed investigation than could be quoted above) and the average cerebral ATP is about 2 μmol g^{-1}. This concentration falls rapidly on excitation to half its original value in about 10 s (Fig. 2.) Greatest depletion of ATP is to be expected at points of Na entry, that is, at the post-synaptic regions just specified. Indeed the earliest and greatest depletion may be highly localized; there are features in the fall in ATP and phosphocreatine with small Na$^+$ entry which leads to the conclusion [33] that the Na,K-ATPase of the cation pump is acting close to the points of Na$^+$ entry and before the entering Na becomes a general cytoplasmic constituent even in the neuronal components of the tissue. Correspondingly the [ATP] likely to be critical in cyclic AMP formation is again that close to the membrane-sited adenyl cyclase and Na,K-ATPase. The Na,K-ATPase gives half-maximal velocity at about 0.3 mM ATP [34]; with optimum Na$^+$ it has enzyme capacity about 1000 times that of the cerebral adenyl cyclase, and can thus deplete the cyclase of its substrate.

(ii) In these circumstances a precursor for ATP, provided locally at the membrane-sites where a transmitter has caused Na entry and depolarization, can be expected to have disproportionately large effects. The adenosine released by excitation could play such a role. In experiments [19] which allowed 40 min for uptake of [^{14}C]-adenine or [^{3}H]-adenosine, or both, solutions of 3 μM were used with cortical tissues. Substrate quantities of adenosine, about 100 μM were needed for maximum stimulation of cyclic AMP formation in such tissues, which without further addition then contained 1.4-2.5% of the isotopes as cyclic AMP. About 10 min was needed for this action of adenosine, a time which can be judged (Fig. 2) to be ample for phosphorylation of adenosine derivatives.

(iii) A broad biological parallel may be noted. Strains of *Escherichia coli* increase in cyclic AMP content when depleted of glucose; this is followed by induction of galactokinase, and β-galactosidase, enzymes capable of metabolizing a substrate alternative to glucose [35]. The cyclic AMP is intermediary and can itself induce these and certain other enzymes. Possibly the liberation of adenosine together with a neurotransmitter indicates that this general property of cyclic AMP as an inducing agent is being applied in the brain for securing, in specified instances, long-term effects of neural excitation [36]. The specified instances appear to involve synapses activated by catecholamines and serotonin rather than by acetylcholine.

Grahame-Smith (St Mary's Hospital)

1. How can you be sure that the changes in cyclic AMP concentrations that you see in brain slices after electrical stimulation or treatment with neurohumoral agents are taking place in neuronal tissue? Dr Peter Isaac and I, at St Mary's Hospital Medical School have recently studied synaptosomal preparations and we find that none of the putative neurotransmitting agents that we have studied (which include 5HT, noradrenaline, dopamine and histamine) stimulate the adenyl cyclase in the membrane of intact synaptosomes, and at the moment it seems that if the neurotransmitters have an effect on adenyl cyclase that this effect occurs at a post-synaptic site.

2. You seem to have suggested that the rise in the cyclic AMP contained by brain slices after treatment with adenosine is due to adenosine being converted to ATP and, as it were, spilling over of ATP on to adenyl cyclase with uncontrolled production of cyclic AMP. I must say I find that very difficult to accept because it takes away the whole concept of the regulator action of adenyl cyclase.

McIlwain (Institute of Psychiatry)

We are not certain, but regard a localized neuronal site as most likely. Events caused by stimulation begin in the neuronal components: these are the excitable cells, liberating on stimulation neurotransmitters of which the immediate action is postsynaptic. The stimulation, and the separate addition of the neurotransmitters, augment the tissue's cyclic AMP. So also does veratridine, which is not a general depolarizing agent but shows specificity for action at excitable tissues. To propose action at glial cells is thus not impossible but involves more indirectness. Certainly glia are involved secondarily in effects of excitation: they appear to assimilate temporarily the K^+ released from cerebral neurons on excitation. They may take up adenosine and experiments to show such phenomena would be valuable. I agree with your conclusion from your experiments with serotonin, noradrenaline, dopamine and histamine. The postsynaptic fragments carried by synaptosomes are not part of polarized cells and this can be seen as a reason for their not reacting to the neurotransmitters; nor can these fragments assimilate adenosine.

2. Adenosine and neurotransmitters stand in synergistic relation in their actions on the formation of cyclic AMP. The additional ATP formed by large additions of adenosine, giving maximal response, can still be augmented by addition of noradrenaline or histamine [3]. Under normal conditions it is pictured that adenosine is liberated in limited quantities on excitation possibly together with noradrenaline, and that the two compounds have characteristically different fashions of augmenting the tissue's cyclic AMP.

References

1. Kakiuchi, S., Rall, T. W. and McIlwain, H.; *J. Neurochem.*; **16**, (1969) 485.
2. McIlwain, H. and Bachelard, H. S.; *Biochemistry and the Central Nervous System*; Churchill, London, (1971) p. 41, 67.
3. Sattin, A. and Rall, T. W.; *Mol. Pharmacol.*; **6**, (1970) 13.
4. Rall, T. W. and Gilman, A. G.; *Neurosci. Res. Progr. Bull.*; **8**, (1970) 221.
5. Thomas, J.; *Biochem. J.*; **66**, (1957) 655.
6. Santos, J. N., Hempstead, K. W., Kopp, L. E. and Miech, R. P.; *J. Neurochem.*; **15**, (1968) 367.
7. Shimizu, H., Daly, J. W. and Crevling, C. R.; *J. Neurochem.*; **16**, (1969) 1609.
8. Ditzion, B. R., Paul, M. I. and Pauk, G. L.; *Pharmacology*; **3**, (1970) 25.
9. Paul, M. I., Pauk, G. L. and Ditzion, B. R.; *Pharmacology*; **3**, (1970) 148.
10. Lowry, O. H., Passonneau, J. V., Hasselberger, F. X. and Schultz, D. W.; *J. biol. Chem.*; **239**, (1964) 18.
11. McIlwain, H. and Snyder, H. S.; *J. Neurochem.*; **17**, (1970) 521.
12. Chase, T. N., Katz, R. I. and Kopin, I. J.; *J. Neurochem.*; **16**, (1969) 607.
13. Srinivasan, V., Neal, M. J. and Mitchell, J. F.; *J. Neurochem.*; **16**, (1969) 1235.
14. Kakiuchi, S. and Rall, T. W.; *Mol. Pharmacol.*; **4**, (1968) 367.
15. Kakiuchi, S. and Rall, T. W.; *Mol. Pharmacol.*; **4**, (1968) 379.
16. Gibson, I. and McIlwain, H.; *J. Physiol.*; **176**, (1965) 261.
17. McIlwain, H.; *Br. med. Bull.*; **24**, (1968) 174.
18. Shimizu, H., Creveling, C. R. and Daly, J.; *Proc. Nat. Acad. Sci. U.S.A.*; **65**, (1970) 1033.
19. Shimizu, H. and Daly, J.; *Biochim. biophys. Acta.*; **222**, (1970) 465.
20. Minard, F. N. and Davis, R. V.; *J. biol. Chem.*; **237**, (1962) 1283.
21. Hillman, H. H., Campbell, W. J. and McIlwain, H.; *J. Neurochem.*; **10**, (1971) 325.
22. Butcher, R. W. and Sutherland, E. W.; *J. biol. Chem.*; **237**, (1962) 1244.
23. Cheung, W. Y.; *Biochemistry*; **6**, (1967) 1079.

24. Brooker, G., Thomas, L. J. and Appleman, M. M.; *Biochemistry*; **7**, (1968) 4177.
25. Cheung, W. Y.; *Biochem. biophys. Res. Comm.*; **38**, (1970) 533.
26. Rall, T. W. and Sutherland, E. W.; *J. biol. Chem.*; **232**, (1968) 1065.
27. Pull, I. and McIlwain, H.; (1971) Unpublished work.
28. Douglas, W. W., Poisner, A. M. and Rubin, R. P.; *J. Physiol.*; **179**, (1965) 130.
29. Douglas, W. W. and Poisner, A. M.; *J. Physiol.*; **183**, (1966) 249.
30. Siggins, G. R., Hoffer, B. J. and Bloom, F. E.; *Science*; **165**, (1969) 1018; ibid.; **166**, (1969) 519.
31. Hoffer, B. J., Siggins, G. R. and Bloom, F. E.; *Brain Res.*; **25**, (1971) 523.
32. Haynes, R. C., Koritz, S. B. and Peron, F. G.; *J. biol. Chem.*; **234**, (1959) 1421.
33. McIlwain, H.; 'Chemical Exploration of the Brain'; Amsterdam, Elsevier (1963) p. 78-9.
34. Swanson, P. D.; *J. Neurochem.*; **13**, (1966) 229.
35. Tao, M. and Schweiger, M.; *J. Bact.*; **102**, (1970) 138.
36. McIlwain, H.; *Essays in Biochemistry*; **7**, (1971) in press.

INDEX